WHO
monographs on selected medicinal plants

VOLUME 1

World Health Organization
Geneva
1999

WHO Library Cataloguing in Publication Data
WHO monographs on selected medicinal plants.—Vol. 1.
1.Plants, Medicinal   2.Herbs   3.Traditional medicine
ISBN 92 4 154517 8   (NLM Classification: QV 766)

The World Health Organization welcomes requests for permission to reproduce or translate its publications, in part or in full. Applications and enquiries should be addressed to the Office of Publications, World Health Organization, Geneva, Switzerland, which will be glad to provide the latest information on any changes made to the text, plans for new editions, and reprints and translations already available.

The designations employed and the presentation of the material in this publication do not imply the expression of any opinion whatsoever on the part of the Secretariat of the World Health Organization concerning the legal status of any country, territory, city or area or of its authorities, or concerning the delimitation of its frontiers or boundaries.

The mention of specific companies or of certain manufacturers' products does not imply that they are endorsed or recommended by the World Health Organization in preference to others of a similar nature that are not mentioned. Errors and omissions excepted, the names of proprietary products are distinguished by initial capital letters.

Designed by WHO Graphics
Typeset in Hong Kong
Printed in Malta
97/11795-Best-set/Interprint-6500

Contents

Contents

Acknowledgements

Special acknowledgement is due to Professors Norman R. Farnsworth, Harry H. S. Fong, and Gail B. Mahady of the WHO Collaborating Centre for Traditional Medicine, College of Pharmacy, University of Illinois at Chicago, USA, for drafting and revising the monographs.

WHO also acknowledges with thanks the members of the advisory group that met in Beijing, China, in 1994, to draw up a list of medicinal plants for which monographs should be prepared, the more than 100 experts who provided comments and advice on the draft texts, and those who participated in the WHO Consultation held in Munich, Germany, in 1996 to review the monographs (see Annex). Finally, WHO would like to thank the Food and Agriculture Organization of the United Nations and the United Nations Industrial Development Organization for their contributions and all those who submitted comments through the World Self-Medication Industry, a nongovernmental organization in official relations with WHO.

Introduction

During the past decade, traditional systems of medicine have become a topic of global importance. Current estimates suggest that, in many developing countries, a large proportion of the population relies heavily on traditional practitioners and medicinal plants to meet primary health care needs. Although modern medicine may be available in these countries, herbal medicines (phytomedicines) have often maintained popularity for historical and cultural reasons. Concurrently, many people in developed countries have begun to turn to alternative or complementary therapies, including medicinal herbs.

Few plant species that provide medicinal herbs have been scientifically evaluated for their possible medical application. Safety and efficacy data are available for even fewer plants, their extracts and active ingredients, and the preparations containing them. Furthermore, in most countries the herbal medicines market is poorly regulated, and herbal products are often neither registered nor controlled. Assurance of the safety, quality, and efficacy of medicinal plants and herbal products has now become a key issue in industrialized and in developing countries. Both the general consumer and health-care professionals need up-to-date, authoritative information on the safety and efficacy of medicinal plants.

During the fourth International Conference of Drug Regulatory Authorities (ICDRA) held in Tokyo in 1986, WHO was requested to compile a list of medicinal plants and to establish international specifications for the most widely used medicinal plants and simple preparations. Guidelines for the assessment of herbal medicines were subsequently prepared by WHO and adopted by the sixth ICDRA in Ottawa, Canada, in 1991.[1] As a result of ICDRA's recommendations and in response to requests from WHO's Member States for assistance in providing safe and effective herbal medicines for use in national health-care systems, WHO is now publishing this first volume of 28 monographs on selected medicinal plants; a second volume is in preparation.

Preparation of the monographs

The medicinal plants featured in this volume were selected by an advisory group in Beijing in 1994. The plants selected are widely used and important in

---

[1] Guidelines for the assessment of herbal medicines. In: *Quality assurance of pharmaceuticals: a compendium of guidelines and related materials. Volume 1*. Geneva, World Health Organization, 1997:31–37.

all WHO regions, and for each sufficient scientific information seemed available to substantiate safety and efficacy. The monographs were drafted by the WHO Collaborating Centre for Traditional Medicine at the University of Illinois at Chicago, United States of America. The content was obtained by a systematic review of scientific literature from 1975 until the end of 1995: review articles; bibliographies in review articles; many pharmacopoeias—the International, African, British, Chinese, Dutch, European, French, German, Hungarian, Indian, and Japanese; as well as many other reference books.

Draft monographs were widely distributed, and some 100 experts in more than 40 countries commented on them. Experts included members of WHO's Expert Advisory Panels on Traditional Medicine, on the International Pharmacopoeia and Pharmaceutical Preparations, and on Drug Evaluation and National Drug Policies; and the drug regulatory authorities of 16 countries.

A WHO Consultation on Selected Medicinal Plants was held in Munich, Germany, in 1996. Sixteen experts and drug regulatory authorities from Member States participated. Following extensive discussion, 28 of 31 draft monographs were approved. The monograph on one medicinal plant was rejected because of the plant's potential toxicity. Two others will be reconsidered when more definitive data are available. At the subsequent eighth ICDRA in Bahrain later in 1996, the 28 model monographs were further reviewed and endorsed, and Member States requested WHO to prepare additional model monographs.

Purpose and content of the monographs

The purpose of the monographs is to:

*   provide scientific information on the safety, efficacy, and quality control/ quality assurance of widely used medicinal plants, in order to facilitate their appropriate use in Member States;
*   provide models to assist Member States in developing their own monographs or formularies for these or other herbal medicines; and
*   facilitate information exchange among Member States.

Readers will include members of regulatory authorities, practitioners of orthodox and of traditional medicine, pharmacists, other health professionals, manufacturers of herbal products, and research scientists.

Each monograph contains two parts. The first part consists of pharmacopoeial summaries for quality assurance: botanical features, distribution, identity tests, purity requirements, chemical assays, and active or major chemical constituents. The second part summarizes clinical applications, pharmacology, contraindications, warnings, precautions, potential adverse reactions, and posology.

In each pharmacopoeial summary, the *Definition* section provides the Latin binomial pharmacopoeial name, the most important criterion in quality assurance. Latin pharmacopoeial synonyms and vernacular names, listed in the sections *Synonyms* and *Selected vernacular names*, are those names used in commerce or by local consumers. The monographs place outdated botanical nomenclature in the synonyms category, based on the International Rules of Nomenclature.

For example, *Aloe barbadensis* Mill. is actually *Aloe vera* (L.) Burm. *Cassia acutifolia* Delile and *Cassia angustifolia* Vahl., often treated in separate monographs, are now believed to be the same species, *Cassia senna* L. *Matricaria chamomilla* L., *M. recutita* L., and *M. suaveolens* L. have been used for many years as the botanical name for camomile. However, it is now agreed that the name *Chamomilla recutita* (L.) Rauschert is the legitimate name.

The vernacular names listed are a selection of names from individual countries worldwide, in particular from areas where the medicinal plant is in common use. The lists are not complete, but reflect the names appearing in the official monographs and reference books consulted during preparation of the WHO monographs and in the Natural Products Alert (NAPRALERT) database (a database of literature from around the world on ethnomedical, biological and chemical information on medicinal plants, fungi and marine organisms, located at the WHO Collaborating Centre for Traditional Medicine at the University of Illinois at Chicago).

A detailed botanical description (under *Description*) is intended for quality assurance at the stages of production and collection, whereas the detailed description of the drug material (under *Plant material of interest*) is for the same purpose at the manufacturing and commerce stages. *Geographical distribution* is not normally found in official compendia, but it is included here to provide additional quality assurance information.

General identity tests, *Purity tests*, and *Chemical assays* are all normal compendial components included under those headings in these monographs. Where purity tests do not specify accepted limits, those limits should be set in accordance with national requirements by the appropriate Member State authorities.

Each medicinal plant and the specific plant part used (the drug) contain active or major chemical constituents with a characteristic profile that can be used for chemical quality control and quality assurance. These constituents are described in the section *Major chemical constituents*.

The second part of each monograph begins with a list of *Dosage forms* and of *Medicinal uses* categorized as those uses supported by clinical data, those uses described in pharmacopoeias and in traditional systems of medicine, and those uses described in folk medicine, not yet supported by experimental or clinical data.

The first category includes medical indications that are well established in some countries and that have been validated by clinical studies documented in the world's scientific literature. The clinical trials may have been controlled, randomized, double-blind studies, open trials, or well-documented observations of therapeutic applications. Experts at the Munich Consultation agreed to include Folium and Fructus Sennae, Aloe, Rhizoma Rhei, and Herba Ephedrae in this category because they are widely used and their efficacy is well documented in the standard medical literature.

The second category includes medicinal uses that are well established in many countries and are included in official pharmacopoeias or national monographs. Well-established uses having a plausible pharmacological basis and supported by older studies that clearly need to be repeated are also included. The references cited provide additional information useful in evaluating specific herbal preparations. The uses described should be reviewed by local experts and health workers for their applicability in the local situation.

The third category refers to indications described in unofficial pharmacopoeias and other literature, and to traditional uses. The appropriateness of these uses could not be assessed, owing to a lack of scientific data to support the claims. The possible use of these remedies must be carefully considered in the light of therapeutic alternatives.

The final sections of each monograph cover *Pharmacology* (both experimental and clinical); *Contraindications* such as sensitivity or allergy; *Warnings*; *Precautions*, including discussion of drug interactions, carcinogenicity, teratogenicity and special groups such as children and nursing mothers; *Adverse reactions*; and *Posology*.

Use of the monographs

WHO encourages countries to provide safe and effective traditional remedies and practices in public and private health services.

This publication is not intended to replace official compendia such as pharmacopoeias, formularies, or legislative documents. The monographs are intended primarily to promote harmonization in the use of herbal medicines with respect to levels of safety, efficacy, and quality control. These aspects of herbal medicines depend greatly on how the individual dosage form is prepared. For this reason, local regulatory authorities, experts, and health workers, as well as the scientific literature, should be consulted to determine whether a specific herbal preparation is appropriate for use in primary health care.

The monographs will be supplemented and updated periodically as new information appears in the literature, and additional monographs will be prepared. WHO would be pleased to receive comments and suggestions, to this end, from readers of the monographs.

Finally, I should like to express our appreciation of the support provided for the development of the monographs by Dr H. Nakajima and Dr F. S. Antezana during their time as Director-General and Assistant Director-General, respectively, of WHO.

Dr Xiaorui Zhang
Medical Officer
Traditional Medicine
World Health Organization

Bulbus Allii Cepae

Definition

Bulbus Allii Cepae is the fresh or dried bulbs of *Allium cepa* L. (Liliaceae) or its varieties and cultivars.

Synonyms

Allium esculentum Salisb., *Allium porrum cepa* Rehb. (*1*).

Selected vernacular names

It is most commonly known as "onion". Basal, basl, cebolla, cebolla morada, cepa bulb, cepolla, cipolla, common onion, cu hanh, hom hua yai, hom khaao, hom yai, hu-t'sung, hu t'sung t'song, hua phak bhu, i-i-bsel, kesounni, khtim, Küchenzwiebel, l'oignon, loyon, Madras oignon, oignon, palandu, piyaj, piyaz, pyaz, pyaaz, ralu lunu, red globe onion, sibuyas, Spanish onion, tamanegi, umbi bawang merah, vengayan, yellow Bermuda onion, white globe onion, Zwiebel (*1–5*).

Description

A perennial herb, strong smelling when crushed; bulbs vary in size and shape from cultivar to cultivar, often depressed-globose and up to 20 cm in diameter; outer tunics membranous. Stem up to 100 cm tall and 30 mm in diameter, tapering from inflated lower part. Leaves up to 40 cm in height and 20 mm in diameter, usually almost semicircular in section and slightly flattened on upper side; basal in first year, in second year their bases sheathing the lower sixth of the stem. Spathe often 3-valved, persistent, shorter than the umbel. Umbel 4–9 cm in diameter, subglobose or hemispherical, dense, many-flowered; pedicels up to 40 mm, almost equal. Perianth stellate; segments 3–4.5 × 2–2.5 mm, white, with green stripe, slightly unequal, the outer ovate, the inner oblong, obtuse or acute. Stamens exserted; filaments 4–5 mm, the outer subulate, the inner with an expanded base up to 2 mm wide and bearing short teeth on each side. Ovary whitish. Capsule about 5 mm, $2n = 16$ (*6*).

Plant material of interest: fresh or dried bulbs

General appearance

Macroscopically, Bulbus Allii Cepae varies in size and shape from cultivar to cultivar, 2–20 cm in diameter; flattened, spherical or pear-shaped; white or coloured (*7*).

Organoleptic properties

Odour strong, characteristic alliaceous; taste strong; crushing or cutting the bulb stimulates lachrymation.

Microscopic characteristics

The external dried leaf scales of the bulbs show a large-celled epidermis with lightly spotted cell walls; the cells are elongated longitudinally. The underlying hypodermis runs perpendicular to the epidermis and contains large calcium oxalate crystals bordering the cell walls. The epidermis of the fleshy leaf scales resembles that of the dried leaf scales, and the epidermal cells on the dorsal side are distinctly longer and more elongated than the epidermal cells on the ventral side. Large calcium oxalate crystals are found in the hypodermis; stomata rare; large cell nuclei conspicuous; and spiral vessel elements occur in the leaf mesophyll (*8*).

Powdered plant material

Contains mainly thin-walled cells of the mesophyll with broken pieces of spiral vessel elements; cells containing calcium oxalate crystals are scarce (*8*).

Geographical distribution

Bulbus Allii Cepae ("onion") is probably indigenous to western Asia, but it is commercially cultivated worldwide, especially in regions of moderate climate (*1*).

General identity tests

Macroscopic inspection, microscopic characteristics and microchemical examination for organic sulfur compounds (*9*); and thin-layer chromatographic analysis for the presence of cysteine sulfoxides (*10, 11*).

Purity tests

Microbiology

The test for *Salmonella* spp. in Bulbus Allii Cepae products should be negative. The maximum acceptable limits of other microorganisms are as follows (*12–14*). Preparations for oral use: aerobic bacteria—not more than 10^5/g or ml; fungi—not more than 10^4/g or ml; enterobacteria and certain Gram-negative bacteria—not more than 10^3/g or ml; *Escherichia coli*—0/g or ml.

Total ash

Not more than 6% (*3*).

Acid-insoluble ash
Not more than 1.0% (3).

Water-soluble extractive
Not more than 5.0% (3).

Alcohol-soluble extractive
Not more than 4.0% (3).

Pesticide residues
To be established in accordance with national requirements. Normally, the maximum residue limit of aldrin and dieldrin for Bulbus Allii Cepae is not more than 0.05 mg/kg (*14*). For other pesticides, see WHO guidelines on quality control methods for medicinal plants (*12*) and guidelines for predicting dietary intake of pesticide residues (*15*).

Heavy metals
Recommended lead and cadmium levels are no more than 10 and 0.3 mg/kg, respectively, in the final dosage form of the plant material (*12*).

Radioactive residues
For analysis of strontium-90, iodine-131, caesium-134, caesium-137 and plutonium-239, see WHO guidelines on quality control methods for medicinal plants (*12*).

Other purity tests
Chemical, foreign organic matter, and moisture tests to be established in accordance with national requirements.

Chemical assays
Assay for organic sulfur constituents, cysteine sulfoxides and sulfides by means of high-performance liquid chromatographic (*16*, *17*) or gas–liquid chromatographic (*18*) methods, respectively. Quantitative levels to be established by appropriate national authority.

Major chemical constituents
Sulfur- and non-sulfur-containing chemical constituents have been isolated from Bulbus Allii Cepae; the sulfur compounds are the most characteristic (*1, 4, 7*).

The organic sulfur compounds of Bulbus Allii Cepae, including the thiosulfinates, thiosulfonates, cepaenes, *S*-oxides, *S,S'*-dioxides, monosulfides, disulfides, trisulfides, and zwiebelanes occur only as degradation products of the naturally occurring cysteine sulfoxides (e.g. (+)-S-propyl-L-cysteine sulfoxide). When the onion bulb is crushed, minced, or otherwise processed, the cysteine sulfoxides are released from compartments and contact the enzyme alliinase in adjacent vacuoles. Hydrolysis and immediate condensation of the reactive intermediate (sulfenic acids) form the compounds as indicated below (*1*). The odorous thiosulphonates occur (in low concentrations) only in freshly chopped onions, whereas the sulfides accumulate in stored extracts or steam-distilled oils. Approximately 90% of the soluble organic-bound sulfur is present as γ-glutamylcysteine peptides, which are not acted on by alliinase. They function as storage reserve and contribute to the germination of seeds. However, on prolonged storage or during germination, these peptides are acted on by γ-glutamyl transpeptidase to form alk(en)yl-cysteine sulfoxides, which in turn give rise to other volatile sulfur compounds (*1*).

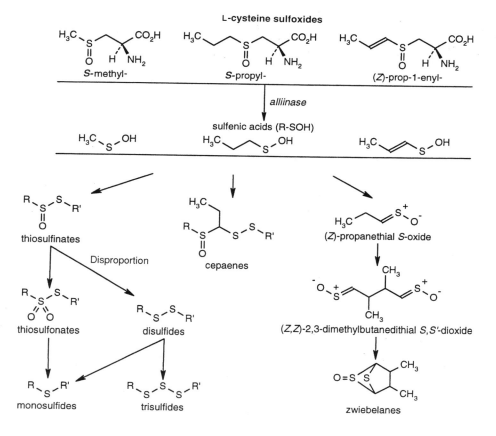

Dosage forms

Fresh juice and 5% and 50% ethanol extracts have been used in clinical studies (*1*). A "soft" extract is marketed in France but is not recognized as a drug by French authorities (*7*). Dried Bulbus Allii Cepae products should be stored in well-closed containers, protected from light, moisture, and elevated temperature. Fresh bulbs and juice should be refrigerated (2–10 °C).

Medicinal uses

Uses supported by clinical data

The principal use of Bulbus Allii Cepae today is to prevent age-dependent changes in the blood vessels, and loss of appetite (*19*).

Uses described in pharmacopoeias and in traditional systems of medicine

Treatment of bacterial infections such as dysentery, and as a diuretic (*2, 7*). The drug has also been used to treat ulcers, wounds, scars, keloids (*3*), and asthma (*20, 21*). Bulbus Allii Cepae has also been used as an adjuvant therapy for diabetes (*4, 22, 23*).

Uses described in folk medicine, not supported by experimental or clinical data

As an anthelminthic, aphrodisiac, carminative, emmenagogue, expectorant, and tonic (*3*), and for the treatment of bruises, bronchitis, cholera, colic, earache, fevers, high blood pressure, jaundice, pimples, and sores (*3*).

Pharmacology

Experimental pharmacology

An aqueous extract or the juice of Bulbus Allii Cepae inhibited the *in vitro* growth of *Escherichia coli, Serratia marcescens, Streptococcus* species, *Lactobacillus odontolyticus, Pseudomonas aeruginosa*, and *Salmonella typhosa* (*24–28*). A petroleum ether extract of Bulbus Allii Cepae inhibited the *in vitro* growth of *Clostridium paraputrificum* and *Staphylococcus aureus* (*24*). The essential oil has activity against a variety of fungi including *Aspergillus niger, Cladosporium werneckii, Candida albicans, Fusarium oxysporium, Saccharomyces cerevisiae, Geotrichum candidum, Brettanomyces anomalus*, and *Candida lipolytica* (*5, 29*).

The hypoglycaemic effects of Bulbus Allii Cepae have been demonstrated *in vivo*. Intragastric administration of the juice, a chloroform, ethanol, petroleum ether (0.25 g/kg) or water extract (0.5 ml), suppressed alloxan-, glucose- and epinephrine-induced hyperglycaemia in rabbits and mice (*30–35*).

Inhibition of platelet aggregation by Bulbus Allii Cepae has been demonstrated both *in vitro* and *in vivo*. An aqueous extract inhibited adenosine diphosphate-, collagen-, epinephrine- and arachidonic acid-induced platelet aggregation *in vitro* (*36, 37*). Platelet aggregation was inhibited in rabbits after administration of the essential oil, or a butanol or chloroform extract of the drug (*38–40*). An ethanol, butanol or chloroform extract or the essential oil (10–60 µg/ml) of the drug inhibited aggregation of human platelets *in vitro* (*41, 42*) by decreasing thromboxane synthesis (*39*). Both raw onions and the essential oil increased fibrinolysis in *ex vivo* studies on rabbits and humans (*1*). An increase in coagulation time was also observed in rabbits (*1*).

Intragastric administration of the juice or an ether extract (100 mg/kg) of the drug inhibited allergen- and platelet activating factor-induced allergic reactions, but not histamine- or acetylcholine-induced allergenic responses in guinea-pigs (*43*). A water extract of the drug was not active (*43*). A chloroform extract of Bulbus Allii Cepae (20–80 mg/kg) inhibited allergen- and platelet aggregation factor-induced bronchial obstruction in guinea-pigs (*44*). The thiosulphinates and cepaenes appear to be the active constituents of Bulbus Allii Cepae (*1*).

Both ethanol and methanol extracts of Bulbus Allii Cepae demonstrated diuretic activity in dogs and rats after intragastric administration (*45, 46*).

Antihyperlipidaemic and anticholesterolaemic activities of the drug were observed after oral administration of minced bulbs, a water extract, the essential oil (100 mg/kg), or the fixed oil to rabbits or rats (*47–52*). However, one study reported no significant changes in cholesterol or lipid levels of the eye in rabbits, after treatment of the animals for 6 months with an aqueous extract (20% of diet) (*53*).

Oral administration of an ethanol extract of the drug to guinea-pigs inhibited smooth muscle contractions in the trachea induced by carbachol and inhibited histamine-, barium chloride-, serotonin-, and acetylcholine-induced contractions in the ileum (*20*).

Topical application of an aqueous extract of Bulbus Allii Cepae (10% in a gel preparation) inhibited mouse ear oedema induced by arachidonic acid (*54*). The active antiallergic and anti-inflammatory constituents of onion are the flavonoids (quercetin and kaempferol) (*55*). The flavonoids act as anti-inflammatory agents because they inhibit the action of protein kinase, phospholipase A2, cyclooxygenase, and lipoxygenase (*56*), as well as the release of mediators of inflammation (e.g. histamine) from leukocytes (*57*).

In vitro, an aqueous extract of Bulbus Allii Cepae inhibited fibroblast proliferation (*58*). A 0.5% aqueous extract of onion inhibited the growth of human fibroblasts and of keloidal fibroblasts (enzymically isolated from keloidal tissue) (*59*). In a comparative study, an aqueous extract of Bulbus Allii Cepae (1–3%) inhibited the proliferation of fibroblasts of varying origin (scar, keloid, embryonic tissue). The strongest inhibition was observed with keloid fibroblasts (65–73%) as compared with the inhibition of scar and embryonic fibroblasts (up to 50%) (*59*). In human skin fibroblasts, both aqueous and chloroform onion extracts, as well as thiosulfinates, inhibited the platelet-derived growth factor-stimulated chemotaxis and proliferation of these cells (*60*). In addition, a protein fraction isolated from an onion extract exhibited antimitotic activity (*61*).

Clinical pharmacology

Oral administration of a butanol extract of Bulbus Allii Cepae (200 mg) to subjects given a high-fat meal prior to testing suppressed platelet aggregation associated with a high-fat diet (*62*).

Administration of a butanol extract to patients with alimentary lipaemia prevented an increase in the total serum cholesterol, β-lipoprotein cholesterol, and β-lipoprotein and serum triglycerides (*63, 64*). A saponin fraction (50 mg) or the bulb (100 mg) also decreased serum cholesterol and plasma fibrinogen levels (*65, 66*). However, fresh onion extract (50 g) did not produce any significant effects on serum cholesterol, fibrinogen, or fibrinolytic activity in normal subjects (*67, 68*).

Antihyperglycaemic activity of Bulbus Allii Cepae has been demonstrated in clinical studies. Administration of an aqueous extract (100 mg) decreased glucose-induced hyperglycaemia in human adults (*69*). The juice of the drug (50 mg) administered orally to diabetic patients reduced blood glucose levels (*22*). Addition of raw onion to the diet of non-insulin-dependent diabetic subjects decreased the dose of antidiabetic medication required to control the disease (*70*). However, an aqueous extract of Bulbus Allii Cepae (200 mg) was not active (*71*).

The immediate and late cutaneous reactions induced by injection of rabbit anti-human IgE-antibodies into the volar side of the forearms of 12 healthy volunteers were reduced after pretreatment of the skin with a 50% ethanol onion extract (*1*). Immediate and late bronchial obstruction owing to allergen inhalation was markedly reduced after oral administration of a 5% ethanol onion extract 1 hour before exposure to the allergen (*1*).

In one clinical trial in 12 adult subjects, topical application of a 45% ethanolic onion extract inhibited the allergic skin reactions induced by anti-IgE (*72*).

Contraindications

Allergies to the plant. The level of safety of Bulbus Allii Cepae is reflected by its worldwide use as a vegetable.

Warnings

No warnings have been reported.

Precautions

Carcinogenesis, mutagenesis, impairment of fertility

Bulbus Allii Cepae is not mutagenic *in vitro* (*73*).

Other precautions

No general precautions have been reported, and no precautions have been reported concerning drug interactions, drug and laboratory test interactions, nursing mothers, paediatric use, or teratogenic or non-teratogenic effects on pregnancy.

Adverse reactions

Allergic reactions such as rhinoconjunctivitis and contact dermatitis have been reported (*74*).

Posology

Unless otherwise prescribed: a daily dosage is 50 g of fresh onion or 20 g of the dried drug; doses of preparations should be calculated accordingly (*14*).

References

1. Breu W, Dorsch W. *Allium cepa* L. (Onion): Chemistry, analysis and pharmacology. In: Wagner H, Farnsworth NR, eds. *Economic and medicinal plants research*, Vol. 6. London, Academic Press, 1994:115–147.
2. Kapoor LD. *Handbook of Ayurvedic medicinal plants*, Boca Raton, FL, CRC Press, 1990.
3. *Materia medika Indonesia*, Jilid VI. Jakarta, Departemen Kesehatan, Republik Indonesia, 1995.
4. Wagner H, Wiesenauer M. *Phytotherapie*. Stuttgart, Gustav Fischer, 1995.
5. Farnsworth NR, ed. *NAPRALERT database*. Chicago, University of Illinois at Chicago, IL, August 8, 1995 production (an on-line database available directly through the University of Illinois at Chicago or through the Scientific and Technical Network (STN) of Chemical Abstracts Services).
6. Tutin TG et al., eds. *Flora Europea*, Vol. 5. Cambridge, Cambridge University Press, 1980.
7. Bruneton J. *Pharmacognosy, phytochemistry, medicinal plants*. Paris, Lavoisier, 1995.
8. Gassner G. *Mikroskopische Untersuchung pflanzlicher Lebensmittel*. Stuttgart, Gustav Fischer, 1973.
9. *African pharmacopoeia*, Vol. *1*, 1st ed. Lagos, Organization of African Unity, Scientific, Technical & Research Commission, 1985.
10. Wagner H, Bladt S, Zgainski EM. *Plant drug analysis*. Berlin, Springer-Verlag, 1984.
11. Augusti KT. Chromatographic identification of certain sulfoxides of cysteine present in onion (*Allium cepa* Linn.) extract. *Current science*, 1976, 45:863–864.
12. *Quality control methods for medicinal plant materials*. Geneva, World Health Organization, 1998.
13. *Deutsches Arzneibuch 1996. Vol. 2. Methoden der Biologie*. Stuttgart, Deutscher Apotheker Verlag, 1996.
14. *European pharmacopoeia*, 3rd ed. Strasbourg, Council of Europe, 1997.
15. *Guidelines for predicting dietary intake of pesticide residues*, 2nd rev. ed. Geneva, World Health Organization, 1997 (unpublished document WHO/FSF/FOS/97.7; available from Food Safety, WHO, 1211 Geneva 27, Switzerland).
16. Bayer T. *Neue schwefelhaltige Inhaltsstoffe aus Allium Cepa L. mit antiasthmatischer und antiallergischer Wirkung* [Thesis]. Germany, University of Munich, 1988.
17. Breu W. *Analytische und pharmakologische Untersuchungen von Allium Cepa L. und neue 5-Lipoxygenase-Inhibitoren aus Arzneipflanzen* [Thesis]. Germany, University of Munich, 1991.
18. Brodnitz MH, Pollock CL. Gas chromatographic analysis of distilled onion oil. *Food technology*, 1970, 24:78–80.

19. German Commission E Monograph, Allii cepae bulbus. *Bundesanzeiger*, 1986, 50:13 March.
20. Dorsch W, Wagner H. New antiasthmatic drugs from traditional medicine? *International archives of allergy and applied immunology*, 1991, 94:262–265.
21. Sharma KC, Shanmugasundram SSK. *Allium cepa* as an antiasthmatic. *RRL jammu newsletter*, 1979:8–10.
22. Sharma KK et al. Antihyperglycemic effect of onion: Effect on fasting blood sugar and induced hyperglycemia in man. *Indian journal of medical research*, 1977, 65:422–429.
23. Mathew PT, Augusti KT. Hypoglycemic effects of onion, *Allium cepa* Linn. on diabetes mellitus: a preliminary report. *Indian journal of physiology and pharmacology*, 1975, 19:213–217.
24. Didry N, Pinkas M, Dubreuil L. Activité antibactérienne d'espèces du genre *Allium. Pharmazie*, 1987, 42:687–688.
25. Arunachalam K. Antimicrobial activity of garlic, onion, and honey. *Geobios*, 1980, 7:46–47.
26. Elnima EI et al. The antimicrobial activity of garlic and onion extracts. *Pharmazie*, 1983, 38:747–748.
27. Sangmachachai K. *Effect of onion and garlic extracts on the growth of certain bacteria* [Thesis]. Bangkok, Chiangmai University, 1978.
28. Abou IA et al. Antimicrobial activities of *Allium sativum, Allium cepa, Raphanus sativus, Capsicum frutescens, Eruca sativa, Allium kurrat* on bacteria. *Qualitas plantarum et materiae vegetabiles*, 1972, 22:29–35.
29. Conner DE, Beuchat LR. Effects of essential oils from plants on growth of food spoilage yeasts. *Journal of food science*, 1984, 49:429–434.
30. El-Ashwah ET et al. Hypoglycemic activity of different varieties of Egyptian onion (*Allium cepa*) in alloxan diabetic rats. *Journal of drug research* (Egypt), 1981, 13:45–52.
31. Karawya MS et al. Diphenylamine, an antihyperglycemic agent from onion and tea. *Journal of natural products*, 1984, 47:775–780.
32. Mossa JS. A study on the crude antidiabetic drugs used in Arabian folk medicine. *International journal of crude drug research*, 1985, 23:137–145.
33. Augusti KT. Studies on the effects of a hypoglycemic principal from *Allium cepa* Linn. *Indian journal of medical research*, 1973, 61:1066–1071.
34. Jain RC, Vyas CR. Hypoglycaemic actions of onion on rabbits. *British medical journal*, 1974, 2:730.
35. Gupta RK, Gupta S. Partial purification of the hypoglycemic principle of onion. *IRCS medical science library compendium*, 1976, 4:410.
36. Srivastava KC. Effects of aqueous extracts of onion, garlic and ginger on platelet aggregation and metabolism of arachidonic acid in the blood vascular system: an *in vitro* study. *Prostaglandins and leukotrienes in medicine*, 1984, 13:227–235.
37. Srivastava KC. Aqueous extracts of onion, garlic and ginger inhibit platelet aggregation and alter arachidonic acid metabolism. *Biomedica biochimica acta*, 1984, 43:S335–S346.
38. Chauhan LS et al. Effect of onion, garlic and clofibrate on coagulation and fibrinolytic activity of blood in cholesterol fed rabbits. *Indian medical journal*, 1982, 76:126–127.
39. Makheja AN, Vanderhoek JY, Bailey JM. Inhibition of platelet aggregation and thromboxane synthesis by onion and garlic. *Lancet*, 1979, i:781.
40. Ariga T, Oshiba S. Effects of the essential oil components of garlic cloves on rabbit platelet aggregation. *Igaku to seibutsugaku*, 1981, 102:169–174.
41. Vanderhoek JY, Makheja AN, Bailey JM. Inhibition of fatty acid oxygenases by onion and garlic oils. Evidence for the mechanism by which these oils inhibit platelet aggregation. *Biochemical pharmacology*, 1980, 29:3169–3173.
42. Weissenberger H et al. Isolation and identification of the platelet aggregation inhibitor present in onion. *Allium cepa. FEBS letters*, 1972, 26:105–108.

43. Dorsch W et al. Antiasthmatic effects of onion extracts—detection of benzyl- and other isothiocyanates (mustard oils) as antiasthmatic compounds of plant origin. *European journal of pharmacology*, 1985, 107:17–24.
44. Dorsch W et al. Anti-asthmatic effects of onions. Alk(en)ylsufinothioc acid al(en)yl-esters inhibit histamine release, leukotriene and thromboxane biosynthesis *in vitro* and counteract PAF and allergen-induced bronchial spasm *in vivo*. *Biochemical pharmacology*, 1988, 37:4479–4486.
45. Kaczmarek F et al. Preparation of a diuretic fraction from dried onion scales. *Bulletin of the Institute of Roslin Leczniczych*, 1961, 7:157–166.
46. De A, Ribeiro R et al. Acute diuretic effects in conscious rats produced by some medicinal plants in the state of São Paulo, Brazil. *Journal of ethnopharmacology*, 1988, 24:19–29.
47. Sharma KK, Chowdhury NK, Sharma AL. Studies on hypocholesterolaemic activity of onion. II. Effect on serum cholesterol in rabbits maintained on high cholesterol diet. *Indian journal of nutrition and diet*, 1975:388–391.
48. Vatsala TM, Singh M. Effects of onion in induced atherosclerosis in rabbits. 2. Reduction of lipid levels in the eye. *Current science*, 1982, 51:230–232.
49. Ahluwalia P, Mohindroo A. Effect of oral ingestion of different fractions of *Allium cepa* on the blood and erythrocyte membrane lipids and certain membrane-bound enzymes in rats. *Journal of nutrition science and vitaminology*, 1989, 35:155–161.
50. Sebastian KL et al. The hypolipidemic effect of onion (*Allium cepa* Linn.) in sucrose fed rabbits. *Indian journal of physiology and pharmacology*, 1979, 23:27–29.
51. Adamu I, Joseph PK, Augusti KT. Hypolipidemic action of onion and garlic unsaturated oils in sucrose fed rats over a two-month period. *Experimentia*, 1982, 38:899–901.
52. Bobboi A, Augusti KT, Joseph PK. Hypolipidemic effects of onion oil and garlic oil in ethanol-fed rats. *Indian journal of biochemistry and biophysics*, 1984, 21:211–213.
53. Vatsala TM, Singh M. Effects of onion in atherosclerosis in rabbits. 4. Maintenance of normal activity of aortic enzymes. *Current science*, 1982, 51:276–278.
54. *Untersuchung von Contractubex® auf antiphlogistische Wirkung.* Münster, Merz, 1989 (internal research report).
55. Alcaraz MJ, Jimenez MJ. Flavonoids as antiinflammatory agents. *Fitoterapia*, 1988, 59:25–38.
56. Middleton E. The flavonoids. *Trends in pharmacological sciences (TIPS)*, 1984, 5:335–338.
57. Amellal M et al. Inhibition of mast cell histamine release by flavonoids and bioflavonoids. *Planta medica*, 1985:16–20.
58. Majewski S, Chadzynska M. Effects of heparin, allantoin and Cepae Extract on the proliferation of keloid fibroblasts and other cells *in vitro*. *Dermatologische Monatsschrift*, 1988, 174:106–129.
59. *Untersuchung der Contractubex®-Inhaltsstoffe auf anti-proliferative Wirkung von humanen Hautfibroblasten.* Münster, Merz, 1989 (internal research report).
60. Dorsch W. *Effect of onion extract and synthetic thiosulfinates on chemotaxis and proliferation of human fibroblasts.* Münster, Merz, 1994 (internal research report).
61. Avuso MJ, Saenz MT. Antimitotic activity of a protein fraction isolated from viscum-cruciatum on the root meristems of *Allium cepa*. *Fitoterapia*, 1985, 56:308–311.
62. Doutremepuich C et al. Action de l'oignon, *Allium cepa* L., sur l'hémostase primaire chez le volontaire sain avant et après absorption d'un repas riche en lipides. [Effects of onion, *Allium cepa* L., on primary haemostasis in healthy voluntary person before and after high fat meal absorption.] *Annales pharmaceutiques françaises*, 1985, 43:273–280.
63. Jain RC, Vyas CR. Onion and garlic in atherosclerotic heart disease. *Medikon*, 1977, 6:12–14.

64. Singhvi S et al. Effect of onion and garlic on blood lipids. *Rajasthan medical journal*, 1984, 23:3–6.
65. Sainani GS et al. Effect of garlic and onion on important lipid and coagulation parameters in alimentary hyperlipidemia. *Journal of the Association of Physicians in India*, 1979, 27:57–64.
66. Sharma KK, Gupta S, Dwivedi KK. Effect of raw and boiled onion on the alterations of blood cholesterol, fibrinogen and fibrinolytic activity in man during alimentary lipaemia. *Indian medical gazette*, 1977, 16:479–481.
67. Sharma KK, Sharma SP. Effect of onion and garlic on serum cholesterol on normal subjects. *Mediscope*, 1979, 22:134–136.
68. Sharma KK, Sharma SP. Effect of onion on blood cholesterol, fibrinogen and fibrinolytic activity in normal subjects. *Indian journal of pharmacology*, 1976, 8:231–233.
69. Jain RC, Vyas CR, Mahatma OP. Hypoglycaemic action of onion and garlic. *Lancet*, 1973, ii:1491.
70. Bhushan S et al. Effect of oral administration of raw onion on glucose tolerance test of diabetics: a comparison with tolbutamide. *Current medical practice*, 1984, 28:712–715.
71. Sharma KK et al. Antihyperglycemic effects of onion: Effect on fasting blood sugar and induced hyperglycemia in man. *Indian journal of medical research*, 1977, 65:422–429.
72. Dorsch W, Ring J. Suppression of immediate and late anti-IgE-induced skin reactions by topically applied alcohol/onion extract. *Allergy*, 1984, 39:43–49.
73. Rockwell P, Raw I. A mutagenic screening of various herbs, spices, and food additives. *Nutrition and cancer*, 1979, 1:10–15.
74. Valdivieso R et al. Bronchial asthma, rhinoconjunctivitis, and contact dermatitis caused by onion. *Journal of allergy and clinical immunology*, 1994, 94:928–930.

Bulbus Allii Sativi

Definition

Bulbus Allii Sativi consists of the fresh or dried bulbs of *Allium sativum* L. (Liliaceae) (*1, 2*).

Synonyms

Porvium sativum Rehb. (*1, 3*).

Selected vernacular names

It is most commonly known as "garlic". Ail, ail commun, ajo, akashneem, allium, alubosa elewe, ayo-ishi, ayu, banlasun, camphor of the poor, dai tóan, dasuan, dawang, dra thiam, foom, Gartenlauch, hom khaao, hom kía, hom thiam, hua thiam, kesumphin, kitunguu-sumu, Knoblauch, kra thiam, krathiam, krathiam cheen, krathiam khaao, l'ail, lahsun, lai, lashun, lasan, lasun, lasuna, Lauch, lay, layi, lehsun, lesun, lobha, majo, naharu, nectar of the gods, ninniku, pa-se-waa, poor man's treacle, rason, rasonam, rasun, rustic treacles, seer, skordo, sluôn, stinking rose, sudulunu, ta-suam, ta-suan, tafanuwa, tellagada, tellagaddalu, thiam, toi thum, tum, umbi bawang putih, vallaip-pundu, velluli, vellulli (*1–13*).

Description

A perennial, erect bulbous herb, 30–60 cm tall, strong smelling when crushed. The underground portion consists of a compound bulb with numerous fibrous rootlets; the bulb gives rise above ground to a number of narrow, keeled, grass-like leaves. The leaf blade is linear, flat, solid, 1.0–2.5 cm wide, 30–60 cm long, and has an acute apex. Leaf sheaths form a pseudostem. Inflorescences are umbellate; scape smooth, round, solid, and coiled at first, subtended by membraneous, long-beaked spathe, splitting on one side and remaining attached to umbel. Small bulbils are produced in inflorescences; flowers are variable in number and sometimes absent, seldom open and may wither in bud. Flowers are on slender pedicels; consisting of perianth of 6 segments, about 4–6 mm long, pinkish; stamens 6, anthers exserted; ovary superior, 3-locular. Fruit is a small loculicidal capsule. Seeds are seldom if ever produced (*8, 9*).

Plant material of interest: fresh or dried bulbs

General appearance

Bulbus Allii Sativi consists of several outer layers of thin sheathing protective leaves which surround an inner sheath. The latter enclose the swollen storage leaves called "cloves". Typically, the bulb possesses a dozen sterile sheathing leaves within which are 6–8 cloves bearing buds making a total of 10–20 cloves and 20–40 well-developed but short and embedded roots. The cloves are asymmetric in shape, except for those near the centre (*1*).

Organoleptic properties

Odour strong, characteristic alliaceous (*1, 6, 8*); taste very persistently pungent and acrid (*1, 6, 8*).

Microscopic characteristics

The bulbs show a number of concentric bulblets; each is 5–10 mm in diameter and consists of an outer scale, an epidermis enclosing a mesophyll free from chlorophyll, a ground tissue and a layer of lower epidermal cells. Dry scales consist of 2 or 3 layers of rectangular cells having end walls with a broadly angular slant. These cells contain many rhomboid crystals of calcium oxalate. The upper epidermal cells next to the dry scale layer consist of a single layer of rectangular to cubical cells next to which are several layers of large parenchymatous cells. Among these cells are interspaced many vascular bundles, each of which consists of xylem and phloem arranged alternately. Lower epidermis consists of cubical cells which are much smaller than the upper epidermal cells. The same arrangement of tissues is met within different bulblets, 2 or 3 of which are arranged concentrically (*1, 6*).

Powdered plant material

Pale buff to greyish or purplish white, with characteristic aromatic alliaceous odour and taste. It is characterized by the presence of sclereids of the epidermis of protective leaves, thin epidermis of storage cells, latex tubes, swollen parenchyma cells with granular contents, and lignified narrow spiral and annular vessels (*1*).

Geographical distribution

Bulbus Allii Sativi is probably indigenous to Asia (*1, 7*), but it is commercially cultivated in most countries.

General identity tests

Macroscopic and microscopic examinations and microchemical analysis are used to identify organic sulfur compounds (*1*), thin-layer chromatographic analysis to determine the presence of alliin (*14*).

Purity tests

Microbiology

The test for *Salmonella* spp. in Bulbus Allii Sativi products should be negative. The maximum acceptable limits of other microorganisms are as follows (*2, 15, 16*). Preparations for internal use: aerobic bacteria—not more than 10^5/g or ml; fungi—not more than 10^4/g or ml; enterobacteria and certain Gram-negative bacteria—not more than 10^3/g or ml; *Escherichia coli*—0/g or ml.

Total ash

Not more than 5.0% (*2*).

Acid-insoluble ash

Not more than 1.0% (*4*).

Water-soluble extractive

Not less than 5.0% (*4*).

Alcohol-soluble extractive

Not less than 4.0% (*4*).

Moisture

Not more than 7% (*2*).

Pesticide residues

To be established in accordance with national requirements. Normally, the maximum residue limit of aldrin and dieldrin for Bulbus Allii Sativi is not more than 0.05 mg/kg (*2*). For other pesticides, see WHO guidelines on quality control methods for medicinal plants (*15*) and guidelines for predicting dietary intake of pesticide residues (*17*).

Heavy metals

Recommended lead and cadmium levels are no more than 10 and 0.3 mg/kg, respectively, in the final dosage form of the plant material (*15*).

Radioactive residues

For analysis of strontium-90, iodine-131, caesium-134, caesium-137, and plutonium-239, see WHO guidelines on quality control methods for medicinal plants (*15*).

Other purity tests

Chemical tests and tests for foreign organic matter to be established in accordance with national requirements.

Chemical assays

Qualitative and quantitative assay for sulfur constituents (alliin, allicin etc.) content by means of high-performance liquid chromatography (*18–22*) or gas chromatography–mass spectroscopy (*23*) methods.

Major chemical constituents

The most important chemical constituents reported from Bulbus Allii Sativi are the sulfur compounds (*7, 9, 24, 25*). It has been estimated that cysteine sulfoxides (e.g. alliin [1]) and the non-volatile γ-glutamylcysteine peptides make up more than 82% of the total sulfur content of garlic (*25*).

The thiosulfinates (e.g. allicin [2]), ajoenes (e.g. *E*-ajoene [3], *Z*-ajoene [4]), vinyldithiins (e.g. 2-vinyl-(4*H*)-1,3-dithiin [5], 3-vinyl-(4*H*)-1,2-dithiin [6]), and sulfides (e.g. diallyl disulfide [7], diallyl trisulfide [8]), however, are not naturally occurring compounds. Rather, they are degradation products from the naturally occurring cysteine sulfoxide, alliin [1]. When the garlic bulb is crushed, minced, or otherwise processed, alliin is released from compartments and interacts with the enzyme alliinase in adjacent vacuoles. Hydrolysis and immediate condensation of the reactive intermediate (allylsulfenic acid) forms allicin [2]. One milligram of alliin is considered to be equivalent to 0.45 mg of allicin (*26*). Allicin itself is an unstable product and will undergo additional reactions to form other derivatives (e.g. products [3]–[8]), depending on environmental and processing conditions (*24–26*). Extraction of garlic cloves with ethanol at <0 °C gave alliin [1]; extraction with ethanol and water at 25 °C led to allicin [2] and no alliin; and steam distillation (100 °C) converted the alliin totally to diallyl sulfides [7], [8] (*24, 25*). Sulfur chemical profiles of Bulbus Allii Sativi products reflected the processing procedure: bulb, mainly alliin, allicin; dry powder, mainly alliin, allicin; volatile oil, almost entirely diallyl sulfide, diallyl disulfide, diallyl trisulfide, and diallyl tetrasulfide; oil macerate, mainly 2-vinyl-[4*H*]-1,3-dithiin, 3-vinyl-[4*H*]-1,3-dithiin, *E*-ajoene, and *Z*-ajoene (*18–22, 24*). The content of alliin was also affected by processing treatment: whole garlic cloves (fresh) contained 0.25–1.15% alliin, while material carefully dried under mild conditions contained 0.7–1.7% alliin (*18–21*).

Gamma-glutamylcysteine peptides are not acted on by alliinase. On prolonged storage or during germination, these peptides are acted on by γ-glutamyl transpeptidase to form thiosulfinates (*25*).

Dosage forms

Fresh bulbs, dried powder, volatile oil, oil macerates, juice, aqueous or alcoholic extracts, aged garlic extracts (minced garlic that is incubated in aqueous alcohol (15–20%) for 20 months, then concentrated), and odourless garlic products (garlic products in which the alliinase has been inactivated by cooking; or in which chlorophyll has been added as a deodorant; or aged garlic preparations that have low concentrations of water-soluble sulfur compounds) (*18, 24*).

The juice is the most unstable dosage form. Alliin and allicin decompose rapidly, and those products must be used promptly (*18*).

Dried Bulbus Allii Sativi products should be stored in well-closed containers, protected from light, moisture, and elevated temperature.

Medicinal uses
Uses supported by clinical data

As an adjuvant to dietetic management in the treatment of hyperlipidaemia, and in the prevention of atherosclerotic (age-dependent) vascular changes (*5, 27–31*). The drug may be useful in the treatment of mild hypertension (*11, 28*).

Uses described in pharmacopoeias and in traditional systems of medicine

The treatment of respiratory and urinary tract infections, ringworm and rheumatic conditions (*1, 4, 7, 9, 11*). The herb has been used as a carminative in the treatment of dyspepsia (*32*).

Uses described in folk medicine, not supported by experimental or clinical data

As an aphrodisiac, antipyretic, diuretic, emmenagogue, expectorant, and sedative, to treat asthma and bronchitis, and to promote hair growth (*6, 9, 13*).

Pharmacology
Experimental pharmacology

Bulbus Allii Sativi has a broad range of antibacterial and antifungal activity (*13*). The essential oil, water, and ethanol extracts, and the juice inhibit the *in vitro* growth of *Bacillus* species, *Staphylococcus aureus*, *Shigella sonnei*, *Erwinia carotovora*, *Mycobacterium tuberculosis*, *Escherichia coli*, *Pasteurella multocida*, *Proteus* species, *Streptococcus faecalis*, *Pseudomonas aeruginosa*, *Candida* species, *Cryptococcus* species, *Rhodotorula rubra*, *Toruloposis* species, *Trichosporon pullulans*, and *Aspergillus niger* (33–40). Its antimicrobial activity has been attributed to allicin, one of the active constituents of the drug (41). However, allicin is a relatively unstable and highly reactive compound (37, 42) and may not have antibacterial activity *in vivo*. Ajoene and diallyl trisulfide also have antibacterial and antifungal activities (43). Garlic has been used in the treatment of roundworm (*Ascaris strongyloides*) and hookworm (*Ancylostoma caninum* and *Necator americanus*) (44, 45). Allicin appears to be the active anthelminthic constituent, and diallyl disulfide was not effective (46).

Fresh garlic, garlic juice, aged garlic extracts, or the volatile oil all lowered cholesterol and plasma lipids, lipid metabolism, and atherogenesis both *in vitro* and *in vivo* (18, 43, 47–64). *In vitro* studies with isolated primary rat hepatocytes and human HepG2 cells have shown that water-soluble garlic extracts inhibited cholesterol biosynthesis in a dose-dependent manner (48–50). Antihypercholesterolaemic and antihyperlipidaemic effects were observed in various animal models (rat, rabbit, chicken, pig) after oral (in feed) or intragastric administration of minced garlic bulbs; water, ethanol, petroleum ether, or methanol extracts; the essential oil; aged garlic extracts and the fixed oil (51–64). Oral administration of allicin to rats during a 2-month period lowered serum and liver levels of total lipids, phospholipids, triglycerides, and total cholesterol (65). Total plasma lipids and cholesterol in rats were reduced after intraperitoneal injection of a mixture of diallyl disulfide and diallyl trisulfide (66). The mechanism of garlic's antihypercholesterolaemic and antihyperlipidaemic activity appears to involve the inhibition of hepatic hydroxymethylglutaryl-CoA (HMG-CoA) reductase and remodelling of plasma lipoproteins and cell membranes (67). At low concentrations (<0.5 mg/ml), garlic extracts inhibited the activity of hepatic HMG-CoA reductase, but at higher concentrations (>0.5 mg/ml) cholesterol biosynthesis was inhibited in the later stages of the biosynthetic pathway (68). Alliin was not effective, but allicin and ajoene both inhibited HMG-CoA reductase *in vitro* (IC_{50} = 7 and 9 mmol/l respectively) (49). Because both allicin and ajoene are converted to allyl mercaptan in the blood and never reach the liver to affect cholesterol biosynthesis, this mechanism may not be applicable *in vivo*. In addition to allicin and ajoene, allyl mercaptan (50 mmol/l) and diallyl disulfide (5 mmol/l) enhanced palmitate-induced inhibition of cholesterol biosynthesis *in vitro* (50). It should be noted that water extracts of garlic probably do not contain any of these compounds; therefore other constituents of garlic, such as nicotinic acid and adenosine, which also inhibit HMG-CoA reductase activity and cholesterol biosynthesis, may be involved (69, 70).

The antihypertensive activity of garlic has been demonstrated *in vivo*. Oral or intragastric administration of minced garlic bulbs, or alcohol or water extracts of the drug, lowered blood pressure in dogs, guinea-pigs, rabbits, and rats (52, 71–73). The drug appeared to decrease vascular resistance by directly relaxing smooth muscle (74). The drug appears to change the physical state functions of the membrane potentials of vascular smooth muscle cells. Both aqueous garlic and ajoene induced membrane hyperpolarization in the cells of isolated vessel strips. The potassium channels opened frequently causing hyperpolarization, which resulted in vasodilation because the calcium channels were closed (*75, 76*). The compounds that produce the hypotensive activity of the drug are uncertain. Allicin does not appear to be involved (*43*), and adenosine has been postulated as being associated with the activity of the drug. Adenosine enlarges the peripheral blood vessels, allowing the blood pressure to decrease, and is also involved in the regulation of blood flow in the coronary arteries; however, adenosine is not active when administered orally. Bulbus Allii Sativi may increase production of nitric oxide, which is associated with a decrease in blood pressure. *In vitro* studies using water or alcohol extracts of garlic or garlic powder activated nitric-oxide synthase (*77*), and these results have been confirmed by *in vivo* studies (*78*).

Aqueous garlic extracts and garlic oil have been shown *in vivo* to alter the plasma fibrinogen level, coagulation time, and fibrinolytic activity (*43*). Serum fibrinolytic activity increased after administration of dry garlic or garlic extracts to animals that were artificially rendered arteriosclerotic (*79, 80*). Although adenosine was thought to be the active constituent, it did not affect whole blood (*43*).

Garlic inhibited platelet aggregation in both *in vitro* and *in vivo* studies. A water, chloroform, or methanol extract of the drug inhibited collagen-, ADP-, arachidonic acid-, epinephrine-, and thrombin-induced platelet aggregation *in vitro* (*81–87*). Prolonged administration (intragastric, 3 months) of the essential oil or a chloroform extract of Bulbus Allii Sativi inhibited platelet aggregation in rabbits (*88–90*). Adenosine, alliin, allicin, and the transformation products of allicin, the ajoenes; the vinyldithiins; and the dialkyloligosulfides are responsible for inhibition of platelet adhesion and aggregation (*4, 42, 91–93*). In addition methyl allyl trisulfide, a minor constituent of garlic oil, inhibited platelet aggregation at least 10 times as effectively than allicin (*94*). Inhibition of the arachidonic acid cascade appears to be one of the mechanisms by which the various constituents and their metabolites affect platelet aggregation. Inhibition of platelet cyclic AMP phosphodiesterase may also be involved (*91*).

Ajoene, one of the transformation products of allicin, inhibited *in vitro* platelet aggregation induced by the platelet stimulators—ADP, arachidonic acid, calcium ionophore A23187, collagen, epinephrine, platelet activating factor, and thrombin (*95, 96*). Ajoene inhibited platelet aggregation in cows, dogs, guinea-pigs, horses, monkeys, pigs, rabbits, and rats (*95, 96*). The antiplatelet activity of ajoene is potentiated by prostacyclin, forskolin, indometacin, and dipyridamole (*95*). The mechanism of action involves the inhibition of the metabolism of arachidonic acid by both cyclooxygenase and lipoxygenase, thereby inhibiting the formation of thromboxane A2 and 12-hydroxyeicosatetraenoic acid (*95*). Two mechanisms have been suggested for ajoene's antiplatelet activity. First, ajoene may interact with the primary agonist–receptor complex with the exposure of fibrinogen receptors through specific G-proteins involved in the signal transduction system on the platelet membrane (*92*). Or it may interact with a haemoprotein involved in platelet activation that modifies the binding of the protein to its ligands (*96*).

Hypoglycaemic effects of Bulbus Allii Sativi have been demonstrated *in vivo*. Oral administration of an aqueous, ethanol, petroleum ether, or chloroform extract, or the essential oil of garlic, lowered blood glucose levels in rabbits and rats (*24, 97–104*). However, three similar studies reported negative results (*105–107*). In one study, garlic bulbs administered orally (in feed) to normal or streptozotocin-diabetic mice reduced hyperphagia and polydipsia but had no effect on hyperglycaemia or hypoinsulinaemia (*107*). Allicin administered orally to alloxan-diabetic rats lowered blood glucose levels and increased insulin activity in a dose-dependent manner (*24*). Garlic extract's hypoglycaemic action appears to enhance insulin production, and allicin has been shown to protect insulin against inactivation (*108*).

Intragastric administration of an ethanol extract of Bulbus Allii Sativi decreased carrageenin-induced rat paw oedema at a dose of 100 mg/kg. The anti-inflammatory activity of the drug appears to be due to its antiprostaglandin activity (*109, 110*).

A water or ethanol extract of the drug showed antispasmodic activity against acetylcholine, prostaglandin E2 and barium-induced contractions in guinea-pig small intestine and rat stomach (*111*). The juice of the drug relaxed smooth muscle of guinea-pig ileum, rabbit heart and jejunum, and rat colon and fundus (*112, 113*). The juice also inhibited norepinephrine-, acetylcholine- and histamine-induced contractions in guinea-pig and rat aorta, and in rabbit trachea (*112, 113*).

Clinical pharmacology

The efficacy of Bulbus Allii Sativi as a carminative has been demonstrated in human studies. A clinical study of 29 patients taking two tablets daily (~1000 mg/day) of a dried garlic preparation demonstrated that garlic relieved epigastric and abdominal distress, belching, flatulence, colic, and nausea, as compared with placebo (*32*). It was concluded that garlic sedated the stomach and intestines, and relaxed spasms, retarded hyperperistalsis, and dispersed gas (*32*).

A meta-analysis of the effect of Bulbus Allii Sativi on blood pressure reviewed a total of 11 randomized, controlled trials (published and unpublished) (*113, 114*). Each of the trials used dried garlic powder (tablets) at a dose of 600–900 mg daily (equivalent to 1.8–2.7 g/day fresh garlic). The median duration of the trials was 12 weeks. Eight of the trials with data from 415 subjects were included in the analysis; three trials were excluded owing to a lack of data. Only three of the trials specifically used hypertensive subjects, and many of the studies suffered from methodological flaws. Of the seven studies that compared garlic with placebo, three reported a decrease in systolic blood pressure, and four studies reported a decrease in diastolic blood pressure (*115*). The results of the meta-analysis led to the conclusion that garlic may have some clinical usefulness in mild hypertension, but there is still insufficient evidence to recommend the drug as a routine clinical therapy for the treatment of hypertension (*115*).

A meta-analysis of the effects of Bulbus Allii Sativi on serum lipids and lipoproteins reviewed 25 randomized, controlled trials (published and unpublished) (*116*) and selected 16 with data from 952 subjects to include in the analysis. Fourteen of the trials used a parallel group design, and the remaining two were cross-over studies. Two of the studies were conducted in an open-label fashion, two others were single-blind, and the remainder were double-blind. The total daily dose of garlic was 600–900 mg of dried garlic powder, or 10 g of raw garlic, or 18 mg of garlic oil, or aged garlic extracts (dosage not stated). The median duration of the therapy was 12 weeks. Overall, the subjects receiving garlic supplementation (powder or non-powder) showed a 12% reduction (average) in total cholesterol, and a 13% reduction (powder only) in serum triglycerides. Meta-analysis of the clinical studies confirmed the lipid-lowering action of garlic. However, the authors concluded that the overall quality of the clinical trials was poor and that favourable results of better-designed clinical studies should be available before garlic can be routinely recommended as a lipid-lowering agent. However, current available data support the hypothesis that garlic therapy is at least beneficial (*116*). Another meta-analysis of the controlled trials of garlic effects on total serum cholesterol reached similar conclusions (*117*). A systematic review of the lipid-lowering potential of a dried garlic powder preparation in eight studies with 500 subjects had similar findings (*118*). In seven of the eight studies reviewed, a daily dose of 600–900 mg of garlic powder reduced serum cholesterol and triglyceride levels by 5–20%. The review concluded that garlic powder preparations do have lipid-lowering potential (*118*).

An increase in fibrinolytic activity in the serum of patients suffering from atherosclerosis was observed after administration of aqueous garlic extracts, the essential oil, and garlic powder (*119*, *120*). Clinical studies have demonstrated that garlic activates endogenous fibrinolysis, that the effect is detectable for several hours after administration of the drug, and that the effect increases as the drug is taken regularly for several months (*43*, *121*). Investigations of the acute haemorheological (blood flow) effect of 600–1200 mg of dry garlic powder demonstrated that the drug decreased plasma viscosity, tissue plasminogen activator activity and the haematocrit level (*118*).

The effects of the drug on haemorheology in conjunctival vessels was determined in a randomized, placebo-controlled, double-blind, cross-over trial. Garlic powder (900 mg) significantly increased the mean diameter of the arterioles (by 4.2%) and venules (by 5.9%) as compared with controls (*122*). In another double-blind, placebo-controlled study, patients with stage II peripheral arterial occlusive disease were given a daily dose of 800 mg of garlic powder for 4 weeks (*123*, *124*). Increased capillary erythrocyte flow rate and decreased plasma viscosity and plasma fibrinogen levels were observed in the group treated with the drug (*123*, *124*). Determinations of platelet aggregation *ex vivo*, after ingestion of garlic and garlic preparations by humans, suffers from methodological difficulties that may account for the negative results in some studies (*24*). In one study in patients with hypercholesterolinaemia treated with a garlic–oil macerate for 3 months, platelet adhesion and aggregation decreased significantly (*125*). In a 3-year intervention study, 432 patients with myocardial infarction were treated with either an ether-extracted garlic oil (0.1 mg/kg/day, corresponding to 2 g fresh garlic daily) or a placebo (*126*). In the group treated with garlic, there were 35% fewer new heart attacks and 45% fewer deaths than in the control group. The serum lipid concentrations of the treated patients were also reduced (*126*).

The acute and chronic effects of garlic on fibrinolysis and platelet aggregation in 12 healthy patients in a randomized, double-blind, placebo-controlled cross-over study were investigated (*30*). A daily dose of 900 mg of garlic powder for 14 days significantly increased tissue plasminogen activator activity as compared with placebo (*30*). Furthermore, platelet aggregation induced by adenosine diphosphate and collagen was significantly inhibited 2 and 4 hours after garlic ingestion and remained lower for 7 to 14 days after treatment (*30*). Another randomized, double-blind, placebo-controlled study investigated the effects of garlic on platelet aggregation in 60 subjects with increased risk of juvenile ischaemic attack (*29*). Daily ingestion of 800 mg of powdered garlic for 4 weeks significantly decreased the percentage of circulating platelet aggregates and spontaneous platelet aggregation as compared with the placebo group (*29*).

Oral administration of garlic powder (800 mg/day) to 120 patients for 4 weeks in a double-blind, placebo-controlled study decreased the average blood glucose by 11.6% (*30*). Another study found no such activity after dosing non-insulin-dependent patients with 700 mg/day of a spray-dried garlic preparation for 1 month (*127*).

Contraindications

Bulbus Allii Sativi is contraindicated in patients with a known allergy to the drug. The level of safety for Bulbus Allii Sativi is reflected by its worldwide use as a seasoning in food.

Warnings

Consumption of large amounts of garlic may increase the risk of postoperative bleeding (*128*, *129*).

Precautions

Drug interactions

Patients on warfarin therapy should be warned that garlic supplements may increase bleeding times. Blood clotting times have been reported to double in patients taking warfarin and garlic supplements (*130*).

Carcinogenesis, mutagenesis, impairment of fertility
Bulbus Allii Sativi is not mutagenic *in vitro* (*Salmonella* microsome reversion assay and *Escherichia coli*) (*131, 132*).

Pregnancy: non-teratogenic effects
There are no objections to the use of Bulbus Allii Sativi during pregnancy and lactation.

Nursing mothers
Excretion of the components of Bulbus Allii Sativi into breast milk and its effect on the newborn has not been established.

Other precautions
No general precautions have been reported, and no precautions have been reported concerning drug and laboratory test interactions, paediatric use, or teratogenic or non-teratogenic effects on pregnancy.

Adverse reactions
Bulbus Allii Sativi has been reported to evoke occasional allergic reactions such as contact dermatitis and asthmatic attacks after inhalation of the powdered drug (*133*). Those sensitive to garlic may also have a reaction to onion or tulip (*133*). Ingestion of fresh garlic bulbs, extracts, or oil on an empty stomach may occasionally cause heartburn, nausea, vomiting, and diarrhoea. Garlic odour from breath and skin may be perceptible (*7*). One case of spontaneous spinal epidural haematoma, which was associated with excessive ingestion of fresh garlic cloves, has been reported (*134*).

Posology
Unless otherwise prescribed, average daily dose is as follows (*7*): fresh garlic, 2–5 g; dried powder, 0.4–1.2 g; oil, 2–5 mg; extract, 300–1000 mg (as solid material). Other preparations should correspond to 4–12 mg of alliin or about 2–5 mg of allicin).

Bulbus Allii Sativi should be taken with food to prevent gastrointestinal upset.

References
1. *African pharmacopoeia, Vol. 1*, 1st ed. Lagos, Organization of African Unity, Scientific, Technical & Research Commission, 1985.
2. *European pharmacopoeia*, 3rd ed. Strasbourg, Council of Europe, 1997.
3. Iwu MM. *Handbook of African medicinal plants*. Boca Raton, FL, CRC Press, 1993:111–113.
4. *Materia medika Indonesia*, Jilid VI. Jakarta, Departemen Kesehatan, Republik Indonesia, 1995.

5. *British herbal pharmacopoeia, Vol. 1.* London, British Herbal Medicine Association. 1990.
6. *The Indian pharmaceutical codex. Vol. I. Indigenous drugs.* New Delhi, Council of Scientific & Industrial Research, 1953:8–10.
7. Bradley PR, ed. *British herbal compendium, Vol. 1.* Bournemouth, British Herbal Medicine Association, 1992.
8. Youngken HW. *Textbook of pharmacognosy,* 6th ed. Philadelphia, Blakiston, 1950: 182–183.
9. Farnsworth NR, Bunyapraphatsara N, eds. *Thai medicinal plants.* Bangkok, Prachachon, 1992:210–287.
10. Kapoor LD. *Handbook of Ayurvedic medicinal plants.* Boca Raton, FL, CRC Press, 1990:26.
11. Hsu HY. *Oriental materia medica, a concise guide.* Long Beach, CA, Oriental Healing Arts Institute, 1986:735–736.
12. Olin BR, ed. Garlic. In: *The Lawrence review of natural products.* St. Louis, MO, Facts and Comparisons, 1994:1–4.
13. *Medicinal plants in Viet Nam.* Manila, World Health Organization, 1990 (WHO Regional Publications, Western Pacific Series, No. 3).
14. Wagner H, Bladt S, Zgainski EM. *Plant drug analysis.* Berlin, Springer-Verlag, 1984:253–257.
15. *Quality control methods for medicinal plant materials.* Geneva, World Health Organization, 1998.
16. *Deutsches Arzneibuch 1996. Vol. 2. Methoden der Biologie.* Stuttgart, Deutscher Apotheker Verlag, 1996.
17. *Guidelines for predicting dietary intake of pesticide residues,* 2nd rev. ed. Geneva, World Health Organization, 1997 (unpublished document WHO/FSF/FOS/97.7; available from Food Safety, WHO, 1211 Geneva 27, Switzerland).
18. Lawson LD et al. HPLC analysis of allicin and other thiosulfinates in garlic clove homogenates. *Planta medica,* 1991, 57:263–270.
19. Iberl B et al. Quantitative determination of allicin and alliin from garlic by HPLC. *Planta medica,* 1990, 56:320–326.
20. Ziegler SJ, Sticher O. HPLC of S-alk(en)yl-L-cysteine derivatives in garlic including quantitative determination of (+)-S-allyl-L-cysteine sulfoxide (alliin). *Planta medica,* 1989, 55:372–378.
21. Mochizuki E et al. Liquid chromatographic determination of alliin in garlic and garlic products. *Journal of chromatography,* 1988, 455:271–277.
22. Freeman F, Kodera Y. Garlic chemistry: Stability of S-(2-propenyl)-2-propene-1-sulfinothioate (allicin) in blood, solvents and simulated physiological fluids. *Journal of agriculture and food chemistry,* 1995, 43:2332–2338.
23. Weinberg DS et al. Identification and quantification of organosulfur compliance markers in a garlic extract. *Journal of agriculture and food chemistry,* 1993, 41:37–41.
24. Reuter HD, Sendl A. *Allium sativum* and *Allium ursinum*: Chemistry, pharmacology, and medicinal applications. In: Wagner H, Farnsworth NR, eds. *Economic and medicinal plants research,* Vol. 6. London, Academic Press, 1994:55–113.
25. Sendl A. *Allium sativum* and *Allium ursinum,* Part 1. Chemistry, analysis, history, botany. *Phytomedicine,* 1995, 4:323–339.
26. Block E. The chemistry of garlic and onions. *Scientific American,* 1985, 252:94–99.
27. German Commission E Monograph, Allii sativi bulbus. *Bundesanzeiger,* 1988, 122:6 June.
28. Auer W, Eiber A, Hertkorn E. Hypertension and hyperlipidemia: garlic helps in mild cases. *British journal of clinical practice,* 1990, 44:3–6.
29. Kiesewetter H et al. Effect of garlic on platelet aggregation in patients with increased risk of juvenile ischaemic attack. *European journal of clinical pharmacology,* 1993, 45:333–336.

30. Kiesewetter H et al. Effect of garlic on thrombocyte aggregation, microcirculation, and other risk factors. *International journal of clinical pharmacology, therapy and toxicology*, 1991, 29:151–155.
31. Legnani C et al. Effects of dried garlic preparation on fibrinolysis and platelet aggregation in healthy subjects. *Arzneimittel-Forschung*, 1993, 43:119–121.
32. Damrau F, Ferguson EA. The modus operandi of carminatives. *Review of gastroenterology*, 1949, 16:411–419.
33. Fitzpatrick FK. Plant substances active against *Mycobacterium tuberculosis*. *Antibiotics and chemotherapy*, 1954, 4:528–529.
34. Sharma VD et al. Antibacterial property of *Allium sativum*. *In vivo* and *in vitro* studies. *Indian journal of experimental biology*, 1980, 15:466–469.
35. Arunachalam K. Antimicrobial activity of garlic, onion and honey. *Geobios*, 1980, 71:46–47.
36. Moore GS, Atkins RD. The antifungistatic effects of an aqueous garlic extract on medically important yeast-like fungi. *Mycologia*, 1977, 69:341–345.
37. Caporaso N, Smith SM, Eng RHK. Antifungal activity in human urine and serum after ingestion of garlic (*Allium sativum*). *Antimicrobial agents and chemotherapy*, 1983, 5:700–702.
38. Abbruzzese MR, Delaha EC, Garagusi VF. Absence of antimycobacterial synergism between garlic extract and antituberculosis drugs. *Diagnosis and microbiology of infectious diseases*, 1987, 8:79–85.
39. Chaiyasothi T, Rueaksopaa V. Antibacterial activity of some medicinal plants. *Undergraduate special project report*, 1975, 75:1–109.
40. Sangmahachai K. *Effect of onion and garlic extracts on the growth of certain bacteria* [Thesis]. Thailand, University of Bangkok, 1978:1–88.
41. Farbman et al. Antibacterial activity of garlic and onions: a historical perspective. *Pediatrics infectious disease journal*, 1993, 12:613–614.
42. Lawson LD, Hughes BG. Inhibition of whole blood platelet-aggregation by compounds in garlic clove extracts and commercial garlic products. *Thrombosis research*, 1992, 65:141–156.
43. Koch HP, Lawson LD, eds. *Garlic, the science and therapeutic application of Allium sativum l. and related species*. Baltimore, Williams and Wilkins, 1996.
44. Kempski HW. Zur kausalen Therapie chronischer Helminthen-Bronchitis. *Medizinische Klinik*, 1967, 62:259–260.
45. Soh CT. The effects of natural food-preservative substances on the development and survival of intestinal helminth eggs and larvae. II. Action on *Ancylostoma duodenale* larvae. *American journal of tropical medicine and hygiene*, 1960, 9:8–10.
46. Araki M et al. Anthelminthics. *Yakugaku zasshi*, 1952, 72:979–982.
47. Mader FH. Treatment of hyperlipidemia with garlic-powder tablets. Evidence from the German Association of General Practitioner's multicentric placebo-controlled, double-blind study. *Arzneimittel-Forschung*, 1990, 40:1111–1116.
48. Gebhardt R. Multiple inhibitory effects of garlic extracts on cholesterol biosynthesis in hepatocytes. *Lipids*, 1993, 28:613–619.
49. Gebhardt R, Beck H, Wagner KG. Inhibition of cholesterol biosynthesis by allicin and ajoene in rat hepatocytes and HepG2 cells. *Biochimica biophysica acta*, 1994, 1213:57–62.
50. Gebhardt R. Amplification of palmitate-induced inhibition of cholesterol biosynthesis in cultured rat hepatocytes by garlic-derived organosulfur compounds. *Phytomedicine*, 1995, 2:29–34.
51. Yeh YY, Yeh SM. Garlic reduces plasma lipids by inhibiting hepatic cholesterol and triacylglycerol synthesis. *Lipids*, 1994, 29:189–193.
52. Petkov V. Pharmacological and clinical studies of garlic. *Deutsche Apotheker Zeitung*, 1966, 106:1861–1867.

53. Jain RC. Onion and garlic in experimental cholesterol induced atherosclerosis. *Indian journal of medical research*, 1976, 64:1509–1515.
54. Qureshi AA et al. Inhibition of cholesterol and fatty acid biosynthesis in liver enzymes and chicken hepatocytes by polar fractions of garlic. *Lipids*, 1983, 18:343–348.
55. Thiersch H. The effect of garlic on experimental cholesterol arteriosclerosis of rabbits. *Zeitschrift für die gesamte experimentelle Medizin*, 1936, 99:473–477.
56. Zacharias NT et al. Hypoglycemic and hypolipidemic effects of garlic in sucrose fed rabbits. *Indian journal of physiology and pharmacology*, 1980, 24:151–154.
57. Gupta PP, Khetrapal P, Ghai CL. Effect of garlic on serum cholesterol and electro-cardiogram of rabbit consuming normal diet. *Indian journal of medical science*, 1987, 41:6–11.
58. Mand JK et al. Role of garlic (*Allium sativum*) in the reversal of atherosclerosis in rabbits. In: *Proceedings of the Third Congress of the Federation of Asian and Oceanian Biochemists*. Bangkok, 1983:79.
59. Sodimu O, Joseph PK, Angusti KT. Certain biochemical effects of garlic oil on rats maintained on high fat–high cholesterol diet. *Experientia*, 1984, 40:78–79.
60. Kamanna VS, Chandrasekhara N. Effect of garlic (*Allium sativum* Linn.) on serum lipoproteins and lipoprotein cholesterol levels in albino rats rendered hyper-cholesteremic by feeding cholesterol. *Lipids*, 1982, 17:483–488.
61. Kamanna VS, Chandrasekhara N. Hypocholesterolic activity of different fractions of garlic. *Indian journal of medical research*, 1984, 79:580–583.
62. Chi MS. Effects of garlic products on lipid metabolism in cholesterol-fed rats. *Proceedings of the Society of Experimental Biology and Medicine*, 1982, 171:174–178.
63. Qureshi AA et al. Influence of minor plant constituents on porcine hepatic lipid metabolism. *Atherosclerosis*, 1987, 64:687–688.
64. Lata S et al. Beneficial effects of *Allium sativum*, *Allium cepa*, and *Commiphora mukul* on experimental hyperlipidemia and atherosclerosis: a comparative evaluation. *Journal of postgraduate medicine*, 1991, 37:132–135.
65. Augusti KT, Mathew PT. Lipid lowering effect of allicin (diallyl disulfide-oxide) on long-term feeding to normal rats. *Experientia*, 1974, 30:468–470.
66. Pushpendran CK et al. Cholesterol-lowering effects of allicin in suckling rats. *Indian journal of experimental biology*, 1980, 18:858–861.
67. Brosche T, Platt D. Garlic. *British medical journal*, 1991, 303, 785.
68. Beck H, Wagnerk G. Inhibition of cholesterol biosynthesis by allicin and ajoene in rat hepatocytes and Hep62 cells. *Biochimica biophysica acta*, 1994, 1213:57–62.
69. Platt D, Brosche T, Jacob BG. Cholesterin-senkende Wirkung von Knoblauch? *Deutsche Medizinische Wochenschrift*, 1992, 117:962–963.
70. Grünwald J. Knoblauch: Cholesterinsenkende Wirkung doppelblind nachgewiesen. *Deutsche Apotheker Zeitung*, 1992, 132:1356.
71. Ogawa H et al. Effect of garlic powder on lipid metabolism in stroke-prone spontaneously hypertensive rats. *Nippon eiyo, shokuryo gakkaishi*, 1993, 46:417–423.
72. Sanfilippo G, Ottaviano G. Pharmacological investigations on *Allium sativum*. I. General action. II. Action on the arterial pressure and on the respiration. *Bollettino Societa Italiana Biologia Sperimentale*, 1944, 19:156–158.
73. Foushee DB, Ruffin J, Banerjee U. Garlic as a natural agent for the treatment of hypertension: A preliminary report. *Cytobios*, 1982:145–152.
74. Ozturk Y et al. Endothelium-dependent and independent effects of garlic on rat aorta. *Journal of ethnopharmacology*, 1994, 44:109–116.
75. Siegel G et al. Potassium channel activation, hyperpolarization, and vascular relaxation. *Zeitschrift für Kardiologie*, 1991, 80:9–24.

76. Siegel G et al. Potassium channel activation in vascular smooth muscle. In: Frank GB, ed. *Excitation-contraction coupling in skeletal, cardiac, and smooth muscle.* New York, Plenum Press, 1992:53–72.

77. Das I, Khan NS, Sooranna SR. Nitric oxide synthetase activation is a unique mechanism of garlic action. *Biochemical Society transactions,* 1995, 23:S136.

78. Das I, Khan NS, Sooranna SR. Potent activation of nitric oxide synthetase by garlic: a basis for its therapeutic applications. *Current medical research opinion,* 1995, 13:257–263.

79. Bordia A et al. Effect of essential oil of onion and garlic on experimental atherosclerosis in rabbits. *Atherosclerosis,* 1977, 26:379–386.

80. Bordia A, Verma SK. Effect of garlic on regression of experimental atherosclerosis in rabbits. *Artery,* 1980, 7:428–437.

81. Mohammad SF et al. Isolation, characterization, identification and synthesis of an inhibitor of platelet function from *Allium sativum. Federation proceedings,* 1980, 39:543A.

82. Castro RA et al. Effects of garlic extract and three pure components from it on human platelet aggregation, arachidonate metabolism, release reaction and platelet ultrastructure. *Thrombosis research,* 1983, 32:155–169.

83. Srivastava KC. Aqueous extracts of onion, garlic and ginger inhibit platelet aggregation and alter arachidonic acid metabolism. *Biomedica biochimica acta,* 1984, 43:S335–S346.

84. Makheja AN, Bailey JM. Antiplatelet constituents of garlic and onion. *Agents and actions,* 1990, 29:360–363.

85. Srivastava KC. Effects of aqueous extracts of onion, garlic and ginger on platelet aggregation and metabolism of arachidonic acid in the blood vascular system: *in vitro* study. *Prostaglandins and leukotrienes in medicine,* 1984, 13:227–235.

86. Srivastava KC, Justesen U. Isolation and effects of some garlic components on platelet aggregation and metabolism of arachidonic acid in human blood platelets. *Wiener Klinische Wochenschrift,* 1989, 101:293–299.

87. Sendl A et al. Comparative pharmacological investigations of *Allium ursinum* and *Allium sativum. Planta medica,* 1992, 58:1–7.

88. Chauhan LS et al. Effect of onion, garlic and clofibrate on coagulation and fibrinolytic activity of blood in cholesterol fed rabbits. *Indian medical journal,* 1982, 76:126–127.

89. Makheja AN, Vanderhoek JY, Bailey JM. Inhibition of platelet aggregation and thromboxane synthesis by onion and garlic. *Lancet,* 1979, i:781.

90. Ariga T, Oshiba S. Effects of the essential oil components of garlic cloves on rabbit platelet aggregation. *Igaku to seibutsugaku,* 1981, 102:169–174.

91. Agarwal KC. Therapeutic actions of garlic constituents. *Medical research reviews,* 1996, 16:111–124.

92. Jain MK, Apitz-Castro R. Garlic: A product of spilled ambrosia. *Current science,* 1993, 65:148–156.

93. Mohammad SM, Woodward SC. Characterization of a potent inhibitor of platelet aggregation and release reaction isolated from *Allium sativum* (garlic). *Thrombosis research,* 1986, 44:793–806.

94. Ariga T, Oshiba S, Tamada T. Platelet aggregation inhibitor in garlic. *Lancet,* 1981, i:150–151.

95. Srivastava KC, Tyagi OD. Effects of a garlic-derived principal (ajoene) on aggregation and arachidonic acid metabolism in human blood platelets. *Prostaglandins, leukotrienes, and essential fatty acids,* 1993, 49:587–595.

96. Jamaluddin MP, Krishnan LK, Thomas A. Ajoene inhibition of platelet aggregation: possible mediation by a hemoprotein. *Biochemical and biophysical research communications,* 1988, 153:479–486.

97. Jain RC, Konar DB. Blood sugar lowering activity of garlic (*Allium sativum* Linn.). *Medikon,* 1977, 6:12–18.

98. Jain RC, Vyas CR, Mahatma OP. Hypoglycaemic action of onion and garlic. *Lancet*, 1973, ii:1491.
99. Jain RC, Vyas CR. Garlic in alloxan-induced diabetic rabbits. *American journal of clinical nutrition*, 1975, 28:684–685.
100. Osman SA. Chemical and biological studies of onion and garlic in an attempt to isolate a hypoglycemic extract. In: *Proceedings of the fourth Asian Symposium of Medicinal Plants and Spices*. Bangkok, 1980:117.
101. Zacharias NT et al. Hypoglycemic and hypolipidemic effects of garlic in sucrose fed rats. *Indian journal of physiology and pharmacology*, 1980, 24:151–154.
102. Srivastana VK, Afao Z. Garlic extract inhibits accumulation of polyols and hydration in diabetic rat lens. *Current science*, 1989, 58:376–377.
103. Farva D et al. Effects of garlic oil on streptozotocin-diabetic rats maintained on normal and high fat diets. *Indian journal of biochemistry and biophysics*, 1986, 23:24–27.
104. Venmadhi S, Devaki T. Studies on some liver enzymes in rats ingesting ethanol and treated with garlic oil. *Medical science research*, 1992, 20:729–731.
105. Kumar CA et al. *Allium sativum*: effect of three weeks feeding in rats. *Indian journal of pharmacology*, 1981, 13:91.
106. Chi MS, Koh ET, Stewart TJ. Effects of garlic on lipid metabolism in rats fed cholesterol or lard. *Journal of nutrition*, 1982, 112:241–248.
107. Swanston-Flatt SK et al. Traditional plant treatments for diabetes. Studies in normal and streptozotocin diabetic mice. *Diabetologia*, 1990, 33:462–464.
108. Mathew PT, Augusti KT. Studies on the effects of allicin (diallyl disulfide-oxide) on alloxan diabetes. Part I. Hypoglycemic action and enhancement of serum insulin effect and glycogen synthesis. *Indian journal of biochemistry and biophysics*, 1973, 10:209–221.
109. Mascolo N et al. Biological screening of Italian medicinal plants for anti-inflammatory activity. *Phytotherapy research*, 1987, 1:28–31.
110. Wagner H, Wierer M, Fessler B. Effects of garlic constituents on arachidonate metabolism. *Planta medica*, 1987, 53:305–306.
111. Gaffen JD, Tavares IA, Bennett A. The effect of garlic extracts on contractions of rat gastric fundus and human platelet aggregation. *Journal of pharmacy and pharmacology*, 1984, 36:272–274.
112. Aqel MB, Gharaibah MN, Salhab AS. Direct relaxant effects of garlic juice on smooth and cardiac muscles. *Journal of ethnopharmacology*, 1991, 33:13–19.
113. Rashid A, Hussain M, Khan HH. Bioassay for prostaglandin-like activity of garlic extract using isolated rat fundus strip and rat colon preparation. *Journal of the Pakistan Medical Association*, 1986, 36:138–141.
114. Neil HA, Silagy CA. Garlic: its cardioprotectant properties. *Current opinions in lipidology*, 1994, 5:6–10.
115. Silagy CA, Neil A. A meta-analysis of the effect of garlic on blood pressure. *Journal of hypertension*, 1994, 12:463–468.
116. Silagy CA, Neil A. Garlic as a lipid lowering agent: a meta-analysis. *Journal of the Royal College of Physicians of London*, 1994, 28:39–45.
117. Warshafsky S, Kamer RS, Sivak SL. Effect of garlic on total serum cholesterol. A meta-analysis. *Annals of internal medicine*, 1993, 119:599–605.
118. Brosche T, Platt D. Garlic as a phytogenic lipid lowering drug: a review of clinical trials with standardized garlic powder preparation. *Fortschritte der Medizin*, 1990, 108:703–706.
119. Harenberg J, Giese C, Zimmermann R. Effects of dried garlic on blood coagulation, fibrinolysis, platelet aggregation, and serum cholesterol levels in patients with hyperlipoproteinemia. *Atherosclerosis*, 1988, 74:247–249.
120. Bordia A et al. Effect of essential oil of garlic on serum fibrinolytic activity in patients with coronary artery disease. *Atherosclerosis*, 1977, 26:379–386.

121. Chutani SK, Bordia A. The effect of fried versus raw garlic on fibrinolytic activity in man. *Atherosclerosis*, 1981, 38:417–421.
122. Wolf S, Reim M. Effect of garlic on conjunctival vessels: a randomised, placebo-controlled, double-blind trial. *British journal of clinical practice*, 1990, 44:36–39.
123. Kiesewetter H, Jung F. Beeinflusst Knoblauch die Atherosklerose? *Medizinische Welt*, 1991, 42:21–23.
124. Jung H, Kiesewetter H. Einfluss einer Fettbelastung auf Plasmalipide und kapillare Hautdurchblutung unter Knoblauch. *Medizinische Welt*, 1991, 42:14–17.
125. Bordia A. Klinische Untersuchung zur Wirksamkeit von Knoblauch. *Apotheken-Magazin*, 1986, 6:128–131.
126. Bordia A. Knoblauch und koronare Herzkrankheit: Wirkungen einer dreijährigen Behandlung mit Knoblauchextrakt auf die Reinfarkt- und Mortalitätsrate. *Deutsche Apotheker Zeitung*, 1989, 129:16–17.
127. Sitprija S et al. Garlic and diabetes mellitus phase II clinical trial. *Journal of the Medical Association of Thailand*, 1987, 70:223–227.
128. Burnham BE. Garlic as a possible risk for postoperative bleeding. *Plastic and reconstructive surgery*, 1995, 95:213.
129. Petry JJ. Garlic and postoperative bleeding. *Plastic and reconstructive surgery*, 1995, 96:483–484.
130. Sunter WH. Warfarin and garlic. *Pharmaceutical journal*, 1991, 246:722.
131. Schimmer O et al. An evaluation of 55 commercial plant extracts in the Ames mutagenicity test. *Pharmazie*, 1994, 49:448–451.
132. Zhang YS, Chen XR, Yu YN. Antimutagenic effect of garlic (*Allium sativum*) on 4NQO-induced mutagenesis in *Escherichia coli* WP2. *Mutation research*, 1989, 227:215–219.
133. Siegers CP. *Allium sativum*. In: De Smet PA et al., eds. *Adverse effects of herbal drugs*, *Vol. 1*. Berlin, Springer-Verlag, 1992:73–76.
134. Rose KD et al. Spontaneous spinal epidural hematoma with associated platelet dysfunction from excessive garlic ingestion: A case report. *Neurosurgery*, 1990, 26:880–882.

Aloe

Definition

Aloe is the dried juice of the leaves of *Aloe vera* (L.) Burm. f. or of *A. ferox* Mill. and its hybrids with *A. africana* Mill. and *A. spicata* Baker (Liliaceae) (*1–6*).

Synonyms

Aloe vera (L.) Burm. f.

Aloe barbadensis Mill., *Aloe chinensis* Bak., *A. elongata* Murray, *A. indica* Royle, *A. officinalis* Forsk., *A. perfoliata* L., *A. rubescens* DC, *A. vera* L. var. *littoralis* König ex Bak., *A. vera* L. var. *chinensis* Berger, *A. vulgaris* Lam. (*7*).

In most formularies and reference books, *Aloe barbadensis* Mill. is regarded as the correct species name, and *Aloe vera* (L.) Burm. f. is considered a synonym. However, according to the International Rules of Botanical Nomenclature, *Aloe vera* (L.) Burm. f. is the legitimate name for this species (*8–10*). The genus *Aloe* has also been placed taxonomically in a family called Aloeaceae.

Aloe ferox Mill.

Aloe horrida Haw., *A. perfoliata* Thunberg., *A. pseudoferox* Salm. Dyck, *A. socotrina* Masson., *A. supralaevis* Haw., *Pachydendron ferox* Humb. & Bonpl., *P. supralaeve* Haw. (*7*).

Selected vernacular names

Aloe capensis, aloe curacao, aloe vera, aloes, aloès, aloès du Cape, aloès fèroce, aloes vrai, aloès vulgaire, alovis, Barbadoes aloe, Barbadoes aloes, Barbados aloe, Bergaalwyn, Bitteraalwyn, Cape aloe, chirukattali, Curacao aloe, Curacao aloes, Curacao alos, Echte Aloe, ghai kunwar, ghai kunwrar, gheekuar, ghikanvar, ghikuar, ghikumar, ghikumari, ghikwar, ghiu kumari, ghrita kumari, ghritakumari, grahakanya, gwar-patha, haang takhe, hlaba, Indian aloe, jadam, korphad, kumari, kumaro, kunvar pata, kunwar, laloi, laluwe, lo-hoei, lo-hoi, lou-houey, lu wei, luchuy, manjikattali, Mediterranean aloe, murr sbarr, musabar, rokai, sabbara, saber, sábila, sabilla, sabr, saibr, savila, savilla, semper vivum, shubiri, sibr, siang-tan, star cactus, tuna, umhlaba, waan haang charakhe, wan-hangchorakhe, yaa dam, yadam, zábila, zambila (*1, 7, 11*).

Description
Aloe vera (L.) Burm. f.

Succulent, almost sessile perennial herb; leaves 30–50 cm long and 10 cm broad at the base; colour pea-green (when young spotted with white); bright yellow tubular flowers 25–35 cm in length arranged in a slender loose spike; stamens frequently project beyond the perianth tube (*12*).

Aloe ferox Mill.

Arborescent perennial shrub with a single stem of 2–3 m in height, crowned by a large rosette of numerous leaves which are glaucous, oval-lanceolate, 40–60 cm in length, thorny on the ridge and the edges; inflorescence an erect raceme 60 cm in height; flowers with perianth 2.5 cm in length, red, yellow, or orange (*2*).

Plant material of interest: dried juice

Solidified juice originating in the cells of the pericycle and adjacent leaf parenchyma, and flowing spontaneously from the cut leaf, allowed to dry with or without the aid of heat.

It is not to be confused with Aloe Vera Gel, which is the colourless mucilaginous gel obtained from the parenchymatous cells in the leaves of *Aloe vera* (L.) Burm. f. (*13*).

General appearance
Curacao or Barbados Aloe, derived from *Aloe vera* (L.) Burm. f.

The dried juice occurs in dark chocolate-brown usually opaque masses; fracture, dull waxy, uneven, and frequently conchoidal (*2, 6*).

Cape Aloe, derived from *A. ferox* Mill. and its hybrids with *A. africana* Mill. and *A. spicata* Baker

The dried juice occurs in dark brown or greenish brown glassy masses, often covered with a yellowish powder; in thin fragments it is transparent and exhibits a yellowish, reddish brown or greenish tinge; fracture, smooth, even, and glassy (*2, 6*).

Organoleptic properties

Aloe is marketed as opaque masses that range from reddish black to brownish black to dark brown in colour. Odour, characteristic and disagreeable; taste, somewhat sour, nauseating and very bitter (*2, 7, 12*).

Microscopic characteristics
See "Powdered plant material" below.

Powdered plant material
Powdered aloes are yellowish brown to dark reddish brown. Microscopically, Cape Aloe appears as transparent brown or greenish brown irregular and angular fragments; Curacao Aloe shows fragments with numerous minute acicular crystals embedded in an amorphous matrix (*1–3, 12, 14*).

Geographical distribution
Native to southern and eastern Africa, and subsequently introduced into northern Africa, the Arabian peninsula, China, Gibraltar, the Mediterranean countries, and the West Indies (*15*). It is commercially cultivated in Aruba, Bonaire, Haiti, India, South Africa, the United States of America, and Venezuela (*2, 7, 12, 14, 15*).

General identity tests
Macroscopic and microscopic examinations (*1–3, 7, 12, 14*); solvent solubility (hot alcohol, boiling water, and ether) determination (*2, 4–6*); chemical reactions (*1–6, 8, 12–14*); and thin-layer chromatographic analysis employing barbaloin as the reference standard (*4–7*).

Purity tests
Microbiology
The test for *Salmonella* spp. in aloe products should be negative. The maximum acceptable limits of other microorganisms are as follows (*16–18*). For preparation of decoction: aerobic bacteria—not more than 10^7/g; fungi—not more than 10^5/g; *Escherichia coli*—not more than 10^2/g. Preparations for internal use: aerobic bacteria—not more than 10^5/g or ml; fungi—not more than 10^4/g or ml; enterobacteria and certain Gram-negative bacteria—not more than 10^3/g or ml; *Escherichia coli*—0/g or ml.

Foreign organic matter
Adulterants: Aloe in commerce may sometimes be adulterated with black catechu, pieces of iron, and stones. These can be detected by examining alcohol-soluble extracts under ultraviolet light which gives a deep brown colour with aloe and a black colour with catechu (*14*).

Total ash
Not more than 2% (*3–5*).

Water-soluble extracts
Not less than 50% (*1*, *2*, *14*).

Alcohol-insoluble extracts
Not more than 10% (*1–3*, *14*).

Moisture
Not more than 10% for Cape Aloe (*6*), and not more than 12% for Curacao or Barbados Aloe (*2–6*, *14*).

Pesticide residues
To be established in accordance with national requirements. Normally, the maximum residue limit of aldrin and dieldrin for Aloe is not more than 0.05 mg/kg (*18*). For other pesticides, see the WHO guidelines on quality control methods for medicinal plants (*16*) and guidelines for predicting dietary intake of pesticide residues (*19*).

Heavy metals
Recommended lead and cadmium levels are not more than 10 and 0.3 mg/kg, respectively, in the final dosage form of the plant material (*16*).

Radioactive residues
For analysis of strontium-90, iodine-131, caesium-134, caesium-137, and plutonium-239, see WHO guidelines on quality control methods for medicinal plants (*16*).

Other tests
Acid-insoluble ash and chemical tests to be established in accordance with national requirements.

Chemical assays
Thin-layer chromatography and microchemical analyses are employed for the qualitative analysis for the presence of anthracene glycosides (*1–7*, *12*, *14*). Quantitative analysis of total anthracene glycosides, calculated as barbaloin, is performed by spectrophotometry (*4*, *5*).

Curacao or Barbados Aloe, derived from Aloe vera (L.) Burm. f.
Contains not less than 28% of hydroxyanthracene derivatives, expressed as barbaloin (*4–6*).

Cape Aloe, derived from A. ferox Miller and its hybrids with A. africana Mill. and A. spicata Baker

Contains not less than 18% of hydroxyanthracene derivatives, expressed as barbaloin (*4, 5*).

Major chemical constituents

Aloe contains as its major and active principles hydroxyanthrone derivatives, mainly of the aloe-emodin-anthrone 10-C-glucoside type. The major constituent is known as barbaloin (aloin) (15–40%) (*8, 13*). It also contains hydroxyaloin (about 3%). Barbaloin (=aloin) is in fact a mixture of aloin A (10S) [1] and B (10R) [2]. *A. ferox* also contains aloinoside A [3] and B [4]. Aloin A and B interconvert through the anthranol form as do aloinoside A and B (*13*).

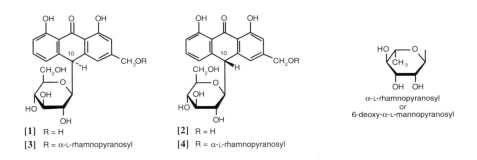

[1] R = H
[3] R = α-L-rhamnopyranosyl

[2] R = H
[4] R = α-L-rhamnopyranosyl

α-L-rhamnopyranosyl
or
6-deoxy-α-L-mannopyranosyl

Dosage forms

Powdered, dried juice and preparations thereof for oral use.

Medicinal uses

Uses supported by clinical data

Short-term treatment of occasional constipation (*2, 12, 13, 15*).

Uses described in pharmacopoeias and in traditional systems of medicine

None.

Uses described in folk medicine, not supported by experimental or clinical data

Treatment of seborrhoeic dermatitis, peptic ulcers, tuberculosis, and fungal infections, and for reduction of blood sugar (glucose) levels (*11, 20*).

Pharmacology
Experimental pharmacology
As shown for senna, Aloe's mechanism of action is twofold. It stimulates colonic motility, augmenting propulsion and accelerating colonic transit, which reduces fluid absorption from the faecal mass. It also increases paracellular permeability across the colonic mucosa probably owing to an inhibition of Na^+, K^+-adenosine triphosphatase or to an inhibition of chloride channels (*8, 21, 22*), which results in an increase in the water content in the large intestine (*21*).

Clinical pharmacology
The laxative effects of Aloe are due primarily to the 1, 8-dihydroxyanthracene glycosides, aloin A and B (formerly designated barbaloin) (*23, 24*). After oral administration aloin A and B, which are not absorbed in the upper intestine, are hydrolysed in the colon by intestinal bacteria and then reduced to the active metabolites (the main active metabolite is aloe-emodin-9-anthrone) (*25, 26*), which like senna acts as a stimulant and irritant to the gastrointestinal tract (*27*). The laxative effect of Aloe is not generally observed before 6 hours after oral administration, and sometimes not until 24 or more hours after.

Toxicity
The major symptoms of overdose are griping and severe diarrhoea with consequent losses of fluid and electrolytes. Treatment should be supportive with generous amounts of fluid. Electrolytes, particularly potassium, should be monitored in all recipients, especially in children and the elderly (*28*).

Contraindications
As with other stimulant laxatives, products containing Aloe should not be used in patients with intestinal obstruction or stenosis, atony, severe dehydration with electrolyte depletion, or chronic constipation (*28*). Aloe should not be administered to patients with inflammatory intestinal diseases, such as appendicitis, Crohn disease, ulcerative colitis, irritable bowel syndrome, or diverticulitis, or to children under 10 years of age. Aloe should not be used during pregnancy or lactation except under medical supervision after evaluating benefits and risks. Aloe is also contraindicated in patients with cramps, colic, haemorrhoids, nephritis, or any undiagnosed abdominal symptoms such as pain, nausea, or vomiting (*28, 29*).

Warnings
Aloe-containing products should be used only if no effect can be obtained through a change of diet or use of bulk-forming products. Stimulant laxative products should not be used when abdominal pain, nausea, or vomiting are present. Rectal bleeding or failure to have a bowel movement within 24 hours

after use of a laxative may indicate a serious condition. Chronic use may cause dependence and need for increased dosages, disturbances of water and electrolyte balance (e.g. hypokalaemia), and an atonic colon with impaired function (*28*).

The use of stimulant laxatives for more than 2 weeks requires medical supervision.

Chronic abuse with diarrhoea and consequent fluid and electrolyte losses (mainly hypokalaemia) may cause albuminuria and haematuria, and may result in cardiac and neuromuscular dysfunction, the latter particularly in the case of concomitant use of cardiac glycosides (digoxin), diuretics, corticosteroids, or liquorice root (see Precautions below).

Precautions
General
Laxatives containing anthraquinone glycosides should not be used continuously for longer than 1–2 weeks, owing to the danger of electrolyte imbalance.

Drug interactions
Decreased intestinal transit time may reduce absorption of orally administered drugs (*30*).

Existing hypokalaemia resulting from long-term laxative abuse can potentiate the effects of cardiotonic glycosides (digitalis, strophanthus) and antiarrhythmic drugs such as quinidine (*30*). The induction of hypokalaemia by drugs such as thiazide diuretics, adrenocorticosteroids, and liquorice root may be enhanced, and electrolyte imbalance may be aggravated (*31*).

Drug and laboratory test interactions
Standard methods may not detect anthranoid metabolites, so measurements of faecal excretion may not be reliable (*26*).

Urinary excretion of certain anthranoid metabolites may discolour the urine, which is not clinically relevant but which may cause false positive results for urinary urobilinogen, and for estrogens when measured by the Kober procedure (*30*).

Carcinogenesis, mutagenesis, impairment of fertility
Data on the carcinogenicity of Aloe are not available. While chronic abuse of anthranoid-containing laxatives was hypothesized to play a role in colorectal cancer, no causal relationship between anthranoid laxative abuse and colorectal cancer has been demonstrated (*32–35*).

In vitro (gene mutation and chromosome aberration tests) and *in vivo* (micronucleus test in murine bone marrow) genotoxicity studies, as well as human and animal pharmacokinetic data, indicate no genotoxic risk from Cape Aloe (*36–38*).

Pregnancy: teratogenic effects

No teratogenic or fetotoxic effects were seen in rats after oral treatment with aloe extract (up to 1000 mg/kg) or aloin A (up to 200 mg/kg) (*39*).

Pregnancy: non-teratogenic effects

Aloe should not be used during pregnancy except under medical supervision after benefits and risks have been evaluated (*40*).

Nursing mothers

Anthranoid metabolites appear in breast milk. *Aloe* should not be used during lactation except under medical supervision, as there are insufficient data available to assess the potential for pharmacological effects in the breast-fed infant (*30, 40*).

Paediatric use

Oral use of Aloe in children under 10 years old is contraindicated.

Adverse reactions

Abdominal spasms and pain may occur after even a single dose. Overdose can lead to colicky abdominal spasms and pain, as well as the formation of thin, watery stools (*28*).

Chronic abuse of anthraquinone stimulant laxatives can lead to hepatitis (*41*). Long-term laxative abuse may lead to electrolyte disturbances (hypokalaemia, hypocalcaemia), metabolic acidosis, malabsorption, weight loss, albuminuria, and haematuria (*30, 42, 43*). Weakness and orthostatic hypotension may be exacerbated in elderly patients when stimulant laxatives are repeatedly used (*31*). Secondary aldosteronism may occur owing to renal tubular damage after aggravated use. Steatorrhoea and protein-losing gastroenteropathy with hypoalbuminaemia have also been observed, as have excessive excretion of calcium in the stools and osteomalacia of the vertebral column (*44, 45*). Melanotic pigmentation of the colonic mucosa (pseudo-melanosis coli) has been observed in individuals taking anthraquinone laxatives for extended time periods (*29, 42*). The pigmentation is clinically harmless and usually reversible within 4 to 12 months after the drug is discontinued (*29, 42*). Conflicting data exist on other toxic effects such as intestinal-neuronal damage after long-term use (*42, 46*).

Posology

The correct individual dose is the smallest amount required to produce a soft-formed stool (*26*). As a laxative for adults and children over 10 years old, 0.04–0.11 g (Curacao or Barbados Aloe) or 0.06–0.17 g (Cape Aloe) of the dried juice (*6, 14*), corresponding to 10–30 mg hydroxyanthraquinones per day, or 0.1 g as a single dose in the evening.

References

1. *The United States pharmacopeia XXIII*. Rockville, MD, US Pharmacopeial Convention, 1996.
2. *African pharmacopoeia, Vol. 1*, 1st ed. Lagos, Organization of African Unity, Scientific, Technical & Research Commission, 1985.
3. *The Japanese pharmacopoeia XIII*. Tokyo, The Society of Japanese Pharmacopoeia, 1996.
4. *Pharmacopée française*. Paris, Adrapharm, 1996.
5. *European pharmacopoeia*, 2nd ed. Strasbourg, Council of Europe, 1995.
6. *British pharmacopoeia*. London, Her Majesty's Stationery Office, 1993.
7. Hänsel R et al., eds. *Hagers Handbuch der Pharmazeutischen Praxis, Vol. 6*, 5th ed. Berlin, Springer, 1994.
8. Bradley PR, ed. *British herbal compendium, Vol. 1*. Bournemouth, British Herbal Medicine Association, 1992:199–203.
9. Newton LE. In defence of the name *Aloe vera*. *The cactus and succulent journal of Great Britain*, 1979, 41:29–30.
10. Tucker AO, Duke JA, Foster S. Botanical nomenclature of medicinal plants. In: Cracker LE, Simon JE, eds. *Herbs, spices and medicinal plants, Vol. 4*. Phoenix, AR, Oryx Press, 1989:169–242.
11. Farnsworth NR, ed. *NAPRALERT database*. Chicago, University of Illinois at Chicago, IL, August 8, 1995 production (an on-line database available directly through the University of Illinois at Chicago or through the Scientific and Technical Network (STN) of Chemical Abstracts Services).
12. Youngken HW. *Textbook of pharmacognosy*, 6th ed. Philadelphia, Blakiston, 1950.
13. Bruneton J. *Pharmacognosy, phytochemistry, medicinal plants*. Paris, Lavoisier, 1995.
14. *The Indian pharmaceutical codex. Vol. I. Indigenous drugs*. New Delhi, Council of Scientific & Industrial Research, 1953.
15. Haller JS. A drug for all seasons, medical and pharmacological history of aloe. *Bulletin of the New York Academy of Medicine*, 1990, 66:647–659.
16. *Quality control methods for medicinal plant materials*. Geneva, World Health Organization, 1998.
17. *Deutsches Arzneibuch 1996. Vol. 2. Methoden der Biologie*. Stuttgart, Deutscher Apotheker Verlag, 1996.
18. *European pharmacopoeia*, 3rd ed. Strasbourg, Council of Europe, 1997.
19. *Guidelines for predicting dietary intake of pesticide residues*, 2nd rev. ed. Geneva, World Health Organization, 1997 (unpublished document WHO/FSF/FOS/97.7; available from Food Safety, WHO, 1211 Geneva 27, Switzerland).
20. Castleman M. *The healing herbs*. Emmaus, PA, Rodale Press, 1991:42–44.
21. de Witte P. Metabolism and pharmacokinetics of anthranoids. *Pharmacology*, 1993, 47(Suppl. 1):86–97.
22. Ishii O, Tanizawa H, Takino Y. Studies of *Aloe* III. Mechanism of laxative effect. *Chemical and pharmaceutical bulletin*, 1990, 38:197–200.
23. Tyler VE, Bradley LR, Robbers JE, eds. *Pharmacognosy*, 9th ed. Philadelphia, Lea & Febiger, 1988:62–63.
24. Tyler VE. *Herbs of choice*. New York, Pharmaceutical Products Press, 1994:155–157.
25. Che QM et al. Isolation of human intestinal bacteria capable of transforming barbaloin to aloe-emodin anthrone. *Planta medica*, 1991, 57:15–19.
26. *Aloe capensis, Cape Aloes: proposal for the summary of product characteristics*. Elburg, Netherlands, European Scientific Committee of Phytotherapy, 1995.
27. Reynolds JEF, ed. *Martindale, the extra pharmacopoeia*, 30th ed. London, Pharmaceutical Press, 1993:903.

28. *Goodman and Gilman's the pharmacological basis of therapeutics*, 8th ed. New York, McGraw Hill, 1990.
29. Bisset NG. *Sennae folium*. In: *Max Wichtl's herbal drugs & phytopharmaceuticals*. Boca Raton, FL, CRC Press, 1994:463–469.
30. *American Hospital Formulary Service*. Bethesda, MD, American Society of Hospital Pharmacists, 1990.
31. *United States pharmacopeia, drug information*. Rockville, MD, United States Pharmacopeial Convention, 1992.
32. Siegers CP et al. Anthranoid laxative abuse—a risk for colorectal cancer. *Gut*, 1993, 34:1099–1101.
33. Siegers CP. Anthranoid laxatives and colorectal cancer. *Trends in pharmacological sciences*, 1992, 13:229–231.
34. Patel PM et al. Anthraquinone laxatives and human cancer. *Postgraduate medical journal*, 1989, 65:216–217.
35. Loew D. Pseudomelanosis coli durch Anthranoide. *Zeitschrift für Phytotherapie*, 1994, 16:312–318.
36. Lang W. Pharmacokinetic–metabolic studies with ^{14}C-aloe emodin after oral administration to male and female rats. *Pharmacology*, 1993, 47(Suppl. 1):73–77.
37. Brown JP. A review of the genetic effects of naturally occurring flavonoids, anthraquinones and related compounds. *Mutation research*, 1980, 75:243–277.
38. Westendorf J et al. Genotoxicity of naturally occurring hydroxyanthraquinones. *Mutation research*, 1990, 240:1–12.
39. Bangel E et al. Tierexperimentelle pharmakologische Untersuchungen zur Frage der abortiven und teratogenen Wirkung sowie zur Hyperämie von Aloe. *Steiner-Informationsdienst*, 1975, 4:1–25.
40. Lewis JH, Weingold AB. The use of gastrointestinal drugs during pregnancy and lactation. *American journal of gastroenterology*, 1985, 80:912–923.
41. Beuers U, Spengler U, Pape GR. Hepatitis after chronic abuse of senna. *Lancet*, 1991, 337:472.
42. Muller-Lissner SA. Adverse effects of laxatives: facts and fiction. *Pharmacology*, 47, 1993, (Suppl. 1):138–145.
43. Godding EW. Therapeutics of laxative agents with special reference to the anthraquinones. *Pharmacology*, 1976, 14(Suppl. 1):78–101.
44. Heizer WD et al. Protein-losing gastroenteropathy and malabsorption associated with factitious diarrhoea. *Annals of internal medicine*, 1968, 68:839–852.
45. *Goodman and Gilman's the pharmacological basis of therapeutics*, 9th ed. New York, McGraw Hill, 1996.
46. Kune GA. Laxative use not a risk for colorectal cancer: data from the Melbourne colorectal cancer study. *Zeitschrift für Gasteroenterologie*, 1993, 31:140–143.

Aloe Vera Gel

Definition

Aloe Vera Gel is the colourless mucilaginous gel obtained from the parenchymatous cells in the fresh leaves of *Aloe vera* (L) Burm. f. (Liliaceae) (*1, 2*).

Synonyms

Aloe barbadensis Mill., *Aloe chinensis* Bak., *A. elongata* Murray, *A. indica* Royle, *A. officinalis* Forsk., *A. perfoliata* L., *A. rubescens* DC, *A. vera* L. var. *littoralis* König ex Bak., *A. vera* L. var. *chinensis* Berger, *A. vulgaris* Lam. (*2–5*). Most formularies and reference books regard *Aloe barbadensis* Mill. as the correct species name, and *Aloe vera* (L.) Burm. f. as a synonym. However, according to the International Rules of Botanical Nomenclature, *Aloe vera* (L.) Burm. f. is the legitimate name for this species (*2–4*). The genus *Aloe* has also been placed taxonomically in a family called Aloeaceae.

Selected vernacular names

Aloe vera gel, aloe gel.

Description

Succulent, almost sessile perennial herb; leaves 30–50 cm long and 10 cm broad at the base; colour pea-green (when young spotted with white); bright yellow tubular flowers 25–35 cm in length arranged in a slender loose spike; stamens frequently project beyond the perianth tube (*6*).

Plant material of interest: liquid gel from the fresh leaf

Aloe Vera Gel is not to be confused with the juice, which is the bitter yellow exudate originating from the bundle sheath cells of the leaf. The drug Aloe consists of the dried juice, as defined on page 33.

General appearance

The gel is a viscous, colourless, transparent liquid.

Organoleptic properties

Viscous, colourless, odourless, taste slightly bitter.

Microscopic characteristics

Not applicable.

Geographical distribution

Probably native to north Africa along the upper Nile in the Sudan, and subsequently introduced and naturalized in the Mediterranean region, most of the tropics and warmer areas of the world, including Asia, the Bahamas, Central America, Mexico, the southern United States of America, south-east Asia, and the West Indies (2).

General identity tests

To be established in accordance with national requirements.

Purity tests

Microbiology

The test for *Salmonella* spp. in Aloe Vera Gel should be negative. Acceptable maximum limits of other microorganisms are as follows (7–9). For external use: aerobic bacteria—not more than 10^2/ml; fungi—not more than 10^2/ml; enterobacteria and certain Gram-negative bacteria—not more than 10^1/ml; *Staphylococcus* spp.—0/ml. (Not used internally.)

Moisture

Contains 98.5% water (10).

Pesticide residues

To be established in accordance with national requirements. For guidance, see WHO guidelines on quality control methods for medicinal plants (7) and guidelines on predicting dietary intake of pesticide residues (11).

Heavy metals

Recommended lead and cadmium levels are not more than 10 and 0.3 mg/kg, respectively, in the final dosage form (7).

Radioactive residues

For analysis of strontium-90, iodine-131, caesium-134, caesium-137, and plutonium-239, see WHO guidelines on quality control methods for medicinal plants (7).

Other tests

Chemical tests for Aloe Vera Gel and tests for total ash, acid-insoluble ash, alcohol-soluble residue, foreign organic matter, and water-soluble extracts to be established in accordance with national requirements.

Chemical assays

Carbohydrates (0.3%) (*12*), water (98.5%) (*10*). Polysaccharide composition analysis by gas–liquid chromatography (*13*).

Major chemical constituents

Aloe Vera Gel consists primarily of water and polysaccharides (pectins, hemi-celluloses, glucomannan, acemannan, and mannose derivatives). It also contains amino acids, lipids, sterols (lupeol, campesterol, and β-sitosterol), tannins, and enzymes (*1*). Mannose 6-phosphate is a major sugar component (*14*).

Dosage forms

The clear mucilaginous gel. At present no commercial preparation has been proved to be stable. Because many of the active ingredients in the gel appear to deteriorate on storage, the use of fresh gel is recommended. Preparation of fresh gel: harvest leaves and wash them with water and a mild chlorine solution. Remove the outer layers of the leaf including the pericyclic cells, leaving a "fillet" of gel. Care should be taken not to tear the green rind which can contaminate the fillet with leaf exudate. The gel may be stabilized by pasteurization at 75–80 °C for less than 3 minutes. Higher temperatures held for longer times may alter the chemical composition of the gel (*2*).

Medicinal uses

Uses supported by clinical data

None.

Uses described in pharmacopoeias and in traditional systems of medicine

Aloe Vera Gel is widely used for the external treatment of minor wounds and inflammatory skin disorders (*1*, *14–17*). The gel is used in the treatment of minor skin irritations, including burns, bruises, and abrasions (*1*, *14*, *18*). The gel is further used in the cosmetics industry as a hydrating ingredient in liquids, creams, sun lotions, shaving creams, lip balms, healing ointments, and face packs (*1*).

Aloe Vera Gel has been traditionally used as a natural remedy for burns (*18*, *19*). Aloe Vera Gel has been effectively used in the treatment of first- and second-degree thermal burns and radiation burns. Both thermal and radiation burns healed faster with less necrosis when treated with preparations containing Aloe Vera Gel (*18*, *19*). In most cases the gel must be freshly prepared because of its sensitivity to enzymatic, oxidative, or microbial degradation. Aloe Vera Gel is not approved as an internal medication, and internal administration of the gel has not been shown to exert any consistent therapeutic effect.

Uses described in folk medicine, not supported by experimental or clinical data

The treatment of acne, haemorrhoids, psoriasis, anaemia, glaucoma, petit ulcer, tuberculosis, blindness, seborrhoeic dermatitis, and fungal infections (*2, 6, 19*).

Pharmacology

Wound healing

Clinical investigations suggest that Aloe Vera Gel preparations accelerate wound healing (*14, 18*). *In vivo* studies have demonstrated that Aloe Vera Gel promotes wound healing by directly stimulating the activity of macrophages and fibroblasts (*14*). Fibroblast activation by Aloe Vera Gel has been reported to increase both collagen and proteoglycan synthesis, thereby promoting tissue repair (*14*). Some of the active principles appear to be polysaccharides composed of several monosaccharides, predominantly mannose. It has been suggested that mannose 6-phosphate, the principal sugar component of Aloe Vera Gel, may be partly responsible for the wound healing properties of the gel (*14*). Mannose 6-phosphate can bind to the growth factor receptors on the surface of the fibroblasts and thereby enhance their activity (*14, 15*).

Furthermore, acemannan, a complex carbohydrate isolated from *Aloe* leaves, has been shown to accelerate wound healing and reduce radiation-induced skin reactions (*20, 21*). The mechanism of action of acemannan appears to be twofold. First, acemannan is a potent macrophage-activating agent and therefore may stimulate the release of fibrogenic cytokines (*21, 22*). Second, growth factors may directly bind to acemannan, promoting their stability and prolonging their stimulation of granulation tissue (*20*).

The therapeutic effects of Aloe Vera Gel also include prevention of progressive dermal ischaemia caused by burns, frostbite, electrical injury and intra-arterial drug abuse. *In vivo* analysis of these injuries demonstrates that Aloe Vera Gel acts as an inhibitor of thromboxane A_2, a mediator of progressive tissue damage (*14, 17*). Several other mechanisms have been proposed to explain the activity of Aloe Vera Gel, including stimulation of the complement linked to polysaccharides, as well as the hydrating, insulating, and protective properties of the gel (*1*).

Because many of the active ingredients appear to deteriorate on storage, the use of fresh gel is recommended. Studies of the growth of normal human cells *in vitro* demonstrated that cell growth and attachment were promoted by exposure to fresh *Aloe vera* leaves, whereas a stabilized Aloe Vera Gel preparation was shown to be cytotoxic to both normal and tumour cells. The cytotoxic effects of the stabilized gel were thought to be due to the addition of other substances to the gel during processing (*23*).

Anti-inflammatory

The anti-inflammatory activity of Aloe Vera Gel has been revealed by a number of *in vitro* and *in vivo* studies (*14, 17, 24, 25*). Fresh Aloe Vera Gel significantly reduced acute inflammation in rats (carrageenin-induced paw oedema), although no effect on chronic inflammation was observed (*25*). Aloe Vera Gel appears to exert its anti-inflammatory activity through bradykinase activity (*24*) and thromboxane B_2 and prostaglandin F_2 inhibition (*18, 26*). Furthermore, three plant sterols in Aloe Vera Gel reduced inflammation by up to 37% in croton oil-induced oedema in mice (*15*). Lupeol, one of the sterol compounds found in *Aloe vera*, was the most active and reduced inflammation in a dose-dependent manner (*15*). These data suggest that specific plant sterols may also contribute to the anti-inflammatory activity of Aloe Vera Gel.

Burn treatment

Aloe Vera Gel has been used for the treatment of radiation burns (*27–30*). Healing of radiation ulcers was observed in two patients treated with *Aloe vera* cream (*27*), although the fresh gel was more effective than the cream (*29, 30*). Complete healing was observed, after treatment with fresh Aloe Vera Gel, in two patients with radiation burns (*30*). Twenty-seven patients with partial-thickness burns were treated with Aloe Vera Gel in a placebo-controlled study (*31*). The Aloe Vera Gel-treated lesions healed faster (11.8 days) than the burns treated with petroleum jelly gauze (18.2 days), a difference that is statistically significant (*t*-test, $P < 0.002$).

Contraindications

Aloe Vera Gel is contraindicated in cases of known allergy to plants in the Liliaceae.

Warnings

No information available.

Precautions

No information available concerning general precautions, or precautions dealing with carcinogenesis, mutagenesis, impairment of fertility; drug and laboratory test interactions; drug interactions; nursing mothers; paediatric use; or teratogenic or non-teratogenic effects on pregnancy.

Adverse reactions

There have been a few reports of contact dermatitis and burning skin sensations following topical applications of Aloe Vera Gel to dermabraded skin (*18, 32*). These reactions appeared to be associated with anthraquinone contaminants in this preparation (*33*). A case of disseminated dermatitis has been reported following application of Aloe Vera Gel to a patient with stasis dermatitis (*34*). An acute bullous allergic reaction and contact urticaria have also been reported to result from the use of Aloe Vera Gel (*35*).

Posology

Fresh gel or preparations containing 10–70% fresh gel.

References

1. Bruneton J. *Pharmacognosy, phytochemistry, medicinal plants*. Paris, Lavoisier, 1995.
2. Grindlay D, Reynolds T. The *Aloe vera* phenomenon: a review of the properties and modern uses of the leaf parenchyma gel. *Journal of ethnopharmacology*, 1986, 16:117–151.
3. Newton LE . In defence of the name *Aloe vera*. *The cactus and succulent journal of Great Britain*, 1979, 41:29–30.
4. Tucker AO, Duke JA, Foster S. Botanical nomenclature of medicinal plants. In: Cracker LE, Simon JE, eds. *Herbs, spices and medicinal plants, Vol. 4*. Phoenix, AR, Oryx Press, 1989:169–242.
5. Hänsel R et al., eds. *Hagers Handbuch der Pharmazeutischen Praxis, Vol. 6*, 5th ed. Berlin, Springer, 1994.
6. Youngken HW. *Textbook of pharmacognosy*, 6th ed. Philadelphia, Blakiston, 1950.
7. *Quality control methods for medicinal plant materials*. Geneva, World Health Organization, 1998.
8. *Deutsches Arzneibuch 1996. Vol. 2. Methoden der Biologie*. Stuttgart, Deutscher Apotheker Verlag, 1996.
9. *European pharmacopoeia*, 3rd ed. Strasbourg, Council of Europe, 1997.
10. Rowe TD, Park LM. Phytochemical study of *Aloe vera* leaf. *Journal of the American Pharmaceutical Association*, 1941, 30:262–266.
11. *Guidelines for predicting dietary intake of pesticide residues*, 2nd rev. ed. Geneva, World Health Organization, 1997 (unpublished document WHO/FSF/FOS/97.7; available from Food Safety, WHO, 1211 Geneva 27, Switzerland).
12. Pierce RF. Comparison between the nutritional contents of the aloe gel from conventional and hydroponically grown plants. *Erde international*, 1983, 1:37–38.
13. Hart LA et al. An anti-complementary polysaccharide with immunological adjuvant activity from the leaf of *Aloe vera*. *Planta medica*, 1989, 55:509–511.
14. Davis RH et al. Anti-inflammatory and wound healing of growth substance in *Aloe vera*. *Journal of the American Pediatric Medical Association*, 1994, 84:77–81.
15. Davis RH et al. *Aloe vera*, hydrocortisone, and sterol influence on wound tensile strength and anti-inflammation. *Journal of the American Pediatric Medical Association*, 1994, 84:614–621.
16. Heggers JP, Pelley RP, Robson MC. Beneficial effects of *Aloe* in wound healing. *Phytotherapy research*, 1993, 7:S48–S52.
17. McCauley R. Frostbite—methods to minimize tissue loss. *Postgraduate medicine*, 1990, 88:67–70.
18. Shelton RM. *Aloe vera*, its chemical and therapeutic properties. *International journal of dermatology*, 1991, 30:679–683.
19. Haller JS. A drug for all seasons, medical and pharmacological history of aloe. *Bulletin of New York Academy of Medicine*, 1990, 66:647–659.
20. Tizard AU et al. Effects of acemannan, a complex carbohydrate, on wound healing in young and aged rats. *Wounds, a compendium of clinical research and practice*, 1995, 6:201–209.
21. Roberts DB, Travis EL. Acemannan-containing wound dressing gels reduce radiation-induced skin reactions in C3H mice. *International journal of radiation oncology, biology and physiology*, 1995, 15:1047–1052.
22. Karaca K, Sharma JM, Norgren R. Nitric oxide production by chicken macrophages

activated by acemannan, a complex carbohydrate extracted from *Aloe vera. International journal of immunopharmacology*, 1995, 17:183–188.

23. Winters WD, Benavides R, Clouse WJ. Effects of aloe extracts on human normal and tumor cells *in vitro. Economic botany*, 1981, 35:89–95.

24. Fujita K, Teradaira R. Bradykininase activity of aloe extract. *Biochemical pharmacology*, 1976, 25:205.

25. Udupa SI, Udupa AL, Kulkarni DR. Anti-inflammatory and wound healing properties of *Aloe vera. Fitoterapia*, 1994, 65:141–145.

26. Robson MC, Heggers J, Hagstrom WJ. Myth, magic, witchcraft or fact? *Aloe vera* revisited. *Journal of burn care and rehabilitation*, 1982, 3:157–162.

27. Collin C. Roentgen dermatitis treated with fresh whole leaf of *Aloe vera. American journal of roentgen*, 1935, 33:396–397.

28. Wright CS. *Aloe vera* in the treatment of roentgen ulcers and telangiectasis. *Journal of the American Medical Association*, 1936, 106:1363–1364.

29. Rattner H. Roentgen ray dermatitis with ulcers. *Archives of dermatology and syphilogy*, 1936, 33:593–594.

30. Loveman AB. Leaf of *Aloe vera* in treatment of roentgen ray ulcers. *Archives of dermatology and syphilogy*, 1937, 36:838–843.

31. Visuthikosol V et al. Effect of *Aloe vera* gel on healing of burn wounds: a clinical and histological study. *Journal of the Medical Association of Thailand*, 1995, 78:403–409.

32. Hormann HP, Korting HC. Evidence for the efficacy and safety of topical herbal drugs in dermatology: Part 1: Anti-inflammatory agents. *Phytomedicine*, 1994, 1:161–171.

33. Hunter D, Frumkin A. Adverse reactions to vitamin E and *Aloe vera* preparations after dermabrasion and chemical peel. *Cutis*, 1991, 47:193–194.

34. Horgan DJ. Widespread dermatitis after topical treatment of chronic leg ulcers and stasis dermatitis. *Canadian Medical Association Journal*, 1988, 138:336–338.

35. Morrow DM, Rappaport MJ, Strick RA. Hypersensitivity to aloe. *Archives of dermatology*, 1980, 116:1064–1065.

Radix Astragali

Definition

Radix Astragali is the dried root of *Astragalus membranaceus* (Fisch.) Bunge and *Astragalus mongholicus* Bunge (Fabaceae) (*1*, *2*).

Synonyms

Fabaceae are also known as Leguminosae.

Astragalus membranaceus (Fisch.) Bunge

A. *propinguus* B. Schischk. (*3*).

Astragalus mongholicus Bunge

A. *membranaceus* (Fisch.) Bunge var. *mongholicus* (Bunge) Hsiao (*3*).

Selected vernacular names

Astragalus root, hoàng ký, huang-chi, huangoi, huangqi, huángqi, hwanggi, membranous milkvetch, milkvetch, Mongolian milk-vetch, neimeng huangqi, ogi, ougi, zhongfengnaomaitong (*1*, *3–9*).

Description

Astragalus membranaceus (Fisch.) Bunge

Perennial herb, 25–40 cm tall. Leaves 3–6 cm long; petiole obsolete; stipules free, cauline, green, triangular ovate, sparingly vested on the outside with white hair. Leaflets oblong-obovate, oval or oblong-oval. Racemes oblong-ovoid to ovoid, 4–5 cm long, 10–15 flowers; bracts lanceolate. Calyx 8–9 mm long, campanulate, strongly oblique, glabrous. Corolla yellowish, 18–20 mm long. Ovary glabrous (*4*). Root cylindrical or nearly cylindrical with small bases of lateral root dispersed on the surface, and usually not branched; greyish yellow to yellowish brown epidermis and fibrous fracture (*2*, *5*).

Astragalus mongholicus Bunge

Perennial herb, 60–150 cm tall. Leaves pinnate, leaflets broadly elliptical. Raceme axillary. Calyx tubular 5 mm long. Corolla yellowish; pod ovate-oblong, glabrous, reticulate. The root is flexible and long and covered with a tough, wrinkled, yellowish brown epidermis, which has a tendency to break up into woolly fibres. The woody interior is yellowish white (*6*).

Plant material of interest: root
General appearance
Radix Astragali is cylindrical, some upper branches relatively thick, 30–90 cm long, 1–3.5 cm in diameter. Externally pale brownish yellow or pale brown, with irregular, longitudinal wrinkles or furrows. Texture hard and tenacious, broken with difficulty, fracture highly fibrous and starchy, bark yellowish white, wood pale yellow, with radiate striations and fissures, the centre part of old root occasionally looking like rotten wood, blackish brown or hollowed (*1*).

Organoleptic properties
Colour, pale yellow to yellow-brown; taste, slightly sweet; odour, slight (*1, 2, 4, 7*).

Microscopic characteristics
The transverse section shows cork consisting of many rows of cells. Phelloderm, 3–5 rows of collenchymatous cells. Outer part of phloem rays often curved and fissured, fibres in bundles, walls thickened and lignified or slightly lignified, arranged alternately with sieve tube groups; stone cells sometimes visible near phelloderm. Cambium in a ring. Xylem vessels scattered singly or 2 or 3 aggregated in groups; wood fibres among vessel stone cells singly or 2–4 in groups, sometimes visible in rays. Parenchymatous cells contain starch granules (*1*).

Powdered plant material
Yellowish white. Fibres in bundles or scattered, 8–30 µm in diameter, thick-walled, with longitudinal fissures on the surface, the primary walls often separated from the secondary walls, both ends often tassel-like, or slightly truncated. Bordered-pitted vessels colourless or orange, bordered pits arranged closely. Stone cells occasionally visible, rounded, oblong or irregular, slightly thick-walled (*1*).

Geographical distribution
Indigenous to China, the Democratic People's Republic of Korea, Mongolia, and Siberia (*5, 6*). Commercially cultivated in northern China and the Democratic People's Republic of Korea (*5*).

General identity tests

Macroscopic and microscopic examination and thin-layer chromatographic analysis for the presence of triterpene saponins (astragaloside I as reference standard) (*1*).

Purity tests

Microbiology

The test for *Salmonella* spp. in Radix Astragali products should be negative. The maximum acceptable limits of other microorganisms are as follows (*10*, *11*). For preparation of decoction: aerobic bacteria—not more than 10^7/g; fungi—not more than 10^5/g; *Escherichia coli*—not more than 10^2/g. Preparations for internal use: aerobic bacteria—not more than 10^5/g or ml; fungi—not more than 10^4/g or ml; enterobacteria and certain Gram-negative bacteria—not more than 10^3/g or ml; *Escherichia coli*—0/g or ml.

Total ash

Not more than 5.0% (*1*, *2*).

Acid-insoluble ash

Not more than 1.0% (*1*, *2*).

Water-soluble extractive

Not less than 17.0% (*1*).

Moisture

Not more than 13.0% (*2*).

Pesticide residues

To be established in accordance with national requirements. Normally, the maximum residue limit of aldrin and dieldrin in Radix Astragali is not more than 0.05 mg/kg (*11*). For other pesticides, see WHO guidelines on quality control methods for medicinal plants (*10*) and WHO guidelines on predicting dietary intake of pesticide residues (*12*).

Heavy metals

Recommended lead and cadmium levels are not more than 10 and 0.3 mg/kg, respectively, in the final dosage form of the plant material (*10*).

Radioactive residues

For analysis of strontium-90, iodine-131, caesium-134, caesium-137, and plutonium-239, see WHO guidelines on quality control methods for medicinal plants (*10*).

Other tests

Chemical tests and tests for alcohol-soluble extractive and foreign organic matter are to be established in accordance with national requirements.

Chemical assays

Determination of triterpene saponins (astragalosides I–X) by thin-layer chromatographic analysis (*1*). Concentration limits and quantitative methods need to be established for the triterpene saponins (e.g. astragalosides), as well as for the polysaccharides.

Major chemical constituents

Major chemical constituents are triterpene saponins (astragalosides I–X and isoastragalosides I–IV), and polysaccharides (e.g. astragalan, astraglucan AMem-P) (*3*, *13*).

	R1	R2	R3	R4	R5
astragaloside I	glc *	H	CH₃CO	CH₃CO	H
astragaloside II	glc *	H	CH₃CO	H	H
astragaloside III	H	H	glc *	H	H
astragaloside IV	glc *	H	H	H	H
astragaloside V	H	glc *	glc *	H	H
astragaloside VI	glc *	H	glc *	H	H
astragaloside VII	glc *	glc *	H	H	H
isoastragaloside I	glc *	H	CH₃CO	H	CH₃CO
isoastragaloside II	glc *	H	H	CH₃CO	H

* glc = β-D-glucopyranosyl

astragaloglucans

Dosage forms

Crude plant material; extracts. Store in a dry environment protected from moisture and insects (*1*).

Medicinal uses
Uses supported by clinical data
None.

Uses described in pharmacopoeias and in traditional systems of medicine
As adjunctive therapy in the treatment of colds and influenza (*1*). The herb is used to enhance the immune system and to increase stamina and endurance (*1*).

Also in the treatment of chronic diarrhoea, oedema, abnormal uterine bleeding, and diabetes mellitus (*1, 4, 14, 15*), and as a cardiotonic agent (*6*).

Uses described in folk medicine, not supported by experimental or clinical data
Treatment of nephritis, chronic bronchitis, postpartum urine retention, leprosy, and the sequelae of cerebrovascular accidents (*4*).

Pharmacology
Experimental pharmacology
Effect on the immune system
Both *in vitro* and *in vivo* investigations have confirmed that *Astragalus membranaceus* enhances the immune system (*14–18*). *In vitro* studies have shown that, at concentrations of 10 mg/ml, polysaccharides isolated from the plant increased the blastization index in mixed lymphocyte cultures and the granulopexis of macrophages or polymorphonucleates (*16*). Using the local xenogenic graft-versus-host reaction (assessed in cyclophosphamide-treated rats) as a model assay for T-cell function, investigators found that mononuclear cells, derived from cancer patients, that were preincubated with a polysaccharide fraction from *A. membranaceus* had significant immunopotentiating activity, and they fully corrected *in vitro* T-cell function deficiency found in cancer patients (*14*). Further investigations of this extract established that the polysaccharide fraction enhanced interleukin-2 activity in the *in vitro* generation of lymphokine-activated killer cell activity (*17*). Intravenous injection of this polysaccharide fraction also reversed cyclophosphamide-induced immunosuppression in rats (*18*).

A decoction of *A. membranaceus* given to mice by gastric lavage, daily or on alternate days for 1–2 weeks, increased the phagocytic activity of the reticuloendothelial system (*4, 5*). The phagocytic index was significantly enhanced even when the rehabilitation of the mouse reticuloendothelial system was disrupted by injection of carbon particles before the *A. membranaceus* extract was administered (*4, 5*). Extracts of the crude drug enhanced antibody response to a T-dependent antigen *in vivo*. Intravenous administration of a crude drug extract to normal mice, or mice immunosuppressed by cyclophosphamide, radiation treatment, or ageing, induced the antibody response to a T-dependent antigen (*19*). Enhancement of this response is associated with an increase in T-helper cell activity in both normal and immunosuppressed mice (*19*). Other *in vivo* studies performed on cyclophosphamide-immunosuppressed mice have further suggested that *A. membranaceus* root extracts may modulate the immune system by activation of macrophages and splenic lymphocytes (*20*).

The immunostimulant activity of *A. membranaceus* has been associated with the polysaccharide fractions of the root extract (*4, 13, 19, 21*). The immune-enhancing polysaccharide molecules have relative molecular masses of approximately 25 000 (*14, 18, 19*). A polysaccharide fraction isolated from *A. membranaceus* reportedly antagonized the effect of cobra venom on the immune function of treated mice and guinea-pigs (*22*). The venom-treated guinea-pigs had decreased levels of complement and neutrophil phagocytotic activity, as well as increased levels of neutrophil granular substances. Treatment of the animals with the polysaccharides antagonized these changes in the venom-treated animals but had no effect in the normal group (*22*). Recently, a new glycan, named AMem-P, isolated from the roots of *A. membranaceus,* was shown by use of an *in vivo* carbon clearance test to significantly potentiate reticuloendothelial system activity in mice (*13*).

Radix Astragali is reported to have cardiovascular activity. Alcohol extracts of the drug enhanced both the contractility and contraction amplitude of isolated frog or toad hearts (*4*). Intraperitoneal injection of the drug to dogs did not produce any immediate effect on heart rate, but 3–4 hours after administration inverted and biphasic T waves and prolonged S–T intervals were noted (*4*). Intravenous administration of the drug produced hypotension in rabbits, dogs, and cats (*4*). Furthermore, saponins isolated from the drug were reported to exert a positive inotropic effect on isolated rat hearts (*23*). The saponins also decreased the resting potential of cultured rat myocardial cells, suggesting that they may exert an inotropic effect through the modulation of Na^+/K^+-exchanging ATPase (*23*).

Toxicology

No adverse effects were observed in mice after oral administration of up to 100 g/kg, a dose several hundred times as high as the effective oral dose in humans (*4*).

Clinical pharmacology

Oral or intranasal administration of an aqueous *A. membranaceus* extract to 1000 human subjects decreased the incidence and shortened the course of the common cold (*4*). Two months of oral administration of the herb significantly increased the levels of IgA and IgG in the nasal secretions of patients susceptible to the common cold (*4*). Details of these studies were not available.

A hot water extract of *A. membranaceus* root taken by human subjects was reported to have a pronounced immunostimulant effect (*24*). Human adults treated with an oral dose of *Astragalus* root (15.6g per person per day for 20 days) significantly increased serum IgM, IgE, and cyclic AMP concentrations (*24*). Extracts of *A. membranaceus* have been further reported to stimulate the production of interferon, a protein with antiviral activity, in both animals and humans in response to viral infections (*21, 25*). A hot water extract of the drug administered intramuscularly for 3–4 months to patients with coxsackievirus B myocarditis enhanced natural killer cells, a response which was mediated through interferon induction (*15*). Furthermore, both natural and recombinant interferons enhanced the antiviral activity of an *A. membranaceus* extract (*26*).

Contraindications

No information available.

Warnings

No information available.

Precautions

Carcinogenesis, mutagenesis, impairment of fertility

Extracts of *A. membranaceus* root were not mutagenic in a modified Ames test using *Salmonella typhimurium* TA 98 and TA 100 (*27*). Furthermore, an aqueous extract of *A. membranaceus* was reported to be antimutagenic in that it inhibited benzo[*a*]pyrene-induced mutagenesis in *Salmonella typhimurium* TA 100 (*28, 29*).

Pregnancy: non-teratogenic effects

No data available; therefore Radix Astragali should not be administered during pregnancy.

Nursing mothers

Excretion of the drug into breast milk and its effects on the newborn infant have not been established; therefore the use of the drug during lactation is not recommended.

Other precautions

No information available describing general precautions or precautions related to drug interactions, drug and laboratory test interactions, paediatric use, or teratogenic effects during pregnancy.

Adverse reactions

No information available.

Posology
Root: 9–30 g/day for oral use (*1*).

References

1. *Pharmacopoeia of the People's Republic of China* (English ed.). Guangzhou, Guangdong Science and Technology Press, 1992.
2. *The pharmacopoeia of Japan XII*. Tokyo, The Society of Japanese Pharmacopoeia, 1991.
3. Leung A, Foster S. *Encyclopedia of common natural ingredients used in food, drugs, and cosmetics*, 2nd ed. New York, John Wiley, 1996.
4. Chang HM, But PPH, eds. *Pharmacology and applications of Chinese materia medica, Vol. 2*. Singapore, World Scientific Publishing, 1987.
5. Morazzoni P, Bombardelli E. *Astragalus membranaceus* (Fish.) Bge. Milan, Indena, 1994.
6. *Medicinal plants in China*. Manila, World Health Organization, 1989 (WHO Regional Publications, Western Pacific Series, No.2).
7. Hsu HY. *Oriental materia medica, a concise guide*. Long Beach, CA, Oriental Healing Arts Institute, 1986.
8. *Vietnam materia medica*. Hanoi, Ministry of Health, 1972.
9. Farnsworth NR, ed. *NAPRALERT database*. Chicago, University of Illinois at Chicago, IL, August 8, 1995 production (an on-line database available directly through the University of Illinois at Chicago or through the Scientific and Technical Network (STN) of Chemical Abstracts Services).
10. *Quality control methods for medicinal plant materials*. Geneva, World Health Organization, 1998.
11. *European pharmacopoeia*, 3rd ed. Strasbourg, Council of Europe, 1997.
12. *Guidelines for predicting dietary intake of pesticide residues*, 2nd rev. ed. Geneva, World Health Organization, 1997 (unpublished document WHO/FSF/FOS/97.7; available from Food Safety, WHO, 1211 Geneva 27, Switzerland).
13. Tomoda M et al. A reticuloendothelial system-activating glycan from the roots of *Astragalus membranaceus. Phytochemistry*, 1992, 31:63–66.
14. Chu DT, Wong WL, Mavligit GM. Immunotherapy with Chinese medicinal herbs I. Immune restoration of local xenogeneic graft-versus-host reactions in cancer patients by fractionated *Astragalus membranaceus in vitro. Journal of clinical laboratory immunology*, 1988, 25:119–123.
15. Yang YZ et al. Effect of *Astragalus membranaceus* on natural killer cell activity and induction of alpha- and gamma-interferon in patients with coxsackie B viral myocarditis. *Chung-hua i hseuh tsa chih* (English Edition), 1990, 103:304–307.
16. Bombardelli E, Pozzi R. Polysaccharides with immunomodulating properties from *Astragalus membranaceus. Europe patent*, 1991, 441:278.
17. Chu DT et al. Fractionated extract of *Astragalus membranaceus*, a Chinese medicinal herb, potentiates LAK cell cytotoxicity generated by a low dose of recombinant interleukin-2. *Journal of clinical laboratory immunology*, 1988, 26:183–187.
18. Chu DT, Wong WL, Mavligit GM. Immunotherapy with Chinese medicinal herbs II. Reversal of cyclophosphamide-induced immune suppression by administration of fractionated *Astragalus membranaceus in vivo. Journal of clinical laboratory immunology*, 1988, 25:125–129.
19. Zhou KS, Mancini C, Doria G. Enhancement of the immune response in mice by *Astragalus membranaceus* extracts. *Immunopharmacology*, 1990, 20:225–233.
20. Jin R et al. Immunomodulative effects of Chinese herbs in mice treated with anti-tumor agent cyclophosphamide. *Yakugaku zasshi*, 1994, 114:533–538.

21. Hou YD et al. Effect of Radix Astragali seu hedysari on the interferon system. *Chinese medical journal*, 1981, 94:35–40.
22. Zhuang MX et al. The effects of polysaccharides of *Astragalus membranaceus*, *Codonopsis pilosula* and *Panax ginseng* on some immune functions in guinea-pigs. *Zhongguo yaoxue zazhi*, 1992, 27:653–655.
23. Wang QL et al. Inotropic action of *Astragalus membranaceus* Bge. saponins and its possible mechanism. *Zhongguo zhongyao zazhi*, 1992, 17:557–559.
24. Institute of Basic Medical Sciences, The Chinese Academy of Medical Sciences. Immunity parameters and blood cAMP changes in normal persons after ingestion of Radix Astragali. *Chung hua i hsueh t'sa chih*, 1979, 59:31–34.
25. Finter NB. *Interferons and interferon-inducers*. Amsterdam, North Holland, 1973:363.
26. Peng JZ et al. Inhibitory effects of interferon and its combination with antiviral drugs on adenovirus multiplication. *Zhongguo yixue kexueyuan xuebao*, 1984, 6:116–119.
27. Yamamoto H, Mizutani T, Nomura H. Studies on the mutagenicity of crude drug extracts. I. *Yakugaku zasshi*, 1982, 102:596–601.
28. Wong BY, Lau BH, Teel RW. Chinese medicinal herbs modulate mutagenesis, DNA binding and metabolism of benzo[a]pyrene. *Phytotherapy research*, 1992, 6:10–14.
29. Liu DX et al. Antimutagenicity screening of water extracts from 102 kinds of Chinese medicinal herbs. *Chung-kuo chung yao tsa chi li*, 1990, 15:617–620.

Fructus Bruceae

Definition

Fructus Bruceae consists of the dried ripe fruits of *Brucea javanica* (L.) Merr. (Simaroubaceae) (*1*, *2*).

Synonyms

Brucea amarissima Desv. ex Gomes, *B. sumatrana* Roxb., *Gonus amarissimus* Lour., *Lussa amarissima* O. Ktze (*2*, *3*).

Selected vernacular names

Biji makassar, bulah makassar, Java brucea, k'u-shen-tzu, kho sam, ko-sam, ku-sheng-tzu, nha dàm tùr, raat cha dat, raat dat, ratchadat, sàu dau rùng, xoan rùng, ya tan tzu, ya-dan-zi, yadǎnzi (*1–7*).

Description

A shrub or small tree, 1–3 m high; younger parts softly pubescent. Leaves compound-paripinnate; leaflets 5–11, oval-lanceolate, 5–10 cm long by 2–4 cm wide; apex acuminate, base broadly cuneate and often somewhat oblique; margin serrate; both surfaces densely pubescent, especially the underside. Flowers minute, purple, in numerous small cymes or clusters collected into axillary panicles. Sepals 4, connate at the base. Petals 4, villous, glandular at the tips. Male flowers, stamens 4, pistil reduced to a stigma; female flowers, stamens 4, much reduced. Ovary with 4 free carpels. Fruit and drupe ovoid, black when ripe. Seeds, compressed, rugose, blackish brown (*3–5*).

Plant material of interest: dried ripe fruit or seed

Fruit also refers to the kernel or seed with the pulp removed (*3*, *4*).

General appearance

The fruit is ovoid, 6–10 mm long by 4–7 mm in diameter. Externally black or brown, with raised reticulate wrinkles, the lumen irregularly polygonal, obviously ribbed at both sides. Apex acuminate, base having a dented fruit stalk scar, shell hard and brittle. Seeds ovoid, 5–6 mm long by 3–5 mm in diameter, externally yellowish white, reticulate; testa thin, cotyledons milky white and oily (*1*, *3*, *4*).

Organoleptic properties
Odour slight; taste, very bitter (*1*, *4*).

Microscopic characteristics
The pulverized pericarp is brown. Epidermal cells polygonal, with brown cellular contents; parenchymatous cells polygonal, containing clusters of calcium oxalate prisms, up to 30 mm in diameter. Stone cells subrounded or polygonal, 14–38 mm in diameter (*1*).

Powdered plant material
Powdered seeds yellowish white. Testa cells polygonal and slightly elongated. Endosperm and cotyledon cells contain aleurone grains (*1*).

Geographical distribution
Indigenous to China, India, Indonesia, and Viet Nam (*3*, *4*).

General identity tests
Macroscopic and microscopic examinations (*1*, *3*, *4*).

Purity tests
Microbiology
The test for *Salmonella* spp. in Fructus Bruceae products should be negative. The maximum acceptable limits of other microorganisms are as follows (*8–10*). For preparation of decoction: aerobic bacteria—not more than 10^7/g; fungi—not more than 10^5/g; *Escherichia coli*—not more than 10^2/g. Preparations (capsules) for internal use: aerobic bacteria—not more than 10^5/g; fungi—not more than 10^4/g; enterobacteria and certain Gram-negative bacteria—not more than 10^3/g; *Escherichia coli*—0/g.

Foreign organic matter
Not more than 2% (*2*).

Total ash
Not more than 6% (*2*).

Acid-insoluble ash
Not more than 0.6% (*2*).

Water-soluble extractive
Not less than 18% (*2*).

Dilute ethanol-soluble extractive
Not less than 26% (*2*).

Pesticide residues
To be established in accordance with national requirements. Normally, the maximum residue limit of aldrin and dieldrin in Fructus Bruceae is not more than 0.05 mg/kg (*10*). For other pesticides, see WHO guidelines on quality control methods for medicinal plants (*8*) and guidelines on predicting dietary intake of pesticide residues (*11*).

Heavy metals
Recommended lead and cadmium levels are no more than 10.0 and 0.3 mg/kg, respectively, in the final dosage form of the plant material (*8*).

Radioactive residues
For analysis of strontium-90, iodine-131, caesium-134, caesium-137, and plutonium-239, see WHO guidelines on quality control methods for medicinal plants (*8*).

Other purity tests
Chemical and moisture tests to be established in accordance with national requirements.

Chemical assays
Contains bruceosides and related quassinoids. Quantitative content requirement to be established. Quantitative determination of quassinoid triterpenes by a high-performance liquid chromatographic method developed for the determination of bruceoside A (*12*).

Major chemical constituents
Quassinoid triterpenes, including bruceantin, bruceantinol, bruceantinoside A, bruceins A–G and Q, brucein E 2-*O*-β-D-glucoside, bruceolide, bruceosides A–C, brusatol, dehydrobruceantinol, dehydrobruceins A and B, dehydrobrusatol, dihydrobrucein A, yadanzigan, yadanziolides A–D, and yadanziosides A–P predominate as the secondary metabolite constituents (*13*, *14*). Representative quassinoid structures are presented in the figure.

Dosage forms

Seeds for decoction, or capsules (*1*, *3*, *4*). Store in airtight container, protected from light and moisture (*1*).

Medicinal uses

Uses supported by clinical data

None.

Uses described in pharmacopoeias and in traditional systems of medicine

Treatment of amoebic dysentery and malaria (*1*, *3*, *14*, *15*).

Uses described in folk medicine, not supported by experimental or clinical data

As a poultice on boils, to treat ringworm, whipworm, roundworm and tape-worm, scurf, centipede bites, haemorrhoids, and enlarged spleen (*3–6*). The seed and seed oil have been used in the treatment of warts and corns (*1*, *4*). Fructus Bruceae has been used in the treatment of trichomoniasis, corns and verrucae (*6*).

Pharmacology
Experimental pharmacology
Amoebicidal and antibacterial activity

A number of *in vitro* studies have indicated that extracts of *Brucea javanica* kernels are effective amoebicides. In one such study, a crude butanol extract of *B. javanica* was highly active against *Entamoeba histolytica* (*16*). This amoebicidal activity was associated with two polar compounds isolated from the extract, bruceantin and brucein C, which are quassinoid constituents (*16*). (*Brucea* quassinoids were active against *E. histolytica* and other protozoa *in vitro* (*17, 18*).) The quassinoids were potent inhibitors of protein synthesis both in mammalian cells and in malaria parasites, and it has been suggested that this effect accounts for their amoebicidal activity (*17*). In one other investigation, brusatol, another quassinoid isolated from the seeds of *B. javanica*, was also reported to be effective in the treatment of dysentery (*19*). Extracts from the kernels of *B. javanica* have also been reported to possess antibacterial activity against *Shigella shiga, S. flexneri, S. boydii, Salmonella lexington, Salmonella derby, Salmonella typhi* type II, *Vibrio cholerae inaba* and *Vibrio cholerae ogawa* (*20*).

Antimalarial activity

Numerous *in vitro* and *in vivo* studies have demonstrated the antiplasmodial activity of Fructus Bruceae extracts. *In vitro* studies have determined that bruceantin, a quassinoid constituent of the drug, exhibited significant anti-plasmodial activity against *Plasmodium falciparum* (*21, 22*). Extracts of the drug were also active *in vitro* against chloroquine-resistant *P. falciparum* (*23, 24*) and *in vivo* against *P. berghei* (mice) (*23, 25*). Nine quassinoid constituents of the drug had *in vitro* IC_{50} values of 0.046–0.0008 mg/ml against chloroquine-resistant *P. falciparum* strain K-1 (*23*). Four of these compounds were also active *in vivo* against *P. berghei* infections in mice after oral dosing (*23*), and three of the compounds, bruceins A–C, had *in vitro* activity comparable to that of the antimalarial drug mefloquine (*24*). Bruceolide, another quassinoid constituent of *B. javanica*, was also effective *in vivo* (mice) against *P. berghei*, and was reported to be more effective than chloroquine (*25*). A recent *in vitro* screening of quassinoids against various protozoa showed that brucein D and brusatol have very selective inhibitory activity against *P. falciparum* (*17*).

Quassinoids isolated from *B. javanica* are reported to have cytotoxic activity *in vitro* (*17, 26, 27*). Bruceantin was tested in phase I clinical cancer trials, but no tumour regression was observed (*28, 29*).

Clinical pharmacology

Brucea javanica fruit extracts have been used clinically in the treatment of amoebic dysentery (*14, 15*). These investigations indicated that the antidysenteric activity of the *Brucea* extract was less effective than that of emetine (*14, 15*).

Contraindications

Fructus Bruceae should not be administered to children or pregnant women (*6*).

Warnings

No information available.

Precautions

Pregnancy: teratogenic and non-teratogenic effects

No data available. Preparations containing Fructus Bruceae must not be administered to pregnant women (*6*).

Nursing mothers

Excretion of Fructus Bruceae into breast milk and its effects on infants have not been established; therefore this drug should not be administered to nursing women.

Paediatric use

Fructus Bruceae should not be administered to young children (*6*).

Other precautions

No information available about general precautions or precautions concerning carcinogenesis, mutagenesis, or impairment of fertility; drug interactions; or drug and laboratory test interactions.

Adverse reactions

Some cases of anaphylaxis have been reported after external applications of the fruits of *B. javanica* (*30*).

Posology

Daily dose to treat amoebiasis, 4–16 g as a decoction or powder in three divided doses for 3–7 days (*3*); to treat malaria, 3–6 g in three divided doses after meals for 4 or 5 days (*3*).

References

1. *Pharmacopoeia of the People's Republic of China* (English ed.). Guangzhou, Guangdong Science and Technology Press, 1992.
2. *Materia medika Indonesia*, Jilid I. Jakarta, Departemen Kesehatan, Republik Indonesia, 1977.

3. *Medicinal plants in Viet Nam.* Manila. World Health Organization Regional Office for the Western Pacific, 1990 (WHO Regional Publications, Western Pacific Series, No. 3).

4. *Medicinal plants in China.* Manila, World Health Organization, 1989 (WHO Regional Publications, Western Pacific Series, No. 2).

5. Keys JD. *Chinese herbs, their botany, chemistry and pharmacodynamics.* Rutland, VT, CE Tuttle, 1976.

6. Hsu HY. *Oriental materia medica, a concise guide.* Long Beach, CA, Oriental Healing Arts Institute, 1986.

7. Farnsworth NR, ed. *NAPRALERT database.* Chicago, University of Illinois at Chicago, IL, August 8, 1995 production (an on-line database available directly through the University of Illinois at Chicago or through the Scientific and Technical Network (STN) of Chemical Abstracts Services).

8. *Quality control methods for medicinal plant materials.* Geneva, World Health Organization, 1998.

9. *Deutsches Arzneibuch 1996. Vol. 2. Methoden der Biologie.* Stuttgart, Deutscher Apotheker Verlag, 1996.

10. *European Pharmacopoeia,* 3rd ed. Strasbourg, Council of Europe, 1997.

11. *Guidelines for predicting dietary intake of pesticide residues,* 2nd rev. ed. Geneva, World Health Organization, 1997 (unpublished document WHO/FSF/FOS/97.7; available from Food Safety, WHO, 1211 Geneva 27, Switzerland).

12. Chi H, Wang YP, Zhou TH. Determination of the anticancer drug bruceoside A in the Chinese drug, Yadanzi (*Brucea javanica* Merr.). *Journal of chromatography,* 1991, 543:250–256.

13. Polonsky J. Quassinoid bitter principles, II. In: Herz W et al., eds. *Progress in the chemistry of organic natural products, Vol. 47.* Berlin, Springer-Verlag, 1972.

14. Tang W, Eisenbrand G. *Chinese drugs of plant origin, chemistry, pharmacology and use in traditional and modern medicine.* Berlin, Springer-Verlag, 1992:207–222.

15. Steak EA. *The chemotherapy of protozoan diseases, Vol. 1.* Washington, DC, US Government Printing Office, 1972.

16. Keene AT et al. *In vitro* amoebicidal testing of natural products, Part I. Methodology. *Planta medica,* 1986, 52:278–285.

17. Wright CW et al. Quassinoids exhibit greater selectivity against *Plasmodium falciparum* than against *Entamoeba histolytica, Giardia intestinalis* or *Toxoplasma gondii in vitro. Journal of eukaryotic microbiology,* 1993, 40:244–246.

18. Wright CW et al. Use of microdilution to assess *in vitro* antiamoebic activities of *Brucea javanica* fruit, *Simarouba amara* stem, and a number of quassinoids. *Antimicrobial agents and chemotherapy,* 1988, 32:1725–1729.

19. Sato Y, Hasegawa M, Suto N. Identity of brusatol and yatansin, an antidysenteric agent. *Agricultural and biological chemistry,* 1980, 44:951–952.

20. Wasuwat S et al. Study on antidysentery and antidiarrheal properties of extracts of *Brucea amarissima.* Bangkok, Applied Science Research Center of Thailand, 1971:14 (Research Project Report 17/10, 2).

21. O'Neill MJ et al. Plants as sources of antimalarial drugs: *in vitro* antimalarial activities of some quassinoids. *Antimicrobial agents and chemotherapy,* 1986, 30:101–104.

22. Ayudhaya T et al. Study on the *in vitro* antimalarial activity of some medicinal plants against *Plasmodium falciparum. Bulletin of the Department of Medical Sciences (India),* 1987, 9:33–38.

23. O'Neill MJ. Plants as sources of antimalarial drugs, Part 4. Activity of *Brucea javanica* fruits against chloroquine-resistant *Plasmodium falciparum in vitro* and against *Plasmodium berghei in vivo. Journal of natural products,* 1987, 50:41–48.

24. Pavanand K et al. *In vitro* antimalarial activity of *Brucea javanica* against multi-drug resistant *Plasmodium falciparum. Planta medica,* 1986, 2:108–111.

25. Ngo VT et al. Effectiveness of *Brucea sumatrana* plant against malaria. *Duoc hoc*, 1979, 4:15–17.
26. Darwish FA, Evan FJ, Phillipson JD. Cytotoxic bruceolides from *Brucea javanica*. *Journal of pharmacy and pharmacology*, 1979, 31:10.
27. Ohnishi S et al. Bruceosides D, E and F, three new cytotoxic quassinoid glycosides from *Brucea javanica*. *Journal of natural products*, 1995, 58:1032–1038.
28. Liesmann J et al. Phase I study on Bruceantin administered on a weekly schedule. *Cancer treatment report*, 1981, 65:883–885.
29. Bedikian AY et al. Initial clinical studies with bruceantin. *Cancer treatment report*, 1979, 63:1843–1847.
30. Zheng GQ et al. A report on three cases of anaphylaxis caused by external application of the fruit of *Brucea javanica*. *Bulletin of the Chinese materia medica*, 1986:11–12.

Radix Bupleuri

Definition

Radix Bupleuri consists of the dried root of *Bupleurum falcatum* L. or *B. falcatum* L. var. *scorzonerifolium* (Willd.) Ledeb. (Apiaceae) (*1, 2*).

Synonyms

Bupleurum chinense D.C. and *B. scorzonerifolium* Willd. have been treated as different species (*1*) but are actually synonyms of *B. falcatum* L. var. *scorzonerifolium* (*3*). Apiaceae are also referred to as Umbelliferae.

Selected vernacular names

Beichaihu, bupleurum root, ch'ai hu, chaifu, chaihu, chaiku-saiko, Chinese thorowax root, juk-siho, kara-saiko, mishima-saiko, nanchaihu, northern Chinese thorowax root, radix bupleur, saiko, shi ho, shoku-saiko, wa-saiko, Yama-saiko (*1–5*).

Description

A perennial herb up to 1 m tall; base woody and the rhizome branching. Stem slender, flexuous, branches spreading. Basal leaves lanceolate, upper lamina broad, lower narrowed into a petiole, veins 7, apex acute, mucronate; middle and upper leaves linear to lanceolate, gradually shorter, falcate, veins 7–9, base slightly amplexicaul, apex acuminate. Involucre of 1–3 minute bracts or lacking. Rays 5–8. Involucel of 5 minute, 3-veined bractlets, shorter than the flowering umbellet. Pedicels shorter than the fruits. Fruit oblong, 3–4 mm long; furrows 3-vittate (*4, 6*).

Plant material of interest: dried roots

General appearance

Single or branched root, of long cone or column shape, 10–20 cm in length, 0.5–1.5 cm in diameter; occasionally with remains of stem on crown; externally light brown to brown and sometimes with deep wrinkles; easily broken, and fractured surface somewhat fibrous (*2*).

Organoleptic properties

Odour, characteristic, slightly aromatic to rancid; taste, slightly bitter (*1, 2*).

Microscopic characteristics

Transverse section reveals often tangentially extended clefts in cortex, the thickness reaching a third to a half of the radius, and cortex scattered with a good many intercellular schizogenous oil canals 1.5–3.5 cm in diameter; vessels lined radially or stepwise in xylem, with scattered fibre groups; in the crown pith also contains oil canals; parenchyma cells filled with starch grains and some oil drops. Starch grains composed of simple grains, 2–10 μm in diameter, or compound grains (*2*).

Powdered plant material

Information not available. Description to be established by appropriate national authorities.

Geographical distribution

Indigenous to northern Asia, northern China, and Europe (*4, 6*).

General identity tests

Macroscopic and microscopic examinations (*1, 2*), microchemical detection for saponins (*1, 2*), and thin-layer chromatographic analysis for triterpene saponins with reference to saikosaponins (*2*).

Purity tests

Microbiology

The test for *Salmonella* spp. in Radix Bupleuri should be negative. The maximum acceptable limits of other microorganisms are as follows (*7–9*). For preparation of decoction: aerobic bacteria—not more than $10^7/g$; fungi—not more than $10^5/g$; *Escherichia coli*—not more than $10^2/g$.

Chemical

Contains triterpene saponins (saikosaponins). Quantitative level to be established by appropriate national authorities, but should be not less than 1.5% according to literature data.

Foreign organic matter

Not more than 10% of stems and leaves (*2*). No roots of *B. longiradiantum* Turcz., which is toxic (*1, 5*). Not more than 1% of other foreign matter (*2*).

Total ash

Not more than 6.5% (2).

Acid-insoluble ash

Not more than 2% (2).

Dilute ethanol-soluble extractive

Not less than 11% (2).

Pesticide residues

To be established in accordance with national requirements. Normally, the maximum residue limit of aldrin and dieldrin for Radix Bupleuri is not more than 0.05 mg/kg (9). For other pesticides, see WHO guidelines on quality control methods for medicinal plants (7) and WHO guidelines for predicting dietary intake of pesticide residues (10).

Heavy metals

Recommended lead and cadmium levels are no more than 10 and 0.3 mg/kg, respectively, in the final dosage form of the plant material (7).

Radioactive residues

For analysis of strontium-90, iodine-131, caesium-134, caesium-137, and plutonium-239, see WHO guidelines on quality control methods for medicinal plants (7).

Other tests

Tests for moisture and for water-soluble extractive to be established by national authorities.

Chemical assays

Total saikosaponins determination by colorimetric analysis (11), and high-performance liquid chromatography analysis for saikosaponins A, B_1, B_2, and D (12, 13).

Major chemical constituents

The major constituents are triterpene saponins, including saikosaponins A, B_{1-4}, D, E, F and H and related compounds including saikogenins A–G (5, 14). Two biologically active polysaccharides, bupleurans 2IIb and 2IIc, have also been isolated from the roots of *B. falcatum* (15, 16). Representative structures of saikosaponins are presented in the figure.

saikogenin A   R1 = OH , R2 = H
saikogenin D   R1 = H , R2 = OH

saikogenin F   R1 = OH , R2 = H
saikogenin G   R1 = H , R2 = OH

saikosaponin A   R1 = OH , R2 = H
saikosaponin D   R1 = H , R2 = OH

saikosaponin B₁   R1 = OH , R2 = H
saikosaponin B₂   R1 = H , R2 = OH

saikosaponin B₃   R1 = OH , R2 = H
saikosaponin B₄   R1 = H , R2 = OH

3-*O*-β-D-glucopyranosyl-β-D-fucopyranosyl

or

3-*O*-β-D-glucopyranosyl-6-deoxy-
β-D-galactopyranosyl

Dosage forms

Decoction (*5*). Store crude plant material in a dry environment protected from moths, light, and moisture (*1*, *2*).

Medicinal uses

Uses supported by clinical data

None.

Uses described in pharmacopoeias and in traditional systems of medicine

Treatment of fever, pain, and inflammation associated with influenza, and the common cold (*1*, *2*, *5*). The drug is also used as an analgesic for the treatment of distending pain in the chest and hypochondriac regions, and for amenorrhoea (*1*). Extracts have been used for the treatment of chronic hepatitis, nephrotic syndrome, and autoimmune diseases (*1*, *5*).

Uses described in folk medicine, not supported by experimental or clinical data

Treatment of deafness, dizziness, diabetes, wounds, and vomiting (5).

Pharmacology

Experimental pharmacology

Antipyretic and analgesic activity

A number of *in vivo* studies have confirmed the antipyretic activity of Radix Bupleuri in the treatment of induced fevers in animals. Oral administration of a *Bupleurum* decoction (5 g/kg) to rabbits with a heat-induced fever decreased body temperature to normal levels within 1.5 hours (5). Subcutaneous injection of an aqueous ethanol extract of *Bupleurum* roots (2.2 ml/kg, 1.1 g crude drug/ml) significantly reduced fevers in rabbits injected with *Escherichia coli* (17).

Oral administration of saikosaponins to rats produced hypothermic and antipyretic effects (5). Furthermore, intraperitoneal injection of the volatile oil (300 mg/kg) or saponins (380 and 635 mg/kg) isolated from *B. chinense* (*B. falcatum*) roots effectively decreased fever in mice induced by yeast injections (18). Oral administration of 200–800 mg/kg of a crude saponin fraction to mice produced sedative, analgesic, and antipyretic effects, but no anticonvulsant effect or reduction in muscle tone was observed (14). Saikosaponins are believed to be the major active antipyretic constituents in Radix Bupleuri extracts.

Analgesic activity of *Bupleurum* extracts is also supported by *in vivo* studies. Injections of a crude *Bupleurum* extract or purified sapogenin A inhibited writhing induced by intraperitoneal injection of acetic acid in mice (5). The saikosaponins appear to be the active analgesic constituents of the drug. Intraperitoneal injection of mice with a total saponin fraction derived from *B. chinense* (*B. falcatum*) produced a marked analgesic effect on the pain induced by electroshock (5). Moreover, orally administered saikosaponins were reported to have an analgesic effect in mice (tail pressure test) (5).

Sedative effects

In vivo studies have also confirmed the sedative effects of Radix Bupleuri. Both the crude saikosaponin fraction and saikogenin A are reported to have significant sedative effects (5). *In vivo* studies, using the rod climbing test, demonstrated that the sedative effect of the saikosaponins (200–800 mg/kg) in mice was similar to that of meprobamate (100 mg) (5). Oral administration of saikosides extracted from *B. chinense* (*B. falcatum*) or saikosaponin A has also been reported to prolong cyclobarbital sodium-induced sleep (5). Furthermore, intraperitoneal injection of saikogenin A inhibited rod climbing in mice and antagonized the stimulant effects of metamfetamine and caffeine (5).

Anti-inflammatory activity

Anti-inflammatory activity of Radix Bupleuri has been demonstrated by *in vivo* studies. Intraperitoneal injection of the saponin fraction, the volatile oil, or a crude extract from *B. chinense* (*B. falcatum*) significantly inhibited carrageenin-induced rat paw oedema (*5*). The saikosaponins are the active anti-inflammatory constituents of the drug (*19, 20*). Oral administration of a crude saikosaponin fraction (2 g/kg) from *B. falcatum* inhibited dextran-, serotonin-, or croton oil-induced rat paw oedema (*5, 21*). Structure–activity correlations have revealed that saikosaponins A and D both have anti-inflammatory activity, while saikosaponin C does not (*22*). The potency of anti-inflammatory activity of the saikosaponins is similar to that of prednisolone (*5*).

Immune regulation activity

In vitro studies have demonstrated that a hot-water extract from the root of *B. falcatum* enhanced the antibody response and inhibited mitogen-induced lymphocyte transformation (*23*). An acidic pectic polysaccharide, bupleuran 2IIb, isolated from the roots of *B. falcatum,* was found to be a potent enhancer of immune complex binding to macrophages (*24*). The activity of this polysaccharide appeared to be due to its ability to enhance the Fc receptor function of macrophages. This study has shown that the binding of glucose oxidase–antiglucose oxidase complexes (a model of immune complexes) to murine peritoneal macrophages was stimulated by treatment with the polysaccharide (*24*). Bupleuran 2IIb appears to up-regulate both FcRI and FcRII receptor expression on the macrophage surface in a dose-dependent manner (*25*). The up-regulation of the Fc receptor by bupleuran 2IIb depends on an increase in intracellular calcium and activation of calmodulin (*25*). Only saikosaponin D has been shown to enhance Fc receptor expression of thioglycollate-elicited murine peritoneal macrophages *in vitro* (*26*). This activity appears to be due to the translocation of FcR from the internal pool to the cell surface. *In vitro* studies with saikosaponin D have shown that this compound was able to control bidirectionally the growth response of T lymphocytes stimulated by concanavalin A, anti-CD3 monoclonal antibody, and calcium ionophore A23187 plus phorbol 12-myristate 13-acetate (*27*). Saikosaponin D also promoted interleukin-2 production and receptor expression, as well as c-fos gene transcription (*28*). The results of this study suggest that saikosaponin D exerts its immunostimulant effects by modification of T lymphocyte function (*28*).

Antiulcer activity

Antiulcer activity of Radix Bupleuri has been demonstrated both *in vivo* and *in vitro*. A polysaccharide fraction of a hot-water extract of the root of *B. falcatum* was reported to inhibit significantly hydrochloric acid- or ethanol-induced ulcerogenesis in mice (*15*). The polysaccharide fraction (BR-2, 100mg/kg) had potent antiulcer activity, and its activity was similar to that of sucralfate (100mg/kg) (*29*). BR-2 significantly protected against a variety of gastric lesions, water-immersion stress ulcer and pylorus-ligation ulcer in mice and rats (*29*). By oral, intraperitoneal, or subcutaneous administration, BR-2 was further found to be effective against hydrochloric acid- or ethanol-induced gastric lesions suggesting that BR-2 acted both locally and systemically (*29*). The mechanism of antiulcer action appears to be due to a reinforcement of the protective mucosal barrier as well as an antisecretory action on acid and pepsin (*30*). Saponins isolated from *B. falcatum* root have also been reported to have weak antiulcer activity in the pylorus-ligation ulcer model (*30*).

Hepatoprotectant activity

Crude saponins of *B. falcatum*, administered orally to rats at a daily dose of 500 mg/kg for 3 days, normalized liver functions as determined by serum alkaline phosphatase levels in rats treated with carbon tetrachloride (*31*). Treatment of rats with saikosaponins 2 hours before treatment with D-galactosamine inhibited the increase in serum aspartate aminotransferase and alanine aminotransferase levels produced by damage of liver tissues (*31*). Conversely, saikosaponins did not affect an increase in serum alanine aminotransferase and experimental cirrhosis in rats caused by carbon tetrachloride intoxication (*32*).

Clinical pharmacology

Antipyretic activity

The antipyretic activity of *B. chinense* (*B. falcatum*) has been investigated in patients with fevers caused by the common cold, influenza, malaria, and pneumonia (*5*). In one clinical study of 143 patients treated with the herb, fevers subsided within 24 hours in 98.1% of all cases of influenza, and in 87.9% of all cases of the common cold (*5*, *33*). In another study, 40 patients with fever of pathological origin had a significant reduction in fever (1–2 °C), but the antipyretic effect of Radix Bupleuri in these patients was transient unless combined with antibiotic therapy (*5*, *34*).

Contraindications

No information available.

Warnings

Radix Bupleuri causes sedation when used in large doses (*5*); therefore, patients should be cautious when operating a motor vehicle or hazardous machinery.

Precautions

Drug interactions

The use of alcohol, sedatives and other central nervous system depressants in conjunction with Radix Bupleuri may cause synergistic sedative effects. No clinical studies have evaluated this possible interaction; however, patients should be cautioned about taking the drug with alcohol, sedatives, or other drugs known to cause depression of the central nervous system.

Carcinogenesis, mutagenesis, impairment of fertility

Methanolic extracts of *B. chinense* (*B. falcatum*) were not mutagenic in the modified Ames test using *Salmonella typhimurium* TA 98 and TA 100, in the presence or absence of rat liver S-9 mix (*35, 36*). Furthermore, hot-water extracts of *Bupleurum* were shown to have antimutagenic activity in AFB1-induced mutagenesis in the mouse *Salmonella typhi*/mammalian microsomal system (Ames test) (strain TA 98) and in the *in vivo* mouse bone marrow cell chromosome aberration and mouse bone marrow eosinophil micronucleus test (*37*). There is one report that a hot-water extract of *B. falcatum* enhanced the mutagenic activity of Trp-P-1 with S9 mix in *Salmonella typhimurium* (*38*).

Pregnancy: teratogenic and non-teratogenic effects

No data available; therefore, *B. falcatum* should not be administered during pregnancy.

Nursing mothers

Excretion of the drug into breast milk and its effects on the newborn infant have not been established; therefore, *Bupleurum* should not be administered to nursing women.

Paediatric use

Guidelines for the administration of the drug to children are not available.

Other precautions

No information available concerning general precautions or drug and laboratory test interactions.

Adverse reactions

Mild lassitude, sedation, and drowsiness have been reported as frequent side-effects (*5*). Large doses have also been reported to decrease appetite and cause pronounced flatulence and abdominal distension. Three incidents of allergic reactions were reported in patients given intramuscular injections of the drug (*5*).

Posology

Generally, doses of 3–9 g/day (*1*).

References

1. *Pharmacopoeia of the People's Republic of China* (English ed.). Guangzhou, Guangdong Science and Technology Press, 1992.

74

2. *The Pharmacopoeia of Japan XII*. Tokyo, The Society of Japanese Pharmacopoeia, 1991.
3. Wolf H. Umbelliferae—Apioideae—*Bupleurum*, Trinia et reliqceae Ammineae hecteroclitae. In: Engler A, ed. *Pflanzenreich IV*. Leipzig, Verlag von Wilhelm Engelmann, 1910.
4. Keys JD. T, *Chinese herbs, their botany, chemistry and pharmacodynamics*. Rutland, VT, CE Tuttle, 1976.
5. Chang HM, But PPH, eds. *Pharmacology and applications of Chinese materia medica, Vol. 2*. Singapore, World Scientific Publishing, 1987.
6. Nasir E. Umbelliferae. In: Nasir E, Ali SI, eds. *Flora of West Pakistan*. Karachi, Pakistan, Stewart Herbarium, 1972:60.
7. *Quality control methods for medicinal plant materials*. Geneva, World Health Organization, 1998.
8. *Deutsches Arzneibuch 1996. Vol. 2. Methoden der Biologie*. Stuttgart, Deutscher Apotheker Verlag, 1996.
9. *European Pharmacopoeia*, 3rd ed. Strasbourg, Council of Europe, 1997.
10. *Guidelines for predicting dietary intake of pesticide residues*, 2nd rev. ed. Geneva, World Health Organization, 1997 (unpublished document WHO/FSF/FOS/97.7; available from Food Safety, WHO, 1211 Geneva 27, Switzerland).
11. Hiai S et al. A simultaneous colorimetric estimation of biologically active and inactive saikosaponins in *Bupleurum falcatum* extracts. *Planta medica*, 1976, 29:247–257.
12. Shimizu K, Amagaya S, Ogihara Y. Separation and quantitative analysis of saikosaponins by high-performance liquid chromatography. *Journal of chromatography*, 1986, 268:85–91.
13. Han DS, Lee DK. Separation and determination of saikosaponins in Bupleuri Radix with HPLC. *Korean journal of pharmacognosy*, 1985, 16:175–179.
14. Tang W, Eisenbrand G, eds. *Chinese drugs of plant origins, chemistry, pharmacology and use in traditional and modern medicine*. Berlin, Springer-Verlag, 1992.
15. Yamada H. Purification of anti-ulcer polysaccharides from the roots of *Bupleurum falcatum*. *Planta medica*, 1991, 57:555–559.
16. Yamada H, Hirano M, Kiyohara H. Partial structure of an anti-ulcer pectic polysaccharide from the roots of *Bupleurum falcatum* L. *Carbohydrate research*, 1991, 219:173–192.
17. Zhu Y. *Pharmacology and applications of Chinese medicinal materials*. Beijing, People's Medical Publishing House, 1958.
18. Zhou ZC et al. *Chinese pharmaceutical bulletin*, 1979, 14:252 (article in Chinese).
19. Yamamoto M, Kumagai A, Yamamura Y. Structure and actions of saikosaponins isolated from *Bupleurum falcatum* L. I. Anti-inflammatory action of saikosaponins. *Arzneimittel-Forschung*, 1974, 25:1021–1023.
20. Abe H et al. Pharmacological actions of saikosaponins isolated from *Bupleurum falcatum*. 1. Effects of saikosaponins on liver function. *Planta medica*, 1980, 40:366–372.
21. Shibata M et al. Pharmacological studies on the Chinese crude drug saiko, *Bupleurum falcatum*. *Hoshi yakka daigaku kiyo*, 1974, 16:77.
22. Shibata S. Medicinal chemistry of triterpenoid saponins and sapogenins. *Proceedings of the 4th Asian Symposium on Medicinal Plants and Spices*. Bangkok, Mahidol University, 1981:59–70.
23. Mizoguchi Y et al. Effects of saiko on antibody response and mitogen-induced lymphocyte transformation *in vitro*. *Journal of medical and pharmaceutical society for WAKAN-YAKU*, 1985, 2:330–336.
24. Matsumoto T et al. The pectic polysaccharide from *Bupleurum falcatum* L. enhances immune-complexes binding to peritoneal macrophages through Fc receptor expression. *International journal of immunopharmacology*, 1993, 15:683–693.

25. Yamada H. Pectic polysaccharides from Chinese herbs—structure and biological activity. *Carbohydrate polymers*, 1994, 25:269–276.
26. Matsumoto T, Yamada H. Regulation of immune complex binding of macrophages by pectic polysaccharide from *Bupleurum falcatum* L.—pharmacological evidence for the requirement of intracellular calcium/calmodulin on Fc receptor up-regulation by bupleuran 2iib. *Journal of pharmacy and pharmacology*, 1995, 47:152–156.
27. Ushio Y, Abe H. Effects of saikosaponin-D on the functions and morphology of macrophages. *International journal of immunopharmacology*, 1991, 13:493–499.
28. Kato M et al. Characterization of the immunoregulatory action of saikosaponin D. *Cellular immunology*, 1994, 159:15–25.
29. Sun XB, Matsumoto T, Yamada H. Effects of a polysaccharide fraction from the roots of *Bupleurum falcatum* L. on experimental gastric ulcer models in rats and mice. *Journal of pharmacy and pharmacology*, 1991, 43:699–704.
30. Shibata M et al. Some pharmacological studies on the crude drugs possessing anti-inflammatory properties of the *Bupleurum* and the leaves of fig. *Shoyakugaku zasshi*, 1976, 30:62–66.
31. Arichi S, Konishi H, Abe H. Studies on the mechanism of action of saikosaponin. I. Effects of saikosaponin on hepatic injury induced by D-galactosamine. *Kanzo*, 1978, 19:430–435.
32. Zhao MQ et al. Preventive and therapeutic effects of glycyrrhizin, glycyrrhetic acid and saikosides on experimental cirrhosis in rats. *Yao hsueh hsueh pao*, 1983, 18:325–331.
33. Nanjing Medical College. *Encyclopedia of Chinese materia medica*, Vol. 2. Shanghai, Shanghai People's Publishing House, 1978:3763.
34. Wuxi First People's Hospital. *Wuxi yiyao [Wuxi medical journal]*, 1973, 1:42 (article in Chinese).
35. Yamamoto H, Mizutani T, Nomura H. Studies on the mutagenicity of crude drug extracts. I. *Yakugaku zasshi*, 1982, 102:596–601.
36. Sakai Y et al. Effects of medicinal plant extracts from Chinese herbal medicines on the mutagenic activity of benzo[a]pyrene. *Mutation research*, 1988, 206:327–334.
37. Liu DX. Antimutagenicity screening of water extracts from 102 kinds of Chinese medicinal herbs. *Chung-kuo tung yao tsa chih*, 1990, 15:640–642.
38. Niikawa M et al. Enhancement of the mutagenicity of TRP-P-1, TRP-P-2 and benzo[alpha]pyrene by Bupleuri radix extract. *Chemical and pharmaceutical bulletin*, 1990, 38:2035–2039.

Herba Centellae

Definition

Herba Centellae consists of the dried aerial parts or the entire plant of *Centella asiatica* (L.) Urban. (Apiaceae) (*1–5*).

Synonyms

Centella coriacea Nannfd., *Hydrocotyle asiatica* L., *Hydrocotyle lunata* Lam. and *Trisanthus cochinchinensis* Lour. (*1, 3, 6*). Apiaceae are also known as Umbelliferae.

Selected vernacular names

Artaniyae-hindi, Asiatic pennywort, barmanimuni, barmi, bhram buti, boa-bok, bodila-ba-dinku, bokkudu, brahma manduki, brahmi ghi, brahmi-buti, brahmi, bua bok, bua-bok, centella, chhota mani-muni, chi-hsueh-ts'ao, ghi brahmi, ghod tapre, ghodtapre, ghortapre, gotu kola, gotukola, herba pegagan, herba kakikuda, hydrocotyle, hydrocotyle asiatique, idrocotile, imsen korokla, Indian pennywort, Indian water navelwort, Indischer Wassernabel, karinga, karivana, kudangal, luei gong gen, lièn tièn tháo, mandooka parni, mandukaparni, mandukparni, manimuni, marsh pepperwort, matoyahuho, matoyahuhu, mrang-khua, mtwigahuwu, pa-na-e-khaa-doh, phác chèn, phaknok, phalwaen, rau má, saraswathiaaku, takip-kohol, thalkuri, thankuni, thol-kuri, tilkushi, titjari, tono'itahi, tsubo-kusa, tungchian, vallari, vallarei, vitovitolenge, water pennywort, waternavel, yahon-yahon, yerba de chavos (*3–11*).

Description

A slender trailing herb, rooting at the nodes. Leaves 1.3–6.3 cm diameter, or-bicular reniform, more or less cupped, entire, crenate or lobulate, glabrous; leaf stalks 2–5 cm long; peduncle about 6 mm, often 2–3 nates; pedicels nil; bracts small, embracing the flowers; inflorescence in single umbel, bearing 1–5 flowers, sessile, white or reddish; fruit small, compressed, 8 mm long, mericarps longer than broad, curved, rounded at top, 7–9-ridged, secondary ridges as prominent as the primary, reticulate between them; pericarp much thickened; seed compressed laterally (*1, 4, 7*).

Plant material of interest: aerial part or entire plant

General appearance

A slender herb. Stems long, prostrate, emerging from the leaf-axils of a vertical rootstock, filiform, often reddish, with long internodes and rooting at the nodes; leaves thin, long-petioled, several from the rootstock and 1–3 from each node of the stems, 1.3–6.3 cm diameter, orbicular reniform, more or less cupped, entire, crenate or lobulate, glabrous; petioles very variable in length, 7.5–15 cm long or more, channelled; stipules short, adnate to the petioles forming a sheathing base (*4, 5*).

Organoleptic properties

Colour, greyish green; odour, characteristic; taste, slightly bittersweet (*4, 5*).

Microscopic characteristics

Greyish green with stomata on both surfaces of the leaf, 30 by 28 μm, mostly rubiaceous type. Palisade cells differentiated into 2 layers of cells, 45 by 25 μm; spongy parenchyma of about 3 layers of cells with many intercellular spaces, some with crystals of calcium oxalate; midrib region shows 2 or 3 layers of parenchymatous cells without chloroplastids; petiole shows epidermis with thickened inner walls; collenchyma of 2 or 3 layers of cells; a broad zone of parenchyma; 7 vascular bundles within parenchymatous zone, 2 in projecting arms and 5 forming the central strand; vessels 15–23 μm in diameter. Some parenchymatous cells contain crystals of calcium oxalate. Fruits, epidermis of polygonal cells, trichomes similar to the leaves, sheets of elongated parquetry layer cells, bundles of narrow annular vessels, and parenchymatous cells contain single large prisms of calcium oxalate (*4*).

Geographical distribution

The plant is indigenous to the warmer regions of both hemispheres, including Africa, Australia, Cambodia, Central America, China, Indonesia, the Lao People's Democratic Republic, Madagascar, the Pacific Islands, South America, Thailand, southern United States of America, and Viet Nam. It is especially abundant in the swampy areas of India, the Islamic Republic of Iran, Pakistan, and Sri Lanka up to an altitude of approximately 700 m (*1, 4, 6, 8, 10, 11*).

General identity tests

Macroscopic and microscopic examinations; and microchemical tests for the presence of triterpenes and reducing sugars (*1, 4*).

Purity tests
Microbiology
The test for *Salmonella* spp. in Herba Centellae products should be negative. The maximum acceptable limits of other microorganisms are as follows (*12–14*). For preparation of decoction: aerobic bacteria—not more than 10^7/g; fungi—not more than 10^5/g; *Escherichia coli*—not more than 10^2/g. Preparations for internal use: aerobic bacteria—not more than 10^5/g or ml; fungi—not more than 10^4/g or ml; enterobacteria and certain Gram-negative bacteria—not more than 10^3/g or ml; *Escherichia coli*—0/g or ml.

Foreign organic matter
Not more than 2% (*4*).

Total ash
Not more than 19% (*2, 3*).

Acid-insoluble ash
Not less than 6% (*2*).

Water-soluble extractive
Not less than 6% (*2, 3*).

Alcohol-soluble extractive
Not less than 9.5% (*2, 3*).

Pesticide residues
To be established in accordance with national requirements. Normally, the maximum residue limit of aldrin and dieldrin in Herba Centellae is not more than 0.05 mg/kg (*14*). For other pesticides, see WHO guidelines on quality control methods for medicinal plants (*12*) and guidelines for predicting dietary intake of pesticide residues (*15*).

Heavy metals
Recommended lead and cadmium levels are not more than 10 and 0.3 mg/kg, respectively, in the final dosage form of the plant material (*12*).

Radioactive residues
For analysis of strontium-90, iodine-131, caesium-134, caesium-137, and plutonium-239, see WHO guidelines on quality control methods for medicinal plants (*12*).

Other purity tests

Chemical tests, and tests for drug interactions and moisture to be established by national authorities.

Chemical assays

Contains not less than 2% triterpene ester glycosides (asiaticoside and madecassoside) (*10*). Determination of asiaticoside and related triterpene ester glycosides by thin-layer chromatography (*16*) and spectroscopic analysis (*17*).

Major chemical constituents

The major principles in Herba Centellae are the triterpenes asiatic acid and madecassic acid, and their derived triterpene ester glycosides, asiaticoside and madecassoside (*8, 10, 11*).

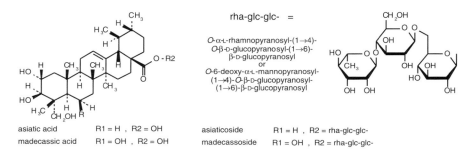

rha-glc-glc- =

O-α-L-rhamnopyranosyl-(1→4)-
O-β-D-glucopyranosyl-(1→6)-
β-D-glucopyranosyl
or
O-6-deoxy-α-L-mannopyranosyl-
(1→4)-*O*-β-D-glucopyranosyl-
(1→6)-β-D-glucopyranosyl

asiatic acid	R1 = H , R2 = OH	
madecassic acid	R1 = OH , R2 = OH	
asiaticoside	R1 = H , R2 = rha-glc-glc-	
madecassoside	R1 = OH , R2 = rha-glc-glc-	

Dosage forms

Dried drug for infusion (*18*); galenic preparations for oral administration (*10*). Powder or extract (liquid or ointment) for topical application (*1, 4*). Package in well-closed, light-resistant containers.

Medicinal uses

Uses supported by clinical data

Treatment of wounds, burns, and ulcerous skin ailments, and prevention of keloid and hypertrophic scars (*10, 18–21*). Extracts of the plant have been employed to treat second- and third-degree burns (*19*). Extracts have been used topically to accelerate healing, particularly in cases of chronic postsurgical and post-trauma wounds (*19*). Extracts have been administered orally to treat stress-induced stomach and duodenal ulcers (*10*).

Uses described in pharmacopoeias and in traditional systems of medicine

Herba Centellae is reported to be used in the treatment of leprous ulcers and venous disorders (*5, 6, 8, 10, 22*).

Studies suggest that extracts of *Centella asiatica* cause regression of inflammatory infiltration of the liver in cirrhosis patients (*10, 23*). Further experimentation is needed to confirm these findings.

Uses described in folk medicine, not supported by experimental or clinical data

Therapy of albinism, anaemia, asthma, bronchitis, cellulite, cholera, measles, constipation, dermatitis, diarrhoea, dizziness, dysentery, dysmenorrhoea, dysuria, epistaxis, epilepsy, haematemesis, haemorrhoids, hepatitis, hypertension, jaundice, leukorrhoea, nephritis, nervous disorders, neuralgia, rheumatism, smallpox, syphilis, toothache, urethritis, and varices; and as an antipyretic, analgesic, anti-inflammatory, and "brain tonic" agent (*4, 5, 7*). Poultices have been used to treat contusions, closed fractures, sprains, and furunculosis (*7*).

Pharmacology
Experimental pharmacology

The pharmacological activity of *Centella asiatica* is thought to be due to several saponin constituents, including asiaticoside, asiatic acid, and madecassic acid (*10*). *In vitro*, each of these compounds stimulated the production of human collagen I, a protein involved in wound healing (*24*). Stimulation of collagen synthesis in foreskin fibroblast monolayer cultures by an extract from Herba Centellae has also been reported (*25*). Asiaticoside accelerated the healing of superficial postsurgical wounds and ulcers by accelerating cicatricial action (*21*). Asiaticoside stimulates the epidermis by activating the cells of the malpighian layer in porcine skin, and by keratinization *in vitro* (*26*). Topical application of asiaticoside promoted wound healing in rats and significantly increased the tensile strength of newly formed skin (*21, 27*).

Extracts of *C. asiatica*, and in particular its major triterpene ester glycoside, asiaticoside, are valuable in the treatment of hypertrophic scars and keloids (*21*). Asiaticoside has been reported to decrease fibrosis in wounds, thus preventing new scar formation (*21*). The mechanism of action appears to be twofold: by increasing the synthesis of collagen and acidic mucopolysaccharides, and by inhibiting the inflammatory phase of hypertrophic scars and keloids. It has further been proposed that asiaticoside interferes with scar formation by increasing the activity of myofibroblasts and immature collagen (*21*).

Extract of Herba Centellae effectively treated stress-induced stomach and duodenal ulcers in humans (*10, 28*). Oral administration of *C. asiatica* extract to rats produced a dose-dependent reduction in stress-induced gastric ulceration, and the antiulcer activity was similar to that of famotidine (*29*). The mechanism of action appears to be associated with a central nervous system-depressant activity of *C. asiatica*, owing to an increase in the concentration of GABA (γ-aminobutyric acid) in the brain (*29*).

A 70% ethanol extract of the drug administered intraperitoneally to mice produced anticonvulsant activity (*30*).

Clinical pharmacology

In clinical trials, an extract of *C. asiatica* in a 1% salve or 2% powder accelerated healing of wounds (*31*). A formulation containing asiaticoside as the main ingredient healed 64% of soiled wounds and chronic or recurrent atony that was resistant to usual treatment (*21*). In an open clinical study, treatment of 20 patients with soiled wounds and chronic or recurrent atony with a galenical formulation containing 89.5% *C. asiatica* healed 64% and produced improvement in another 16% of the lesions studied (*20*). Local application of an extract of the drug to second- and third-degree burns expedited healing, prevented the shrinking and swelling caused by infection, and further inhibited hypertrophic scar formation (*11*).

Twenty-two patients with chronic infected skin ulcers were treated with a cream containing a 1% extract of *C. asiatica* (*32*). After 3 weeks of treatment, 17 of the patients were completely healed and the ulcer size in the remaining 5 patients was decreased (*32*). Another trial using the same cream preparation demonstrated similar results (*33*). A standardized extract of Herba Centellae was reported to treat ulcus cruris (indolent leg ulcers) effectively in clinical trials (*34, 35*). In a double-blind study, no significant effect on healing was observed in patients with ulcus cruris after oral treatment with asiaticoside (*36*).

Oral administration of *C. asiatica* or asiaticoside and potassium chloride capsules was reported to be as effective as dapsone therapy in patients with leprosy (*37*). In a controlled study of 90 patients with perforated leg lesions owing to leprosy, application of a salve of the plant produced significantly better results than a placebo (*11, 22, 38*).

Clinical trials of the drug have demonstrated its antiulcer activity after oral administration (*28, 39, 40*). Fifteen patients with peptic or duodenal ulcer were treated with a titrated extract of Herba Centellae (60.0 mg/person). Approximately 93% of the patients exhibited a definite improvement in subjective symptoms and 73% of the ulcers were healed as measured by endoscopic and radiological observations (*28*).

Clinical studies of Herba Centellae in the treatment of various venous disorders has demonstrated a positive therapeutic effect (*11*). In patients suffering from venous insufficiency who were treated with a titrated extract of the drug, venous distension and oedema improved significantly, as compared with controls (*41*).

Contraindications

Allergy to plants of the Apiaceae family.

Warnings
No information available.

Precautions
Carcinogenesis, mutagenesis, impairment of fertility
Asiaticoside has been implicated as a possible skin carcinogen in rodents after repeated topical application (42). Further experimentation is needed to substantiate this claim.

Other precautions
No information was available concerning drug interactions, drug and laboratory test interactions, teratogenic or non-teratogenic effects on pregnancy, nursing mothers, or paediatric use.

Adverse reactions
Allergic contact dermatitis has been associated with topical application of *C. asiatica* (21, 43, 44). However, further testing revealed that these reactions may be due to other ingredients in the preparations (45).

Posology
Oral dose: 0.33–0.68 g or by oral infusion of a similar amount three times daily (4–6).

References
1. *African pharmacopoeia*, 1st ed. Lagos, Organization of African Unity, Scientific, Technical & Research Commission, 1985.
2. *Materia medika Indonesia*, Jilid I. Jakarta, Departemen Kesehatan, Republik Indonesia, 1977.
3. *Vietnam materia medica*. Hanoi, Ministry of Health, 1972.
4. *The Indian pharmaceutical codex. Vol. I. Indigenous drugs*. New Delhi, Council of Scientific & Industrial Research, 1953.
5. *British herbal pharmacopoeia, Part 2*. London, British Herbal Medicine Association, 1979.
6. Iwu MM. *Handbook of African medicinal plants*. Boca Raton, FL, CRC Press, 1993.
7. *Medicinal plants in Viet Nam*. Manila, World Health Organization, 1990 (WHO Regional Publications, Western Pacific Series, No. 3).
8. Tyler VE, Brady LR, Robbers JE, eds. *Pharmacognosy*, 9th ed. Philadelphia, Lea & Febiger, 1988.
9. *Medicinal plants of India, Vol. 1*. New Delhi, Indian Council of Medical Research, 1976.
10. Kartnig T. Clinical applications of *Centella asiatica* (L.) Urb. In: Craker LE, Simon JE, eds., *Herbs, spices, and medicinal plants: recent advances in botany, horticulture, and pharmacology, Vol. 3*. Phoenix, AZ, Oryx Press, 1988:145–173.

11. Farnsworth NR, Bunyapraphatsara N, eds. *Thai medicinal plants*. Bangkok, Prachachon, 1992.
12. *Quality control methods for medicinal plant materials*. Geneva, World Health Organization, 1998.
13. *Deutsches Arzneibuch 1996. Vol. 2. Methoden der Biologie*. Stuttgart, Deutscher Apotheker Verlag, 1996.
14. *European pharmacopoeia*, 3rd ed. Strasbourg, Council of Europe, 1997.
15. *Guidelines for predicting dietary intake of pesticide residues*, 2nd rev. ed. Geneva, World Health Organization, 1997 (unpublished document WHO/FSF/FOS/97.7; available from Food Safety, WHO, 1211 Geneva 27, Switzerland).
16. Meng ZM, Zheng YN. Determination of asiaticoside contained in sanjinplan. *Zhongguo yaoke daxue xuebao*, 1988, 19:205–206.
17. Castellani C, Marai A,Vacchi P. The *Centella asiatica*. *Bolletin chimica farmacia*, 1981, 120:570–605.
18. Reynolds JEF, ed. *Martindale, the extra pharmacopoeia*, 30th ed. London, Pharmaceutical Press, 1993:756.
19. Gravel JA. Oxygen dressings and asiaticoside in the treatment of burns. *Laval medicine*, 1965, 36:413–415.
20. Bosse JP et al. Clinical study of a new antikeloid agent. *Annals of plastic surgery*, 1979, 3:13–21.
21. Morisset R et al. Evaluation of the healing activity of Hydrocotyle tincture in the treatment of wounds. *Phytotherapy research*, 1987, 1:117.
22. Chaudhuri S et al. Use of common Indian herb Mandukaparni in the treatment of leprosy (preliminary report). *Journal of the Indian Medical Association*, 1978, 70:177–180.
23. Darnis F et al. Use of a titrated extract of *Centella asiatica* in chronic hepatic disorders. *Semaine hospitaux de Paris*, 1979, 55:1749–1750.
24. Bonte F et al. Influence of asiatic acid, madecassic acid, and asiaticoside on human collagen I synthesis. *Planta medica*, 1994, 60:133–135.
25. Maquart FX et al. Stimulation of collagen synthesis in fibroblast cultures by triterpene extracted from *Centella asiatica*. *Connective tissue research*, 1990, 24:107–120.
26. May A. The effect of asiaticoside on pig skin in organ culture. *European journal of pharmacology*, 1968, 4:177–181.
27. Rosen H, Blumenthal A, McCallum J. Effect of asiaticoside on wound healing in the rat. *Proceedings of the Society of Experimental Biology and Medicine*, 1972, 125:279.
28. Shin HS et al. Clinical trials of madecassol (*Centella asiatica*) on gastrointestinal ulcer patients. *Korean journal of gastroenterology*, 1982, 14:49–56.
29. Chatterjee TK, Chakraborty A, Pathak M. Effects of plant extract *Centella asiatica* L. on cold restraint stress ulcer in rats. *Indian journal of experimental biology*, 1992, 30:889–891.
30. Adesina SK. Studies on some plants used as anticonvulsants in Amerindian and African traditional medicine. *Fitoterapia*, 1982, 53:147–162.
31. Kiesewetter H. Erfahrungsbericht über die Behandlung von Wunden mit Asiaticosid (Madecassol). *Wiener medizinische Wochenschrift*, 1964, 114:124–126.
32. Boiteau P, Ratsimamanga AR. Asiaticoside extracted from *Centella asiatica*, its therapeutic uses in healing of experimental or refractory wounds, leprosy, skin tuberculosis, and lupus. *Therapie*, 1956, 11:125–149.
33. Boiteau P, Ratsimamanga AR. Cicatrizants of vegetable origin and the biostimulins. *Bulletin de la Société Scientifique de CASSI*, 1957, 32:28.
34. Huriez C. Action of the titrated extract of *Centella asiatica* in the cicatrization of leg ulcers (10 mg tablets). Apropos of 50 cases. *Lille medicale*, 1972, 17(Suppl. 3):574–579.
35. Bourde C, Bourde J. The place of cicatrizing agents in leg ulcers. *Semaine des hôpitaux de Paris*, 1952, 2:105–113.

36. Mayall RC et al. U'lceras troficas-Acbo cicatricial do extrato titulad da *Centella asiatica*. *Review of Brasilian medicine*, 1975, 32:26–29.
37. Chakrabarty T, Deshmukh S. *Centella asiatica* in the treatment of leprosy. *Science and culture*, 1976, 42:573.
38. Nebout M. Résultats d'un essai controlé de l'extrait titre de *Centella asiatica* (E.T.C.A.) (I) dans une population lepreuse presentant des maux perforants plantaires. *Bulletin de la Société de Pathologie exotique*, 1974, 67:471–478.
39. Rhee JC, Choi KW. Clinical effect of the titrated extract of *Centella asiatica* (madecassol) on peptic ulcer. *Korean journal of gastroenterology*, 1981, 13:35–40.
40. Cho KH et al. Clinical experiences of madecassol (*Centella asiatica*) in the treatment of peptic ulcer. *Korean journal of gastroenterology*, 1981, 13:49–56.
41. Lythgoe B, Trippett S. Derivatives of *Centella asiatica* used against leprosy. Centelloside. *Nature*, 1949, 163:259–260.
42. Laerum OD, Iversen OH. Reticuloses and epidermal tumors in hairless mice after topical skin applications of cantharidin and asiaticoside. *Cancer research*, 1972, 32:1463–1469.
43. Izu R et al. Allergic contact dermatitis from a cream containing *Centella asiatica* extract. *Contact dermatitis*, 1992, 26:192–193.
44. Danese P, Carnevali C, Bertazzoni MG. Allergic contact dermatitis due to *Centella asiatica* extract. *Contact dermatitis*, 1994, 31:201.
45. Hausen BM. *Centella asiatica* (Indian pennywort), an effective therapeutic but a weak sensitizer. *Contact dermatitis*, 1993, 29:175–179.

Flos Chamomillae

Definition

Flos Chamomillae consists of the dried flowering heads of *Chamomilla recutita* (L.) Rauschert (Asteraceae) (*1–4*).

Synonyms

Matricaria chamomilla L., *M. recutita* L., *M. suaveolens* L. (*3*).

In most formularies and reference books, *Matricaria chamomilla* L. is regarded as the correct species name. However, according to the International Rules of Botanical Nomenclature, *Chamomilla recutita* (L.) Rauschert is the legitimate name for this species (*5*). Asteraceae are also known as Compositae.

Selected vernacular names

Baboonig, babuna, babunah camomile, babunj, bunga kamil, camamilla, camomile, chamomile, camomilla, chamomille allemande, campomilla, chamomille commune, camomille sauvage, fleurs de petite camomille, flos chamomillae, german chamomile, hungarian chamomile, Kamille, Kamillen, kamitsure, kamiture, manzanilla, manzanilla chiquita, manzanilla comun, manzanilla dulce, matricaire, matricaria flowers, pin heads, sweet false chamomille, sweet feverfew, wild chamomile (*3, 6–9*).

Description

Herbaceous annual; 10–30 cm in height, with erect, branching stems and alternate, tripinnately divided leaves below and bipinnately divided leaves above, both types having almost filiform lobes; the capitulum (to 1.5 cm in diameter) comprises 12–20 white ligulate florets surrounding a conical hollow receptacle on which numerous yellow tubular (disk) florets are inserted; the inflorescence is surrounded by a flattened imbricated involucre; fruit small, smooth, yellowish (*3, 7, 10*).

Plant material of interest: flower heads

General appearance

Flos Chamomillae consists of conical flower heads, each bearing a few white ligulate florets and numerous yellowish orange to pale yellow tubular or disk florets on conical, narrow hollow receptacles with a short peduncle; disk florets perfect and without a pappus; ray florets pistillate, white, 3-toothed and 4-veined; involucre hemispherical, composed of 20–30 imbricate, oblanceolate and pubescent scales; peduncles weak brown to dusky greenish yellow, longitudinally furrowed, more or less twisted and up to 2.5 cm long; achenes more or less obovoid and faintly 3- to 5-ribbed; pappus none, or slightly membranous crown (*7, 11*).

Organoleptic properties
Odour, pleasant, aromatic; taste, aromatic and slightly bitter (*1–3*).

Microscopic characteristics
Receptacle and bracteoles with schizogenous secretory ducts; vascular bundles with phloem fibres; spiral, annular and reticulate but pitted vessels; lignified cells at the bases of the ovaries absent; nearly all parts of florets bear composite-type glandular hairs with short, biseriate stalk and enlarged head, formed of several tiers, each of two cells; ovary with longitudinal bands of small mucilage cells; stigma with elongated papillae at the apex; pollen grains, spherical or triangular, with numerous short spines (*3*).

Powdered plant material
Powdered Flos Chamomillae is greenish yellow to yellowish brown; spiny pollen grains numerous, 18–25 μm in diameter; fragments of yellow or white corolla, with polygonal, small epidermal cells having straight or slightly wavy walls, sometimes papillosed, and sometimes bearing glandular hairs of composite type; fragments of the fibrous layer of anther; fragments from ovary, with glandular hairs and rows of small mucilage cells; green fragments of parenchyma of involucre; stigma with papillae; cells of the achenes with sclariform perforations in walls; fragments of fibrovascular bundles with spiral, annular and reticulate vessels and sclerenchyma fibres; fragments of involucral bracts with epidermis having elliptical stomata up to 30 μm in length, also vessels and fibres; occasional fibre from the stems; minute cluster crystals of calcium oxalate, up to 10 μm in diameter; fragments of lignified parenchyma of the filaments and occasional fragments of vessels (*3, 7, 10*).

Geographical distribution
The plant is indigenous to northern Europe and grows wild in central European countries; it is especially abundant in eastern Europe. Also found in western Asia, the Mediterranean region of northern Africa, and the United States of America. It is cultivated in many countries (*3, 7–13*).

General identity tests
The drug is identified by its macroscopic and microscopic characteristics, and by thin-layer chromatography (*1–3*).

Purity tests
Microbiology

The test for *Salmonella* spp. in Flos Chamomillae products should be negative. The maximum acceptable limits of other microorganisms are as follows (*1, 14, 15*). For preparation of decoction: aerobic bacteria—not more than 10^7/g; fungi—not more than 10^5/g; *Escherichia coli*—not more than 10^2/g. Preparations for internal use: aerobic bacteria—not more than 10^5/g or ml; fungi—not more than 10^4/g or ml; enterobacteria and certain Gram-negative bacteria—not more than 10^3/g or ml; *Escherichia coli*—0/g or ml. Preparations for external use: aerobic bacteria—not more than 10^2/g or ml; fungi—not more than 10^2/g or ml; enterobacteria and certain Gram-negative bacteria—not more than 10^1/g or ml.

Foreign organic matter

Not more than 10% stems and not more than 2% foreign organic matter (*3*). No flowering heads of *Anthemis cotula* L. or *A. nobilis* L. (*7*).

Total ash

Not more than 13% (*2*).

Acid-insoluble ash

Not more than 4% (*11*).

Moisture

Not more than 12% (*12*).

Pesticide residues

To be established in accordance with national requirements. Normally, the maximum residue limit of aldrin and dieldrin for Flos Chamomillae is not more than 0.05 mg/kg (*1*). For other pesticides, see WHO guidelines on quality control methods for medicinal plants (*14*) and guidelines for predicting dietary intake of pesticide residues (*16*).

Heavy metals

Recommended lead and cadmium levels are no more than 10 and 0.3 mg/kg, respectively, in the final dosage form of the plant material (*14*).

Radioactive residues

For analysis of strontium-90, iodine-131, caesium-134, caesium-137, and plutonium-239, see WHO guidelines on quality control methods for medicinal plants (*14*).

Other tests

Chemical, dilute ethanol-soluble extractive, and water-soluble extractive tests to be established in accordance with national requirements.

Chemical assays

Contains not less than 0.4% v/w of essential oil (*1–3*). Total volatile oil content is determined by pharmacopoeial methods (*1–3*).

Thin-layer (*1, 2*) and gas–liquid (*17*) chromatography for volatile oil constituents, and high-performance liquid chromatography for flavonoids (*18, 19*).

Major chemical constituents

Flos Chamomillae contains an essential oil (0.4–1.5%), which has an intense blue colour owing to its chamazulene content (1–15%). Other major constituents include α-bisabolol and related sesquiterpenes (up to 50% of the oil). Apigenin and related flavonoid glycosides constitute up to 8% (dry weight) of the drug (*10, 18*).

chamazulene   (−)-α-bisabolol   apigenin

Dosage forms

Dried flower-heads, liquid extract (1:1 in 45% alcohol), tinctures and other galenicals (*11*). Store in well-closed containers, protected from light (*1–3*).

Medicinal uses
Uses supported by clinical data
Internal use

Symptomatic treatment of digestive ailments such as dyspepsia, epigastric bloating, impaired digestion, and flatulence (*3, 7, 8, 10, 11, 20, 21*). Infusions of camomile flowers have been used in the treatment of restlessness and in mild cases of insomnia due to nervous disorders (*21, 22*).

External use

Inflammation and irritations of the skin and mucosa (skin cracks, bruises, frostbite, and insect bites) (*10, 23*), including irritations and infections of the mouth and gums, and haemorrhoids (*10, 11, 20, 21, 23*).

Inhalation

Symptomatic relief of irritations of the respiratory tract due to the common cold (24).

Uses described in pharmacopoeias and in traditional systems of medicine

Adjuvant in the treatment of minor inflammatory conditions of the gastrointestinal tract (24).

Uses described in folk medicine, not supported by experimental or clinical data

As an antibacterial and antiviral agent, an emetic, and an emmenagogue. It is also used to relieve eye strain, and to treat urinary infections and diarrhoea (13).

Pharmacology

Experimental pharmacology

Both camomile extract and (−)-α-bisabolol demonstrated antipeptic activity *in vitro* (25, 26). A hydroalcoholic extract of camomile inhibited the growth of *Staphylococcus aureus, Streptococcus mutans*, group B *Streptococcus*, and *Streptococcus salivarius*, and it had a bactericidal effect *in vitro* on *Bacillus megatherium* and *Leptospira icterohaemorrhagiae* (27). *In vitro*, the volatile oil of camomile also inhibited *Staphylococcus aureus* and *Bacillus subtilis* (28). *In vitro*, camomile extracts inhibited both cyclooxygenase and lipoxygenase (29), and thus the production of prostaglandins and leukotrienes, known inducers of inflammation. Both bisabolol and bisabolol oxide have been shown to inhibit 5-lipoxygenase, but bisabolol was the more active of the two compounds (30). Numerous *in vivo* studies have demonstrated the anti-inflammatory effects of the drug. The anti-inflammatory effects of camomile extract, the essential oil, and the isolated constituents have been evaluated in yeast-induced fever in rats and against ultraviolet radiation-induced erythema in guinea-pig models (31). The principal anti-inflammatory and antispasmodic constituents of camomile appear to be the terpene compounds matricin, chamazulene, (−)-α-bisabololoxides A and B, and (−)-α-bisabolol (32–39). While matricin and (−)-α-bisabolol have been isolated from the plant, chamazulene is actually an artefact formed during the heating of the flowers when an infusion or the essential oil is prepared (10). The anti-inflammatory effects of these compounds in various animal models, such as inhibition of carrageenin-induced rat paw oedema, have been demonstrated (30), although their activity was somewhat less than that of salicylamide (39). In the mouse model for croton oil-induced dermatitis, topical application of either the total camomile extract, or the flavonoid fraction only, was very effective in reducing inflammation (34). Apigenin and luteolin were more active than indometacin and phenylbutazone (34). Activity decreased in the following order: apigenin > luteolin > quercetin > myricetin > apigenin-7-glucoside > rutin (*34*). The spasmolytic activity of camomile has been attributed to apigenin, apigenin-7-O-glucoside (*10*, *36*) and (−)-α-bisabolol, which have activity similar to papaverine (*10*, *35*).

Intradermal application of liposomal apigenin-7-glucoside inhibited, in a dose-dependent manner, skin inflammations induced in rats by xanthine oxidase and cumene hydroperoxide (*38*).

Intraperitoneal administration to mice of a lyophilized infusion of camomile decreased basal motility, exploratory and motor activities, and potentiated hexobarbital-induced sleep (*40*). These results demonstrated that in mice camomile depresses the central nervous system (*40*).

Clinical pharmacology

A double-blind study of the therapeutic effects of a camomile extract on re-epithelialization and drying of wound weeping after dermabrasion demonstrated a statistically significant decrease in the wound size and drying tendency (*41*).

In clinical trials, topical application of a camomile extract in a cream base was found to be superior to hydrocortisone 0.25% for reducing skin inflammation (*42*). In an international multicentre trial camomile cream was compared with hydrocortisone 0.25%, fluocortin butyl ester 0.75% and bufexamac 5% in the treatment of eczema of the extremities (*42*). The camomile cream was shown to be as effective as hydrocortisone and superior to the other two treatments, but no statistical analysis was performed. Camomile preparations have also been found to be beneficial in the treatment of radiation mucositis owing to head and neck radiation and systemic chemotherapy (*43*).

Contraindications

Camomile is contraindicated in patients with a known sensitivity or allergy to plants of the Asteraceae (Compositae) such as ragweed, asters, and chrysanthemums (*21*).

Warnings

No information available.

Precautions

Carcinogenesis, mutagenesis, impairment of fertility

No mutagenic effects were found in *Salmonella typhimurium* strains TA 97a, TA 98, TA 100 and TA 104, with or without metabolic activation (*44*).

Pregnancy: teratogenic effects

No adverse effects reported *in vivo* (*45*).

Other precautions

No information available concerning general precautions, drug interactions, drug and laboratory test interactions, non-teratogenic effects on pregnancy, nursing mothers, or paediatric use.

Adverse reactions

The presence of lactones in Flos Chamomillae-based preparations may cause allergic reactions in sensitive individuals and there have been reports of contact dermatitis due to camomile preparations (*46–48*). It should be noted that very few cases of allergy were specifically attributed to German camomile (*49*). A few cases of anaphylactic reactions to the ingestion of Flos Chamomillae have also been reported (*50–52*).

Posology

Internal use

Adult dose of flower head: average daily dose 2–8 g, 3 times a day (*7, 8, 11*); of fluid extract 1 : 1 in 45% ethanol: dose 1–4 ml, 3 times a day (*6, 11*). Child dose of flower head: 2 g, 3 times daily; of fluid extract (ethanol 45–60%): single dose 0.6–2 ml (*11*). Should not be used by children under 3 years old.

External use

For compresses, rinses or gargles: 3–10% (30–100 g/l) infusion or 1% fluid extract or 5% tincture (*11*). For baths: 5 g/l of water or 0.8 g/l of alcoholic extract. For semisolid preparations: hydroalcoholic extracts corresponding to 3–10% (30–100 g/kg) of the drug. For vapour inhalation: 6 g of the drug or 0.8 g of alcoholic extract per litre of hot water (*11*).

References

1. *European pharmacopoeia*, 3rd ed. Strasbourg, Council of Europe, 1997.
2. *Pharmacopée française*. Paris, Adrapharm, 1996.
3. *African pharmacopoeia*, 1st ed. Lagos, Organization of African Unity, Scientific, Technical & Research Commission, 1985.
4. *Estra farmakope Indonesia*. Jakarta, Cetakan Kedua, Hal 152, Departemen Kesehatan, Republik Indonesia, 1974.
5. Rauschert S. Nomenklatorische Probleme in der Gattung *Matricaria* L. *Folia geobotanica phytotaxonomica*, 1990, 9:249–260.
6. Farnsworth NR, ed. *NAPRALERT database*. Chicago, University of Illinois at Chicago, IL, August 8, 1995 production (an on-line database available directly through the University of Illinois at Chicago or through the Scientific and Technical Network (STN) of Chemical Abstracts Services).
7. Youngken HW. *Textbook of pharmacognosy*, 6th ed. Philadelphia, Blakiston, 1950.
8. *The Indian Pharmaceutical Codex. Vol. I. Indigenous drugs*. New Delhi, Council of Scientific & Industrial Research, 1953.
9. Leung A, Foster S. *Encyclopedia of common natural ingredients used in food, drugs, and cosmetics*, 2nd ed. New York, John Wiley, 1996.

10. Bruneton J. *Pharmacognosy, phytochemistry, medicinal plants*. Paris, Lavoisier, 1995.
11. *British herbal pharmacopoeia*. London, British Herbal Medicine Association, 1990.
12. *Polish pharmacopoeia*. Warsaw, 1965.
13. Tyler VE, Brady LR, Robbers JE, eds. *Pharmacognosy*, 9th ed. Philadelphia, Lea & Febiger, 1988.
14. *Quality control methods for medicinal plant materials*. Geneva, World Health Organization, 1998.
15. *Deutsches Arzneibuch 1996. Vol. 2. Methoden der Biologie*. Stuttgart, Deutscher Apotheker Verlag, 1996.
16. *Guidelines for predicting dietary intake of pesticide residues*, 2nd rev. ed. Geneva, World Health Organization, 1997 (unpublished document WHO/FSF/FOS/97.7; available from Food Safety, WHO, 1211 Geneva 27, Switzerland).
17. Carle R, Fleischhauer I, Fehr D. Qualitätsbeurteilung von Kamillenölen. *Deutsche Apotheker Zeitung*, 1987, 127:2451–2457.
18. Dölle B, Carle R, Müller W. Flavonoidbestimmung in Kamillenextraktpräparaten. *Deutsche Apotheker Zeitung*, 1985, 125(Suppl. I):14–19.
19. Redaelli C, Formentini L, Santaniello E. Reversed-phase high-performance liquid chromatography analysis of apigenin and its glucosides in flowers of *Matricaria chamomilla* and chamomille extracts. *Planta medica*, 1981, 42:288–292.
20. Carle R, Isaac O. Die Kamille—Wirkung and Wirksamkeit. *Zeitschrift für Phytotherapie*, 1987, 8:67–77.
21. Carle R, Gomaa K. Chamomile: a pharmacological and clinical profile. *Drugs of today*, 1992, 28:559–565.
22. Gould L, Reddy CVR, Gomprecht RF. Cardiac effect of chamomile tea. *Journal of clinical pharmacology*, 1973, 13:475–479.
23. Hormann HP, Korting HC. Evidence for the efficacy and safety of topical herbal drugs in dermatology. Part 1. Anti-inflammatory agents. *Phytomedicine*, 1994, 1:161–171.
24. Weiß RF. Kamille—"Heilpflanze 1987". *Kneipp-Blätter*, 1987, 1:4–8.
25. Thiemer VK, Stadler R, Isaac O. Biochemische Untersuchungen von Kamilleninhaltsstoffen. *Arzneimittel-Forschung*, 1972, 22:1086–1087.
26. Isaac O, Thiemer K. Biochemische Untersuchungen von Kamilleninhaltsstoffen. *Arzneimittel-Forschung*, 1975, 25:1086–1087.
27. Cinco M et al. A microbiological survey on the activity of a hydroalcoholic extract of chamomile. *International journal of crude drug research*, 1983, 21:145–151.
28. Aggag ME, Yousef RT. Study of antimicrobial activity of chamomile oil. *Planta medica*, 1972, 22:140–144.
29. Wagner H, Wierer M, Bauer R. *In vitro* inhibition of prostaglandin biosynthesis by essential oils and phenolic compounds. *Planta medica*, 1986:184–187.
30. Ammon HPT, Kaul R. Pharmakologie der Kamille und ihrer Inhaltsstoffe. *Deutsche Apotheker Zeitung*, 1992, 132(Suppl. 27):3–26.
31. Jakovlev V et al. Pharmacological investigations with compounds of chamomile. II. New investigations on the antiphlogistic effects of (−)-α-bisabolol and bisabolol oxides. *Planta medica*, 1979, 35:125–240.
32. Jakovlev V, Isaac O, Flaskamp E. Pharmakologische Untersuchungen von Kamilleninhaltsstoffen. VI. Untersuchungen zur antiphlogistischen Wirkung von Chamazulen und Matricin. *Planta medica*, 1983, 49:67–73.
33. Tubaro A et al. Evaluation of anti-inflammatory activity of chamomile extract after topical application. *Planta medica*, 1984, 51:359.
34. Della Loggia R. Lokale antiphlogistische Wirkung der Kamillen-Flavone. *Deutsche Apotheker Zeitung*, 1985, 125(Suppl. 1):9–11.
35. Della Loggia R et al. Evaluation of the anti-inflammatory activity of chamomile preparations. *Planta medica*, 1990, 56:657–658.

36. Lang W, Schwandt K. Untersuchung über die glykosidischen Bestandteile der Kamille. *Deutsche Apotheker Zeitung*, 1957, 97:149–151.
37. Mann C, Staba J. The chemistry, pharmacology, and commercial formulations of chamomile. In: Craker LE, Simon JE, eds., *Herbs, spices, and medicinal plants: recent advances in botany, horticulture and pharmacology*, Vol. I. Phoenix, AZ, Oryx Press, 1986:233–280.
38. Fuchs J, Milbradt R. Skin anti-inflammatory activity of apigenin-7-glucoside in rats. *Arzneimittel-Forschung*, 1993, 43:370–372.
39. Albring M et al. The measuring of the anti-inflammatory effect of a compound on the skin of volunteers. *Methods and findings in experimental and clinical pharmacology*, 1983, 5:75–77.
40. Della Loggia R et al. Depressive effects of *Chamomilla recutita* (L.) Rausch. tubular flowers, on central nervous system in mice. *Pharmacological research communications*, 1982, 14:153–162.
41. Glowania HJ, Raulin C, Svoboda M. The effect of chamomile on wound healing—a controlled clinical-experimental double-blind study. *Zeitschrift für Hautkrankheiten*, 1986, 62:1262–1271.
42. Aertgeerts P et al. Vergleichende Prüfung von Kamillosan® Creme gegenüber steroidalen (0.25% Hydrocortison, 0.75% Fluocortinbutylester) und nichtsteroidalen (5% Bufexamac) Externa in der Erhaltungstherapie von Ekzemerkrankungen. *Zeitschrift für Hautkrankheiten*, 1985, 60:270–277.
43. Carl W, Emrich LS. Management of oral mucositis during local radiation and systemic chemotherapy: a study of 98 patients. *Journal of prosthetic dentistry*, 1991, 66:361–369.
44. Rivera IG et al. Genotoxicity assessment through the Ames test of medicinal plants commonly used in Brazil. *Environmental toxicology and water quality*, 1994, 9:87–93.
45. Leslie GB, Salmon G. Repeated dose toxicity studies and reproductive studies on nine Bio-Strath herbal remedies. *Swiss medicine*, 1979, 1:1–3.
46. Dstychova E, Zahejsky J. Contact hypersensitivity to camomile. *Ceskoslovenska dermatologie*, 1992, 67:14–18.
47. Subiza J et al. Allergic conjunctivitis to chamomile tea. *Annals of allergy*, 1990, 65:127–132.
48. Paulsen E, Andersen KE, Hausen BM. Compositae dermatitis in a Danish dermatology department in one year. *Contact dermatitis*, 1993, 29:6–10.
49. Hausen BM, Busker E, Carle R. Über das Sensibilisierungsvermögen von Compositenarten. VII. Experimentelle Untersuchungen mit Auszügen und Inhaltsstoffen von *Chamomilla recutita* (L.) Rauschert und *Anthemis cotula* L. *Planta medica*, 1984:229–234.
50. Benner MH, Lee HJ. Anaphylactic reaction to chamomile tea. *Journal of allergy and clinical immunology*, 1973, 52:307–308.
51. Casterline CL. Allergy to chamomile tea. *Journal of the American Medical Association*, 1980, 244:330–331.
52. Subiza J et al. Anaphylactic reaction after the ingestion of chamomile tea: a study of cross-reactivity with other composite pollens. *Journal of allergy and clinical immunology*, 1989, 84:353–358.

Cortex Cinnamomi

Definition

Cortex Cinnamomi consists of the dried inner bark of the shoots grown on cut stock of *Cinnamomum verum* J.S. Presl. (*1–5*) or of the trunk bark, freed of cork, of *Cinnamomum cassia* Blume (*6–8*) (Lauraceae).

Synonyms

Cinnamomum verum J.S. Presl.

Cinnamomum zeylanicum Nees (*9–11*), *Laurus cinnamomum* L. (*4*).

Cinnamomum verum J.S. Presl. is the correct botanical name according to the International Rules of Botanical Nomenclature (*11*).

Cinnamomum cassia Blume

Cinnamomum aromaticum Nees (*7, 12, 13*).

Selected vernacular names

Cinnamomum verum J.S. Presl.

Abdalasini, blood-giving drops, canela, canela en raja, cannalavanga pattai, cannelle de ceylan, cannelle dite de Ceylan, cannelier, Ceylon celonzimi cinnamon, Ceylon cinnamon, cinnamon, cinnamon bark, cinnamon tree, cortex cinnamomi ceylanici, dalchini, dalochini, dar sini quirfa, darchini, daruchini, darusila, ecorce de cannelier de Ceylan, echter Kanel, gujerati-dalchini, kannel, kuei-pi, kurundu, kurundu-potu, kulit kayumanis, ob choei, tamalpatra, wild cinnamon, Zimtrinde (*2–4, 10, 14, 15*).

Cinnamomum cassia Blume

Annan cinnamon, cassia, cassia bark, cassia bark tree, cassia lignea, chinazimt, Chinese cassia, Chinese cinnamon, ching hua yu-kuei, cinnamomi cassiae cortex, cinnamon, cinnamon bark, dalchini, guipi, guizhi, kannan keihi, keihi, keishi, kuei-chíi, lavanga-pattai, lavanga-patti, lurundu, macrophyllos cassia bark tree, rou gui, róugì, Saigon cinnamon, saleekha, taj, toko keihi, Viet Nam cinnamon (*6, 7, 12–17*).

Description
Cinnamomum verum J.S. Presl.

A moderate-sized evergreen tree; bark rather thick, smooth, pale; twigs often compressed; young parts glabrous except the buds which are finely silky. Leaves opposite or subopposite (rarely alternate), hard and coriaceous, 7.5–20 by 3.8–7.5 cm, ovate or ovate-lanceolate, subacute or shortly acuminate, glabrous and shining above, slightly paler beneath, base acute or rounded; main nerves 3–5 from the base or nearly so, strong, with fine reticulate venation between; petioles 1.3–2.5 cm long, flattened above. Flowers numerous, in silky pubescent, lax panicles usually longer than the leaves; peduncles long, often clustered, glabrous or pubescent; pedicels long. Perianth 5–6 mm long; tube 2.5 mm long; segments pubescent on both sides, oblong or somewhat obovate, usually obtuse. Fruit 1.3–1.7 cm long, oblong or ovoid-oblong, minutely apiculate, dry or slightly fleshy, dark purple, surrounded by the enlarged campanulate perianth that is 8 mm in diameter (*14*).

Cinnamomum cassia Blume

An evergreen tree, up to 10 m high. Leaves alternate, coriaceous, petiolate, oblong, elliptical-oval or oblong-lanceolate, 8–15 cm long by 3–4 cm wide, tip acuminate, base rounded, entire, 3-nerved; glabrous or underside lightly pubescent; petiole 10 mm long, lightly pubescent. Inflorescence a densely hairy panicle as long as the leaves; panicles cymose, terminal and axillary. Flowers yellowish white, small, in cymes of 2–5. Perianth 6-lobed. No petals. Stamens 6, pubescent. Ovary free, 1-celled. Fruit a globular drupe, 8 mm long, red. The bark is used in either channelled pieces or simple quills, 30–40 cm long by 3–10 cm wide and 0.2–0.8 cm in thickness. The surface is greyish brown, slightly coarse, with irregularly fine wrinkles and transverse lenticels. Here and there are found scars of holes, indicating the insertion of leaves or lateral shoots; the inner surface is rather darker than the outer, with fine longitudinal striae. The fracture is short, the section of the thicker pieces showing a faint white line (pericyclic sclerenchyma) sometimes near the centre, sometimes near and parallel to the outer margin (*14*).

Plant material of interest: dried bark, free from the outer cork
General appearance
Cinnamomum verum J.S. Presl.

The bark is about 0.2–0.8 mm thick and occurs in closely packed compound quills made up of single or double quills. The outer surface is smooth, yellowish brown with faint scars marking the positions of leaves and axillary buds and has fine, whitish and wavy longitudinal striations. The inner surface is slightly darker and longitudinally striated. The fracture is short and fibrous (*1*).

Cinnamomum cassia **Blume**

The drug is channelled or quilted, 30–40 cm long, 3–10 cm in diameter, 2–8 mm thick. Outer surface greyish brown, slightly rough, with irregular fine wrinkles and transverse raised lenticels, some showing greyish white streaks; inner surface reddish brown, with fine longitudinal striations and exhibiting oily trace on scratching. Texture hard and fragile, easily broken, fracture uneven, outer layer brown and relatively rough, inner layer reddish brown and oily and showing a yellowish brown line between two layers (*6*).

Organoleptic properties

Odour, characteristic and aromatic (*2*, *3*, *4*, *6*); taste, characteristic, slightly sweet and fragrant (*3*, *4*, *6*).

Microscopic characteristics

Cinnamomum verum **J.S. Presl.**

The outside shows a few discontinuous layers of cortical parenchyma within which is a wide, continuous layer of pericyclic sclerenchyma composed of groups of isodiametric or tangentially elongated sclereids with thickened and pitted walls, and occasional groups of fibres. The phloem is composed of sieve tissue and parenchyma with large secretion cells containing essential oil or mucilage and phloem fibres occurring singly or in small groups, individual fibres 15–25 µm in diameter with thickened walls; medullary rays uniseriate or biseriate. Some of the cells contain small acicular crystals of calcium oxalate; the remainder, together with the phloem parenchyma, contain starch granules, simple or 2–4 compound, rarely more than 10 µm in diameter (*1*, *3*).

Cinnamomum cassia **Blume**

The transverse section shows the cork being composed of several layers of cells, the innermost layer with thickened and lignified outer walls. Cortex scattered with stone cells and secretory cells. Pericycle stone cells in groups arranged in an interrupted ring, accompanied by fibre bundles at outer side, the outer walls of stone cells usually thinner. Phloem rays 1 or 2 rows of cells wide, containing minute needle crystals of calcium oxalate; usually 2 or 3 fibres in bundles; oil cells scattered throughout. Parenchymatous cells contain starch granules (*6*).

Powdered plant material

Cinnamomum verum **J.S. Presl.**

The powdered drug is yellowish to reddish brown and consists of groups of rounded sclereids with pitted, channelled and moderately thickened walls; numerous colourless fibres, often whole with narrow lumen and thickened, lignified walls and few pits; rarely small acicular crystals of calcium oxalate; abundant starch granules. Cork fragments are absent or very rare (*1*, *3*).

Cinnamomum cassia Blume

Reddish brown. Most fibres singly scattered, long fusiform, 195–920 μm long, up to 50 μm in diameter, with thickened and lignified wall, pits indistinct. Stone cells subsquare or sub-rounded, 32–88 μm in diameter, the walls thickened, some thin at one side. Oil cells sub-rounded or oblong, 45–108 μm in diameter. Needle crystals minute, scattered in ray cells. Cork cells polygonal, containing reddish brown contents (1).

Geographical distribution

Cinnamomum verum J.S. Presl.

Native to India and Sri Lanka (4, 11, 14); cultivated in parts of Africa, south-eastern India, Indonesia, the Seychelles, South America, Sri Lanka, and the West Indies (4, 10, 11).

Cinnamomum cassia Blume

Found in China, Indonesia, the Lao People's Democratic Republic, and Viet Nam, (12, 13, 16); mostly cultivated (12).

General identity tests

Macroscopic and microscopic examinations (1–6); and thin-layer chromatographic analysis for the presence of cinnamaldehyde (1–6, 8).

Purity tests

Microbiology

The test for *Salmonella* spp. in Cortex Cinnamomi products should be negative. The maximum acceptable limits of other microorganisms are as follows (18–20). For preparation of decoction: aerobic bacteria—not more than 10^7/g; fungi—not more than 10^5/g; *Escherichia coli*—not more than 10^2/g. Preparations for internal use: aerobic bacteria—not more than 10^5/g or ml; fungi—not more than 10^4/g or ml; enterobacteria and certain Gram-negative bacteria—not more than 10^3/g or ml; *Escherichia coli*—0/g or ml.

Foreign organic matter

C. verum: not more than 2% (4, 14). C. cassia: not more than 1% (16).

Total ash

C. verum: not more than 6% (2). C. cassia: not more than 5% (6, 8, 14, 16).

Acid-insoluble ash

C. verum: not more than 4% (4). C. cassia: not more than 2% (14, 16).

Sulfated ash

C. verum: not more than 6% (*1*, *3*). *C. cassia*: to be established in accordance with national requirements.

Alcohol (90%)-soluble extractive

C. verum: 14–16% (*4*). *C. cassia*: to be established in accordance with national requirements.

Pesticide residues

To be established in accordance with national requirements. Normally, the maximum residue limit of aldrin and dieldrin for Cortex Cinnamomi is not more than 0.05 mg/kg (*21*). For other pesticides, see WHO guidelines on quality control methods for medicinal plants (*18*) and guidelines for predicting dietary intake of pesticide residues (*20*).

Arsenic and heavy metals

Recommended lead and cadmium levels are not more than 10 mg/kg and 0.3 mg/kg, respectively, in the final dosage form of the plant material (*18*).

Radioactive residues

For analysis of strontium-90, iodine-131, caesium-134, caesium-137, and plutonium-239, see WHO guidelines on quality control methods for medicinal plants (*18*).

Other tests

Chemical tests to be established in accordance with national requirements.

Chemical assays

Not less than 1.2% v/w of volatile oil derived from C. *verum* (*1–3*) and 1–2% v/w of volatile oil derived from C. *cassia* (*16*), containing 60–80% w/w aldehydes calculated as cinnamaldehyde (*3*, *16*).

Assay for cinnamaldehyde content by means of thin-layer (*1–4*, *6*) or high-performance liquid chromatographic (*21*, *22*) methods.

Major chemical constituents

The major constituent in both C. *verum* and C. *cassia* is cinnamaldehyde, at concentrations of 65–80% (*9*, *10*) and 90% (*9*) of the volatile oil, respectively.

cinnamaldehyde   eugenol   coumarin

Cinnamomum verum also contains *o*-methoxycinnamaldehyde (*10*). *Cinnamomum verum* differs from *C. cassia* in its eugenol and coumarin content. *Cinnamomum verum* volatile oil contains 10% eugenol, whereas in *C. cassia*, only a trace quantity of this compound is found (*9*). Coumarin is present in *C. cassia* (0.45%), but not in *C. verum* (*21*).

Dosage forms

Crude plant material, powder, volatile oil, other galenic preparations. Store in a well-closed glass or metal container (do not use plastic), protected from light and moisture (*1–6, 10*).

Medicinal uses

Uses supported by clinical data

None.

Uses described in pharmacopoeias and in traditional systems of medicine

The treatment of dyspeptic conditions such as mild spastic conditions of the gastrointestinal tract, fullness and flatulence, and loss of appetite (*4, 6, 7, 12*). Also used to treat abdominal pain with diarrhoea, and pain associated with amenorrhoea and dysmenorrhoea (*6, 12*).

Uses described in folk medicine, not supported by experimental or clinical data

The treatment of impotence, frigidity, dyspnoea, inflammation of the eye, leukorrhoea, vaginitis, rheumatism, neuralgia, wounds, and toothache (*15*).

Pharmacology

Experimental pharmacology

Antibacterial and antifungal activities of the essential oil have been demonstrated *in vitro* (*10*). The essential oil of *C. verum* is active *in vitro* against the following bacteria: *Bacillus subtilis* (*23, 24*), *Escherichia coli, Staphylococcus aureus* (*24, 25*), *Salmonella typhimurium* (*26*), and *Pseudomonas aeruginosa* (*24*). It was also active *in vitro* against the following fungi: *Aspergillus* spp., *Cladosporium werneckii* (*27*), *Geotrichum candidum, Kloeckera apivulata, Candida lipolytica* and *C. albicans* (*23, 28*). The antibacterial and fungicidal effects have been attributed to *o*-methoxycinnamaldehyde (*9*).

The essential oil of *C. verum* has carminative activity (*29*) and decreases smooth muscle contractions in guinea-pig trachea and ileum (*30*), and in dog ileum, colon and stomach (*31*). The active antispasmodic constituent of the drug is cinnamaldehyde. A reduction of stomach motility in rats and dogs and intestinal motility in mice and a decrease in the number of stress- and serotonin-induced ulcers in mice have been described (32–36). An ethanol extract of the drug inhibits histamine- and barium-induced contractions in guinea-pig ileum; the hot-water extract was not active (36).

Contraindications

The drug is contraindicated in cases of fever of unknown origin, pregnancy, stomach or duodenal ulcers (7, 9, 12), and in patients with an allergy to cinnamon or Peru balsam (9).

Warnings

No information available.

Precautions

Drug interactions

Cinnamomum cassia bark extract (2 g in 100 ml) markedly decreased the *in vitro* dissolution of tetracycline hydrochloride (37). In the presence of *C. cassia* bark, only 20% of tetracycline was in solution after 30 minutes, in contrast to 97% when only water was used (37). However, the clinical significance of this interaction has not been established. The drug is reported to be incompatible with *Halloysitum rubrum* (6).

Carcinogenesis, mutagenesis, impairment of fertility

There are insufficient data to evaluate the carcinogenic potential of Cortex Cinnamomi (35). Reports concerning the mutagenicity of the drug are contradictory. Extracts of the plant and cinnamaldehyde have been reported to be both mutagenic and non-mutagenic in *Salmonella typhimurium* (Ames assay) and in assays using *Bacillus subtilis* (38, 39). However, the results of these *in vitro* mutagenicity studies are difficult to assess because, at the doses given, the effects may have been due to the antimicrobial effects of the drug (35). Cortex Cinnamomi and cinnamaldehyde gave positive results in chromosomal aberration tests using Chinese hamster cell cultures (35), and in *Drosophila* test systems (40–43). An aqueous extract of the drug was also negative in the *Drosophila* test system (35).

Pregnancy: teratogenic effects

Available data are not sufficient for an adequate benefit/risk assessment. Therefore, Cortex Cinnamomi should not be used during pregnancy. There is one report of teratogenicity of cinnamaldehyde in chick embryos (35), but studies of teratogenicity in chick embryos are of limited usefulness when evaluating the teratogenic potential for humans (35). A methanol extract of the drug given by gastric intubation was not teratogenic in rats (44, 45).

Pregnancy: non-teratogenic effects

Cortex Cinnamomi should not be used during pregnancy. See Contra-indications.

Nursing mothers

Available data are not sufficient for an adequate benefit/risk assessment. There-fore, Cortex Cinnamomi should not be used during lactation.

Paediatric use

The safety and efficacy of the drug in children have not been established.

Other precautions

No information available concerning general precautions, or drug and labora-tory test interactions.

Adverse reactions

Allergic reactions of the skin and mucosa have been reported (7, 46–49).

Posology

Crude drug—average daily dose, 2–4 g (7); volatile oil—average daily dose, 0.05–0.2 g (7); other preparations—average daily dose as above (7).

References

1. *European pharmacopoeia*, 3rd ed. Strasbourg, Council of Europe, 1997.
2. *Pharmacopée française*. Paris, Adrapharm, 1996.
3. *British pharmacopoeia*. London, Her Majesty's Stationery Office, 1988.
4. *African pharmacopoeia*, 1st ed. Lagos, Organization of African Unity, Scientific, Tech-nical & Research Commission, 1985.
5. *Deutsches Arzneibuch 1996*. Stuttgart, Deutscher Apotheker Verlag, 1996.
6. *Pharmacopoeia of the People's Republic of China* (English ed.). Guangzhou, Guangdong Science and Technology Press, 1992.
7. German Commission E Monograph, Cinnamomi cassiae cortex. *Bundesanzeiger*, 1990, 22: 1 February.
8. *The pharmacopoeia of Japan XIII*. Tokyo, The Society of Japanese Pharmacopoeia, 1996.
9. Bisset NG. *Max Wichtl's herbal drugs & phytopharmaceuticals*. Boca Raton, FL, CRC Press, 1994:148–150.
10. Bruneton J. *Pharmacognosy, phytochemistry, medicinal plants*. Paris, Lavoisier, 1995:451–453.
11. Klostermans AJGH. Miscellaneous botanical notes. *Herbarium Bogoriense*, 1965:141–146.
12. *Medicinal plants in China*. Manila, World Health Organization, 1989:78–79 (WHO Regional Publications, Western Pacific Series, No. 2).
13. Keys JD. *Chinese herbs, their botany, chemistry and pharmacodynamics*. Rutland, VT, CE Tuttle, 1976:111.

14. Mukerji B. In: *The Indian Pharmaceutical Codex, Vol. I. Indigenous drugs*. New Delhi, Council of Scientific & Industrial Research, 1953:70–72.
15. Farnsworth NR, ed. *NAPRALERT database*. Chicago, University of Illinois at Chicago, IL, August 8, 1995 production (an on-line database available directly through the University of Illinois at Chicago or through the Scientific and Technical Network (STN) of Chemical Abstracts Services).
16. *British herbal pharmacopoeia, Part 2*. London, British Herbal Medicine Association, 1979:55–57.
17. Chang HM, But PPH, eds. *Pharmacology and applications of Chinese materia medica, Vol. 2*. Singapore, World Scientific Publishing, 1987:949–951.
18. *Quality control methods for medicinal plant materials*. Geneva, World Health Organization, 1998.
19. *Deutsches Arzneibuch 1996. Vol. 2. Methoden der Biologie*. Stuttgart, Deutscher Apotheker Verlag, 1996.
20. *Guidelines for predicting dietary intake of pesticide residues*, 2nd rev. ed. Geneva, World Health Organization, 1997 (unpublished document WHO/FSF/FOS/97.7; available from Food Safety, WHO, 1211 Geneva 27, Switzerland).
21. Archer AW. Determination of cinnamaldehyde, coumarin and cinnamyl alcohol in cinnamon and *Cassia* by high-performance liquid chromatography. *Journal of chromatography*, 1988, 447:272–276.
22. Sagara K et al. Determination of Cinnamomi Cortex by high-performance liquid chromatography. *Journal of chromatography*, 1987, 409:365–370.
23. Raharivelomanana PJ et al. Study of the antimicrobial action of various essential oil extracts from Madagascan plants. II. The Lauraceae. *Archives of the Institute of Pasteur Madagascar*, 1989, 56:261–271.
24. Janssen AM et al. Screening for antimicrobial activity of some essential oils by the agar overlay technique. *Pharmaceutisch Weekblad (Sci. ed.)*, 1986, 8:289–292.
25. George M, Pandalai KM. Investigations on plant antibiotics. Part IV. Further search for antibiotic substances in Indian medicinal plants. *Indian journal of medical research*, 1949, 37:169–181.
26. Sivaswamy SN et al. Mutagenic activity of south Indian food items. *Indian journal of experimental biology*, 1991, 29:730–737.
27. Morozumi S. A new antifungal agent in cinnamon. *Shinkin to shinkinsho*, 1978, 19:172–180.
28. Conner DE, Beuchat LR. Effects of essential oils from plants on growth of food spoilage yeasts. *Journal of food science*, 1984, 49:429–434.
29. Harries N, James KC, Pugh WK. Antifoaming and carminative actions of volatile oils. *Journal of clinical pharmacology*, 1978, 2:171–177.
30. Reiter M, Brandt W. Relaxant effects on tracheal and ileal smooth muscles of the guinea pig. *Arzneimittel-Forschung*, 1985, 35:408–414.
31. Plant OH, Miller GH. Effects of carminative volatile oils on the muscular activity of the stomach and colon. *Journal of pharmacology and experimental therapeutics*, 1926, 27:149.
32. Harada M, Yano S. Pharmacological studies on Chinese cinnamon. II. Effects of cinnamaldehyde on the cardiovascular and digestive systems. *Chemical and pharmaceutical bulletin*, 1975, 23:941–947.
33. Plant OH. Effects of carminative volatile oils on the muscular movements of the intestine. *Journal of pharmacology and experimental therapeutics*, 1921, 22:311–324.
34. Akira T, Tanaka S, Tabata M. Pharmacological studies on the antiulcerogenic activity of Chinese cinnamon. *Planta medica*, 1986, 52:440–443.
35. Keller K. *Cinnamomum* Species. In: DeSmet PAGM, Keller K, Hänsel R, Chandler RF, eds., *Adverse reactions of herbal drugs*. Berlin, Springer-Verlag, 1992:105–114.
36. Itokawa H et al. Studies on the constituents of crude drugs having inhibitory activity

against contraction of the ileum caused by histamine or barium chloride. Screening test for the activity of commercially available crude drugs and the related plant materials. *Shoyakugaku zasshi*, 1983, 37:223–228.

37. Miyazaki S, Inoue H, Nadai T. Effect of antacids on the dissolution behavior of tetracycline and methacycline. *Chemical and pharmaceutical bulletin*, 1977, 27:2523–2527.

38. Mahmoud I, Alkofahi A, Abdelaziz A. Mutagenic and toxic activities of several spices and some Jourdanian medicinal plants. *International journal of pharmacognosy*, 1992, 30:81–85.

39. Kasamaki A et al. Genotoxicity of flavouring agents. *Mutation research*, 1982, 105:387–392.

40. Ishidate M. Primary mutagenicity screening of food additives currently used in Japan. *Food chemistry and toxicology*, 1984, 22:623–636.

41. Venkatasetty R. Genetic variation induced by radiation and chemical agents in *Drosophila melanogaster*. *Dissertation abstracts international B*, 1972, 32:5047–5048.

42. Woodruff RC, Manson JM, Valencia R, Zimmering S. Chemical mutagenesis testing in *Drosophila*. Results of 53 coded compounds tested for the National Toxicology Program. *Environmental mutagenesis*, 1985, 7:677–702.

43. Abraham SK, Kesavan PC. A preliminary analysis of the genotoxicity of a few species in *Drosophila*. *Mutation research*, 1985, 143:219–224.

44. Abramovici A, Rachmuth-Roizman P. Molecular structure–teratogenicity relationships of some fragrance additives. *Toxicology*, 1983, 29:143–156.

45. Lee EB. Teratogenicity of the extracts of crude drugs. *Korean journal of pharmacognosy*, 1982, 13:116–121.

46. Nixon R. Vignette in contact dermatology. Cinnamon allergy in bakers. *Australian journal of dermatology*, 1995, 36:41.

47. Hausen BJM. *Allergiepflanzen-Pflanzenallergene*. Landsberg, Ecomed, 1988:95–96.

48. Calnan CD. Cinnamon dermatitis from an ointment. *Contact dermatitis*, 1976, 2:167–170.

49. Drake TE, Maibach HI. Allergic contact dermatitis and stomatitis caused by cinnamic aldehyde-flavored toothpaste. *Archives of dermatology*, 1976, 112:202–203.

Rhizoma Coptidis

Definition

Rhizoma Coptidis is the dried rhizome of *Coptis chinensis* Franch, *Coptis deltoides* C.Y. Cheng et Hsiao, *Coptis japonica* Makino (Ranunculaceae), or other berberine-containing species of the same genus (*1, 2*).

Synonyms

None.

Selected vernacular names

Coptis chinensis Franch

Chinese goldthread, ch'uan-lien, coptis, coptis rhizome, gold thread, huang lian, huang-lien, huánglián, oren, Perlenschnur, weilian (*1–6*).

Coptis deltoides C.Y. Cheng et Hsiao

Coptis, gold thread, huang lian, huang-lien, huánglián, yalian (*1, 4, 7*).

Coptis japonica Makino

Coptis, coptis rhizome, oren (*2, 5*).

Description

Coptis chinensis Franch

A perennial stemless herb, 20–50 cm high. Leaves basal, long petiolate; blade triangular-ovate, 3–8 cm long by 2.5–7 cm wide, ternatisect; leaflets pinnatifid, lobes incised, the terminal leaflet longer than the others. Peduncles 1–2, 12–25 cm long, bracts resembling leaves. Inflorescence a terminal cyme with 3–8 whitish green flowers; sepals narrow-ovate, 9–12 mm long; petals small, oblanceolate, 5–7 mm long; stamens numerous, 3–6 mm long; carpels 8–12, with carpophores, follicles many-seeded. Seeds with black crustaceous testa. Rhizome shaped like a cockspur, 5–6 cm long, brownish yellow, densely covered with numerous nodes and often with rootlets; interior yellow-orange; in transverse section, the central pith deeper in colour (*4*).

Coptis deltoides C.Y. Cheng et Hsiao and *Coptis japonica Makino*

Descriptions to be established by appropriate national authorities.

Plant material of interest: dried rhizome
General appearance
Coptis chinensis Franch

The rhizome is curved, gathered in a cluster and resembles "chicken feet", 3–6 cm long and 3–8 mm in diameter. Rough, greyish yellow or yellowish brown surface, bearing irregular protrusions, rootlets, and rootlet remnants. Apex often bearing remains of stem or petiole. Texture is hard and fracture uneven. Bark is orange-red or dark brown; wood brightly yellow or orange-yellow. Pith, sometimes hollowed (*1*).

Coptis deltoides C.Y. Cheng et Hsiao

Frequently single, somewhat cylindrical, slightly curved, 4–8 cm long and 0.5–1 cm in diameter. Internodes smooth and relatively long. Apex with some stem remains (*1*).

Coptis japonica Makino

Irregular, cylindrical rhizome, 2–4 cm, rarely up to 10 cm in length, 0.2–0.7 cm in diameter, slightly curved and often branched; externally greyish yellow-brown, with ring nodes, and with numerous remains of rootlets; generally remains of petiole at one end; fractured surface rather fibrous; cork layer light greyish brown, cortex yellow-brown, xylem yellow, and pith yellow-brown in colour (*2*).

Organoleptic properties
Odour, slight; taste, very bitter; colour, greyish yellow to yellowish brown, drug when chewed colours saliva yellow (*1, 2*).

Microscopic characteristics
Coptis chinensis Franch

In transverse section cork cells occupy several layers. Cortex broader than others; stone cells singly or grouped together; pericycle fibres yellow, in bundles or accompanied by stone cells; collateral vascular bundles arranged in a ring. Interfascicular cambium indistinct. Xylem yellow, lignified with well developed fibres. Pith consisting of parenchyma cells and devoid of stone cells (*1*).

Coptis deltoides C.Y. Cheng et Hsiao

Transverse section shows pith with stone cells (*1*).

Coptis japonica Makino

Transverse section reveals a cork layer composed of thin-walled cork cells; cortex parenchyma usually contains groups of stone cells near the cork layer and yellow phloem fibres near the cambium; xylem consists chiefly of vessels, tracheae and wood fibres; medullary ray distinct; pith large; in pith, stone cells or sometimes stone cells with thick and lignified cells are recognized; parenchyma cells contain minute starch grains (2).

Powdered plant material
Coptis japonica Makino

Almost all elements are yellow. The powder shows mainly fragments of vessels, tracheids, and xylem fibres; parenchyma cells containing starch grains; polygonal cork cells. Usually, round to obtuse polygonal stone cells and their groups, and phloem fibres, 10–20 µm in diameter, and fragments of their bundles. Occasionally, polygonal and elongated epidermal cells, originating from the petiole, having characteristic thickened membranes. Starch grains are single grains 1–7 µm in diameter (2).

Coptis chinensis Franch and *Coptis deltoides* C.Y. Cheng et Hsiao

Descriptions to be established by appropriate national authorities.

Geographical distribution
Coptis chinensis Franch. and *Coptis deltoides* C.Y. Cheng et Hsiao

China (3, 4).

Coptis japonica Makino

Japan (2).

Coptis teeta Wall.

Indigenous in India, where it is considered an endangered species (7). *Coptis teeta* Wall. has compendial status in China (1), where it is cultivated commercially (2).

General identity tests

Macroscopic, microscopic, and microchemical examinations; thin-layer chromatographic analysis for the presence of berberine (1, 2).

Purity tests

Microbiological

The test for *Salmonella* spp. in Rhizoma Coptidis products should be negative. The maximum acceptable limits of other microorganisms are as follows (8–10). For preparation of decoction: aerobic bacteria—not more than 10^7/g; fungi—not more than 10^5/g; *Escherichia coli*—not more than 10^2/g. Preparations for internal use: aerobic bacteria—not more than 10^5/g or ml; fungi—not more than 10^4/g or ml; enterobacteria and certain Gram-negative bacteria—not more than 10^3/g or ml; *Escherichia coli*—0/g or ml.

Total ash

Not more than 5.0% (1, 2).

Pesticide residues

To be established in accordance with national requirements. Normally, the maximum residue limit of aldrin and dieldrin for Rhizoma Coptidis is not more than 0.05 mg/kg (10). For other pesticides, see WHO guidelines on quality control methods for medicinal plants (8) and guidelines for predicting dietary intake of pesticide residues (11).

Heavy metals

Recommended lead and cadmium levels are no more than 10 and 0.3 mg/kg, respectively, in the final dosage form of the plant material (8).

Radioactive residues

For analysis of strontium-90, iodine-131, caesium-134, caesium-137, and plutonium-239, see WHO guidelines on quality control methods for medicinal plants (8).

Other purity tests

Chemical tests and tests for acid-insoluble ash, dilute ethanol-soluble extractive, foreign organic matter, moisture and water-soluble extractive are to be established in accordance with national requirements.

Chemical assays

Should contain not less than 4.2% of berberine, calculated as berberine chloride, assayed by means of thin-layer chromatography or high-performance liquid chromatography (2).

Major chemical constituents

The major constituents are berberine and related protoberberine alkaloids (3, 8, 10). Berberine occurs in the range of 4–8% (*C. chinensis*: 5–7%; *C. deltoides*: 4–

berberine

8%; *C. japonica*: 7–9%), followed by palmatine (*C. chinensis*: 1–4%; *C. deltoides*: 1–3%; *C. japonica*: 0.4–0.6%), coptisine (*C. chinensis*: 0.8–2%; *C. deltoides*: 0.8–1%; *C. japonica*: 0.4–0.6%), berberastine (*C. chinensis*: 1%; *C. deltoides*: 1%; *C. japonica*: trace) among others (*12*).

Dosage forms
Crude plant material, decoction, and powder. Store in a well-ventilated dry environment protected from light (*1*).

Medicinal uses
Uses supported by clinical data
None.

Uses described in pharmacopoeias and in traditional systems of medicine
To manage bacterial diarrhoeas (*1*, *4*). The drug is also used in the treatment of acute conjunctivitis, gastroenteritis, boils, and cutaneous and visceral leish-maniasis ("oriental sore") (*1*, *4*, *13*, *14*).

Uses described in folk medicine, not supported by experimental or clinical data
Treatment of arthritis, burns, diabetes, dysmenorrhoea, toothache, malaria, gout, and renal disease (*13*).

Pharmacology
Experimental pharmacology
Numerous reports support the antimicrobial activity of Rhizoma Coptidis. *In vitro* studies have shown that the crude drug and its active constituent, berberine, have a similar spectrum of antibacterial action (*3*, *15*). Both inhibit the *in vitro* growth of staphylococci, streptococci, pneumococci, *Vibrio cholerae*, *Bacillus anthracis*, and *Bacillus dysenteriae*, but they do not inhibit *Escherichia coli*, *Proteus vulgaris*, *Salmonella typhi*, *S. paratyphi*, *Pseudomonas aeruginosa*, and *Shigella sonnei* (*3*). Berberine was also active *in vitro* against *Entamoeba histolytica*, *Giardia lamblia*, and *Trichomonas vaginalis* (*16*).

In vitro studies have demonstrated that *V. cholerae* can grow in a medium containing berberine, but it fails to produce toxins (*17*). It has been hypothesized that the antidysenteric activity of berberine is due to local effects on the intestinal tract and not due to its bactericidal activity. The mechanism by which berberine exerts its antidiarrhoeal effects is thought to be activation of α_2-adrenoceptors and inhibition of cyclic AMP accumulation (*18*), which in turn decrease intestinal motility (*19*). However, *in vitro* studies of the drug on guinea-pig ileum contractility have demonstrated that berberine ($\geq 1\,\mu$mol/l) inhibits acetylcholinesterase, which decreases the breakdown of acetylcholine and increases the contractility of the ileum (*20*). This study suggests that the antidiarrhoeal activity of berberine may be due to its antisecretory (*21*) as well as its antimicrobial actions (*20*). Berberine inhibits *in vivo* and *in vitro* intestinal secretions induced by cholera toxin (*22–24*). In addition, berberine reduces intestinal secretion induced by the heat-labile toxin of *Escherichia coli* in rabbit ileal loop by 70% and it markedly inhibits the secretory response of the heat-stable toxin of *E. coli* in rats (*25, 26*).

Intragastric administration of berberine to mice produces hypoglycaemic effects with doses of 50–100 mg/kg (*27–29*).

Local injection of berberine into lesions caused by *Leishmania braziliensis panamensis* in hamsters reduced lesion size by approximately 50% (*30*).

Clinical pharmacology

Despite the large number of published clinical studies, only two have examined the effect of berberine in comparison with a positive control, such as tetracycline, on fluid loss caused by diarrhoea in patients with cholera or in non-cholera diarrhoea (*14, 31–33*). In the first study, berberine chloride 100 mg was administered orally four times daily. The alkaloid did not have any significant vibriostatic effect; instead it only slightly reduced stool volume, and possibly reduced the vibriostatic effect of tetracycline (*32*). Berberine or tetracycline was no better than a placebo in patients with non-cholera diarrhoea of unspecified etiologies (*32*). A randomized controlled trial of 165 patients utilized a 400 mg single-bolus dose of berberine sulfate for enterotoxigenic *Escherichia coli*-induced diarrhoea and either 400 mg as a single oral dose or 1200 mg of berberine sulfate (400 mg every 8 hours) for the treatment of cholera (*33*). Berberine significantly reduced stool volume during enterotoxigenic *E. coli* (ETEC) diarrhoea regardless of strain and had a slight antisecretory activity in patients with cholera. No adverse effects were observed in the patients receiving berberine. The results of this study indicated that berberine was an effective and safe antisecretory drug for ETEC diarrhoea, but that it had only a modest antisecretory effect in cholera patients, where the activity of tetracycline alone was superior (*33*).

Berberine has been used therapeutically in the treatment of cutaneous leishmaniasis ("oriental sore") by direct injection of the drug into local lesions.

In humans, injection of a preparation containing 2% berberine into lesions caused by *Leishmania tropica* was an effective treatment (34–36).

Contraindications

The safety of berberine or extracts of Rhizoma Coptidis in pregnancy has not been established (14). Therefore, until such data are available the use of berberine during pregnancy is contraindicated.

Warnings

No information available.

Precautions

Carcinogenesis, mutagenesis, impairment of fertility

The safety of berberine or extracts of Rhizoma Coptidis has not been established with respect to fertility (14). There are conflicting reports as to the mutagenicity of Rhizoma Coptidis and berberine (37–43).

Pregnancy: non-teratogenic effects

The safety of berberine or extracts of Rhizoma Coptidis has not been established with respect to pregnancy. See Contraindications, above.

Nursing mothers

Excretion of berberine or Rhizoma Coptidis into breast milk, and its effects on the newborn have not been established; therefore, use of the herb during lactation is not recommended.

Paediatric use

The safety and efficacy of Rhizoma Coptidis or berberine in children have not been established.

Other precautions

No information available concerning general precautions, drug interactions, drug and laboratory test interactions, or teratogenic effects on pregnancy.

Adverse reactions

Berberine was reported to be well tolerated in therapeutic doses of 500 mg, and no serious intoxication was reported in humans (44). One report of nausea, vomiting, enterocinetic sound, abdominal distortion, diarrhoea, polyuria, and erythropenia after administration of oral Rhizoma Coptidis to human adults (*45*) does not state the dosage used. No systematic studies have assessed organ function during acute or chronic administration of berberine salts or extracts of Rhizoma Coptidis (*14*).

Posology

Maximum daily oral dosage of crude plant material: 1.5–6 g (*1, 3*).

References

1. *Pharmacopoeia of the People's Republic of China* (English ed.). Guangzhou, Guangdong Science and Technology Press, 1992.
2. *The pharmacopoeia of Japan XII*. Tokyo, The Society of Japanese Pharmacopoeia, 1991.
3. Chang HM, But PPH, eds. *Pharmacology and applications of Chinese materia medica*, Vol. 2. Singapore, World Scientific Publishing, 1987.
4. *Medicinal plants in China*. Manila, World Health Organization, 1989 (WHO Regional Publications, Western Pacific Series, No. 2).
5. Hsu HY. *Oriental materia medica, a concise guide*. Long Beach, CA, Oriental Healing Arts Institute, 1986.
6. Farnsworth NR, ed. *NAPRALERT database*. Chicago, University of Illinois at Chicago, IL, March 15, 1995 production (an on-line database available directly through the University of Illinois at Chicago or through the Scientific and Technical Network (STN) of Chemical Abstracts Services).
7. Pandit MK, Babu CR. Cytology and taxonomy of *Coptis teeta* Wall. (Ranunculaceae). *Botanical journal of the Linnean Society*, 1993, 111:371–378.
8. *Quality control methods for medicinal plant materials*. Geneva, World Health Organization, 1998.
9. *Deutsches Arzneibuch 1996. Vol. 2. Methoden der Biologie*. Stuttgart, Deutscher Apotheker Verlag, 1996.
10. *European pharmacopoeia*, 3rd ed. Strasbourg, Council of Europe, 1997.
11. *Guidelines for predicting dietary intake of pesticide residues*, 2nd rev. ed. Geneva, World Health Organization, 1997 (unpublished document WHO/FSF/FOS/97.7; available from Food Safety, WHO, 1211 Geneva 27, Switzerland).
12. Ikuta A, Kobayashi A, Itokawa H. Studies on the quantitative analysis of protoberberine alkaloids in Japanese, Chinese and other countries *Coptis* rhizomes by thin-layer chromatography-densitometry. *Shoyakugaku zasshi*, 1984, 38:279–282.
13. Bruneton J. *Pharmacognosy, phytochemistry, medicinal plants*. Paris, Lavoisier, 1995.
14. Lampe KF, Berberine. In: De Smet PAGM et al., eds. *Adverse effects of herbal drugs*, Vol. 1. Berlin, Springer-Verlag, 1992:97–104.
15. Simeon S, Rios JL, Villar A. Pharmacological activities of protoberberine alkaloids. *Plantes médicinales et phytothérapie*, 1989, 23:202–250.
16. Kaneda Y et al. *In vitro* effects of berberine sulfate on the growth and structure of *Entamoeba histolytica, Giardia lamblia,* and *Trichomonas vaginalis. Annals of tropical medicine and parasitology*, 1991, 85:417–425.
17. Hah FE, Ciak J. Berberine. *Antibiotics*, 1975, 3:577.
18. Uebaba K et al. Adenylate cyclase inhibitory activity of berberine. *Japanese journal of pharmacology*, 1984, 36(Suppl. 1):352.

19. Hui KK et al. Interaction of berberine with human platelet alpha-2 adrenoceptors. *Life sciences*, 1989, 49:315–324.
20. Shin DH et al. A paradoxical stimulatory effect of berberine on guinea-pig ileum contractility: possible involvement of acetylcholine release from the postganglionic parasympathetic nerve and cholinesterase inhibition. *Life sciences*, 1993, 53:1495–1500.
21. Sack RB, Froehlich JL. Berberine inhibits intestinal secretory response of *Vibrio cholerae* and *Escherichia coli* enterotoxins. *Infection and immunity*, 1989, 35:471–475.
22. Gaitonde BB, Marker PH, Rao NR. Effect of drugs on cholera toxin induced fluid in adult rabbit ileal loop. *Progress in drug research*, 1975, 19:519–526.
23. Sabir M, Akhter MH, Bhide NK. Antagonism of cholera toxin by berberine in the gastrointestinal tract of adult rats. *Indian journal of medical research*, 1977, 65:305–313.
24. Swabb EA, Tai YH, Jordan L. Reversal of cholera toxin-induced secretion in rat ileum by luminal berberine. *American journal of physiology*, 1981, 241:G248–G252.
25. Tai YH et al. Antisecretory effects of berberine in rat ileum. *American journal of physiology*, 1981, 241:G253–G258.
26. Guandalini S et al. Berberine effects on ion transport in rabbit ileum. *Pediatric research*, 1983, 17:423.
27. Shen ZF, Xie MZ. Determination of berberine in biological specimens by high performance TLC and fluoro-densitometric method. *Yao hsueh hsueh pao*, 1993, 28:532–536.
28. Chen QM, Xie MZ. Studies on the hypoglycemic effect of *Coptis chinensis* and berberine. *Yao hsueh hsueh pao*, 1986, 21:401–406.
29. Chen QM, Xie MZ. Effect of berberine on blood glucose regulation of normal mice. *Yao hsueh hsueh pao*, 1987, 22:161–165.
30. Vennerstrom JL et al. Berberine derivatives as antileishmanial drugs. *Antimicrobial agents and chemotherapy*, 1990, 34:918–921.
31. Lahiri SC, Dutta NK. Berberine and chloramphenicol in the treatment of cholera and severe diarrhea. *Journal of the Indian Medical Association*, 1967, 48:1–11.
32. Khin-Maung U et al. Clinical trial of berberine in acute watery diarrhoea. *British medical journal*, 1986, 291:1601–1605.
33. Rabbani GH et al. Randomized controlled trial of berberine sulfate therapy for diarrhea due to enterotoxigenic *Escherichia coli* and *Vibrio cholerae*. *Journal of infectious diseases*, 1987, 155:979–984.
34. Devi AL. Berberine sulfate in oriental sore. *Indian medical gazette*, 1929, 64:139.
35. Das Gupta BM. The treatment of oriental sore with berberine acid sulfate. *Indian medical gazette*, 1930, 65:683.
36. Das Gupta BM, Dikshit BB. Berberine in the treatment of Oriental boil. *Indian medical gazette*, 1929, 67:70.
37. Lee HK et al. Effect of bacterial growth-inhibiting ingredients on the Ames mutagenicity of medicinal herbs. *Mutation research*, 1987, 192:99–104.
38. Pasqual MS et al. Genotoxicity of the isoquinoline alkaloid berberine in prokaryotic and eukaryotic organisms. *Mutation research*, 1993, 286:243–252.
39. Faddejeva MD et al. Possible intercalative bindings of alkaloids sanguinarine and berberine to DNA. *IRCS medical science and biochemistry*, 1980, 8:612.
40. Nozaka T et al. Mutagenicity of isoquinoline alkaloids, especially the aporphine type. *Mutation research*, 1990, 240:267–279.
41. Morimoto I et al. Mutagenicity screening of crude drugs with *Bacillus subtilis* Rec-assay and *Salmonella*/microsome reversion assay. *Mutation research*, 1982, 97:81–102.
42. Yamamoto K, Mizutani T, Nomura H. Studies on the mutagenicity of crude drug extracts. I. *Yakugaku zasshi*, 1982, 102:596–601.
43. Watanabe F et al. Mutagenicity screening of hot water extracts from crude drugs. *Shoyakugaku zasshi*, 1983, 37:237–240.

44. Roth L, Daunderer M, Kormann K. *Giftpflanzen. Pflanzengifte*, 3rd ed. Landsberg, Ecomed, 1988:145–146, 810.
45. Bao Y. Side effects of *Coptis chinensis* and berberine. *Chinese journal of integrated and traditional western medicine*, 1983, 3:12–13.

Rhizoma Curcumae Longae

Definition

Rhizoma Curcumae Longae is the dried rhizome of *Curcuma longa* L. (Zingiberaceae) (*1*).

Dried rhizomes of *Curcuma wenyujin* Y.H. Lee et C. Ling, *C. kwangsiensis* S. Lee et C.F. Liang. and *C. phaeocaulis* Val. are also official sources of Radix Curcumae or Turmeric Root-Tuber in China (*2*).

Synonyms

Curcuma domestica Valeton., *C. rotunda* L., *C. xanthorrhiza* Naves, *Amomum curcuma* Jacq. (*3–5*).

Selected vernacular names

Acafrao, arqussofar, asabi-e-safr, avea, cago rerega, chiang-huang, common tumeric, curcum, curcuma, dilau, dilaw, Gelbwurzel, gezo, goeratji, haladi, haldi, haldu, haku halu, hardi, haridra, huang chiang, hsanwen, hurid, Indian saffron, jiânghuang, kaha, kakoenji, kalo haledo, khamin chan, khaminchan, kilunga kuku, kitambwe, kiko eea, koening, koenit, koenjet, kondin, kooneit, kunyit, kurcum, kurkum, Kurkumawurzelstock, luyang dilaw, mandano, manjano, manjal, nghe, nisha, oendre, pasupu, rajani, rame, renga, rhizome de curcuma, saffran vert, safran, safran des indes, skyer-rtsa, tumeric, tumeric root, tumeric rhizome, turmeric, ukon, ul gum, wong keong, wong keung, yellow root, yii-chin, zardchob (*1–3, 6–14*).

Description

Perennial herb up to 1.0 m in height; stout, fleshy, main rhizome nearly ovoid (about 3 cm in diameter and 4 cm long). Lateral rhizome, slightly bent (1 cm × 2–6 cm), flesh orange in colour; large leaves lanceolate, uniformly green, up to 50 cm long and 7–25 cm wide; apex acute and caudate with tapering base, petiole and sheath sparsely to densely pubescent. Spike, apical, cylindrical, 10–15 cm long and 5–7 cm in diameter. Bract white or white with light green upper half, 5–6 cm long, each subtending flowers, bracteoles up to 3.5 cm long. Pale yellow flowers about 5 cm long; calyx tubular, unilaterally split, unequally toothed; corolla white, tube funnel shaped, limb 3-lobed. Stamens lateral, petaloid, widely elliptical, longer than the anther; filament united to anther

115

about the middle of the pollen sac, spurred at base. Ovary trilocular; style glabrous. Capsule ellipsoid. Rhizomes orange within (*1, 4, 6, 15*).

Plant material of interest: dried rhizome
General appearance
The primary rhizome is ovate, oblong or pear-shaped round turmeric, while the secondary rhizome is often short-branched long turmeric; the round form is about half as broad as long; the long form is from 2–5 cm long and 1–1.8 cm thick; externally yellowish to yellowish brown, with root scars and annulations, the latter from the scars of leaf bases; fracture horny; internally orange-yellow to orange; waxy, showing a cortex separated from a central cylinder by a distinct endodermis (*1, 9, 13*).

Organoleptic properties
Odour, aromatic; taste, warmly aromatic and bitter (*1, 9, 13*). Drug when chewed colours the saliva yellow (*9*).

Microscopic characteristics
The transverse section of the rhizome is characterized by the presence of mostly thin-walled rounded parenchyma cells, scattered vascular bundles, definite endodermis, a few layers of cork developed under the epidermis and scattered oleoresin cells with brownish contents. The cells of the ground tissue are also filled with many starch grains. Epidermis is thin walled, consisting of cubical cells of various dimensions. The cork cambium is developed from the subepidermal layers and even after the development of the cork, the epidermis is retained. Cork is generally composed of 4–6 layers of thin-walled brick-shaped parenchymatous cells. The parenchyma of the pith and cortex contains curcumin and is filled with starch grains. Cortical vascular bundles are scattered and are of collateral type. The vascular bundles in the pith region are mostly scattered and they form discontinuous rings just under the endodermis. The vessels have mainly spiral thickening and only a few have reticulate and annular structure (*1, 8, 9*).

Powdered plant material
Coloured deep yellow. Fragments of parenchymatous cells contain numerous altered, pasty masses of starch grains coloured yellow by curcumin, fragments of vessels; cork fragments of cells in sectional view; scattered unicellular trichomes; abundant starch grains; fragments of epidermal and cork cells in surface view; and scattered oil droplets, rarely seen (*1, 13*).

Geographical distribution
Cambodia, China, India, Indonesia, Lao People's Democratic Republic, Madagascar, Malaysia, the Philippines, and Viet Nam (*1, 13, 16*). It is exten-

sively cultivated in China, India, Indonesia, Thailand and throughout the tropics, including tropical regions of Africa (*1, 7, 13, 16*).

General identity tests

Macroscopic and microscopic examinations; test for the presence of curcuminoids by colorimetric and thin-layer chromatographic methods (*1*).

Purity tests

Microbiology

The test for *Salmonella* spp. in Rhizoma Curcumae Longae products should be negative. The maximum acceptable limits of other microorganisms are as follows (*17–19*). For preparation of decoction: aerobic bacteria—not more than 10^7/g; fungi—not more than 10^5/g; *Escherichia coli*—not more than 10^2/g. Preparations for internal use: aerobic bacteria—not more than 10^5/g or ml; fungi—not more than 10^4/g or ml; enterobacteria and certain Gram-negative bacteria—not more than 10^3/g or ml; *Escherichia coli*—0/g or ml.

Foreign organic matter

Not more than 2% (*1, 9*).

Total ash

Not more than 8.0% (*1, 15*).

Acid-insoluble ash

Not more than 1% (*1, 9, 15*).

Water-soluble extractive

Not less than 9.0% (*1*).

Alcohol-soluble extractive

Not less than 10% (*1*).

Moisture

Not more than 10% (*1*).

Pesticide residues

To be established in accordance with national requirements. Normally, the maximum residue limit of aldrin and dieldrin in Rhizoma Curcumae Longae is not more than 0.05 mg/kg (*19*). For other pesticides, see WHO guidelines on quality control methods for medicinal plants (*17*) and guidelines for predicting dietary intake of pesticide residues (*20*).

Heavy metals

Recommended lead and cadmium levels are not more than 10 and 0.3 mg/kg, respectively, in the final dosage form of the plant material (*17*).

Radioactive residues

For analysis of strontium-90, iodine-131, caesium-134, caesium-137, and plutonium-239, see WHO guidelines on quality control methods for medicinal plants (*17*).

Other purity tests

Chemical tests to be established in accordance with national requirements.

Chemical assays

Not less than 4.0% of volatile oil, and not less than 3.0% of curcuminoids (*1*). Qualitative analysis by thin-layer and high-performance liquid chromatography (*1, 21*) and quantitative assay for total curcuminoids by spectrophotometric (*1, 22*) or by high-performance liquid chromatographic methods (*23, 24*).

Major chemical constituents

Pale yellow to orange-yellow volatile oil (6%) composed of a number of monoterpenes and sesquiterpenes, including zingiberene, curcumene, α- and β-turmerone among others. The colouring principles (5%) are curcuminoids, 50–60% of which are a mixture of curcumin, monodesmethoxycurcumin and bisdesmethoxycurcumin (*1, 6, 25*). Representative structures of curcuminoids are presented below.

α-turmerone β-turmerone ar-turmerone zingiberene

curcumin   R = OCH₃, R' = OCH₃
desmethoxycurcumin R = OCH₃, R' = H
bisdesmethoxycurcumin R = H, R' = H

Dosage forms

Powdered crude plant material, rhizomes (*1, 2*), and corresponding preparations (*25*). Store in a dry environment protected from light. Air dry the crude drug every 2–3 months (*1*).

Medicinal uses
Uses supported by clinical data
The principal use of Rhizoma Curcumae Longae is for the treatment of acid, flatulent, or atonic dyspepsia (*26–28*).

Uses described in pharmacopoeias and in traditional systems of medicine
Treatment of peptic ulcers, and pain and inflammation due to rheumatoid arthritis (*2, 11, 14, 29, 30*) and of amenorrhoea, dysmenorrhoea, diarrhoea, epilepsy, pain, and skin diseases (*2, 3, 16*).

Uses described in folk medicine, not supported by experimental or clinical data
The treatment of asthma, boils, bruises, coughs, dizziness, epilepsy, haemorrhages, insect bites, jaundice, ringworm, urinary calculi, and slow lactation (*3, 7, 8–10, 14*).

Pharmacology
Experimental pharmacology
Anti-inflammatory activity
The anti-inflammatory activity of Rhizoma Curcumae Longae has been demonstrated in animal models (*3, 30–32*). Intraperitoneal administration of the drug in rats effectively reduced both acute and chronic inflammation in carrageenin-induced paw oedema, the granuloma pouch test, and the cotton pellet granuloma test (*32, 33*). The effectiveness of the drug in rats was reported to be similar to that of hydrocortisone acetate or indometacin in experimentally induced inflammation (*31, 32*). Oral administration of turmeric juice or powder did not produce an anti-inflammatory effect; only intraperitoneal injection was effective (*33*). The volatile oil has exhibited anti-inflammatory activity in rats against adjuvant-induced arthritis, carrageenin-induced paw oedema, and hyaluronidase-induced inflammation (*32*). The anti-inflammatory activity appears to be mediated through the inhibition of the enzymes trypsin and hyaluronidase (*33*). Curcumin and its derivatives are the active anti-inflammatory constituents of the drug (*34–40*). After intraperitoneal administration, curcumin and sodium curcuminate exhibited strong anti-inflammatory activity in the carrageenin-induced oedema test in rats and mice (*41*). Curcumin was also found to be effective after oral administration in the acute carrageenin-induced oedema test in mice and rats (*41*). The anti-inflammatory activity of curcumin may be due to its ability to scavenge oxygen radicals, which have been implicated in the inflammation process (*42*). Furthermore, intraperitoneal injection of a polysaccharide fraction, isolated from the drug, increased phagocytosis capacity in mice in the clearance of colloidal carbon test (*43*).

Activity against peptic ulcer and dyspepsia

Oral administration to rabbits of water or methanol extracts of the drug significantly decreased gastric secretion (44) and increased the mucin contents of gastric juice (45). Intragastric administration of an ethanol extract of the drug to rats effectively inhibited gastric secretion and protected the gastroduodenal mucosa against injuries caused by pyloric ligation, hypothermic-restraint stress, indometacin, reserpine, and mercaptamine administration, and cytodestructive agents such as 80% methanol, 0.6 mol/l hydrochloric acid, 0.2 mol/l sodium hydroxide and 25% sodium chloride (30, 46). The drug stimulated the production of gastric wall mucus, and it restored non-protein sulfides in rats (46, 47). Curcumin, one of the anti-inflammatory constituents of the drug, has been shown to prevent and ameliorate experimentally induced gastric lesions in animal models by stimulation of mucin production (48). However, there are conflicting reports regarding the protective action of curcumin against histamine-induced gastric ulceration in guinea-pigs (41). Moreover, both intraperitoneal and oral administration of curcumin (100 mg/kg) have been reported to induce gastric ulceration in rats (41, 49–51).

Non-specific inhibition of smooth muscle contractions in isolated guinea-pig ileum by sodium curcuminate has been reported (41).

The effect of curcumin on intestinal gas formation has been demonstrated *in vitro* and *in vivo*. Addition of curcumin to *Clostridium perfringens* of intestinal origin *in vitro* and to a chickpea flour diet fed to rats led to a gradual reduction in gas formation (41).

Both the essential oil and sodium curcuminate increase bile secretion after intravenous administration to dogs (41). In addition, gall-bladder muscles were stimulated (39).

Clinical pharmacology

Oral administration of the drug to 116 patients with acid dyspepsia, flatulent dyspepsia, or atonic dyspepsia in a randomized, double-blind study resulted in a statistically significant response in the patients receiving the drug (27). The patients received 500 mg of the powdered drug four times daily for 7 days (27). Two other clinical trials which measured the effect of the drug on peptic ulcers showed that oral administration of the drug promoted ulcer healing and decreased the abdominal pain involved (28, 29).

Two clinical studies have shown that curcumin is an effective anti-inflammatory drug (52, 53). A short-term (2 weeks) double-blind, crossover study of 18 patients with rheumatoid arthritis showed that patients receiving either curcumin (1200 mg/day) or phenylbutazone (30 mg/day) had significant improvement in morning stiffness, walking time and joint swelling (52). In the second study, the effectiveness of curcumin and phenylbutazone on postoperative inflammation was investigated in a double-blind study (53). Both drugs produced a better anti-inflammatory response than a placebo (53), but the degree of inflammation in the patients varied greatly and was not evenly distributed among the three groups.

Contraindications

Obstruction of the biliary tract. In cases of gallstones, use only after consultation with a physician (26). Hypersensitivity to the drug.

Warnings

No information available.

Precautions

Carcinogenesis, mutagenesis, impairment of fertility

Rhizoma Curcumae Longae is not mutagenic *in vitro* (54–56).

Pregnancy: teratogenic effects

Orally administered Rhizoma Curcumae Longae was not tetratogenic in mice or rats (34, 57, 58).

Pregnancy: non-teratogenic effects

The safety of Rhizoma Curcumae Longae during pregnancy has not been established. As a precautionary measure the drug should not be used during pregnancy except on medical advice (59).

Nursing mothers

Excretion of the drug into breast milk and its effects on the newborn have not been established. Until such data are available, the drug should not be used during lactation except on medical advice.

Paediatric use

The safety and effectiveness of the drug in children has not been established.

Other precautions

No information on drug interactions or drug and laboratory test interactions was found.

Adverse reactions

Allergic dermatitis has been reported (60). Reactions to patch testing occurred most commonly in persons who were regularly exposed to the substance or who already had dermatitis of the finger tips. Persons who were not previously exposed to the drug had few allergic reactions (60).

Posology

Crude plant material, 3–9 g daily (*5, 6*); powdered plant material, 1.5–3.0 g daily (*9, 19*); oral infusion, 0.5–1 g three times per day; tincture (1 : 10) 0.5–1 ml three times per day.

References

1. *Standard of ASEAN herbal medicine*, Vol. 1. Jakarta, ASEAN Countries, 1993.
2. *Pharmacopoeia of the People's Republic of China* (English ed.). Guangzhou, Guangdong Science and Technology Press, 1992.
3. Chang HM, But PPH, eds. *Pharmacology and applications of Chinese materia medica, Vol. 1*. Singapore, World Scientific Publishing, 1986.
4. Keys JD. *Chinese herbs, their botany, chemistry and pharmacodynamics*. Rutland, VT, CE Tuttle, 1976.
5. Wren RC. *Potter's new cyclopedia of botanical drugs and preparations*. Saffron Walden, C.W. Daniel, 1988.
6. Bisset NG. *Max Wichtl's herbal drugs & phytopharmaceuticals*. Boca Raton, FL, CRC Press, 1994.
7. Ghazanfar SA. *Handbook of Arabian medicinal plants*. Boca Raton, FL, CRC Press, 1994.
8. Kapoor LD. *Handbook of Ayurvedic medicinal plants*. Boca Raton, FL, CRC Press, 1990.
9. *The Indian pharmaceutical codex, Vol. I. Indigenous drugs*. New Delhi, Council of Scientific & Industrial Research, 1953.
10. Cambie RC, Ash J. *Fijian medicinal plants*. CSIRO, Australia, 1994.
11. Iwu MM. *Handbook of African medicinal plants*. Boca Raton, FL, CRC Press, 1993.
12. Hsu HY. *Oriental materia medica, a concise guide*. Long Beach, CA, Oriental Healing Arts Institute, 1986.
13. Youngken HW. *Textbook of pharmacognosy*, 6th ed. Philadelphia, Blakiston, 1950.
14. *Medicinal plants in Viet Nam*. Manila, World Health Organization, 1990 (WHO Regional Publications, Western Pacific Series, No. 3).
15. *Japanese standards for herbal medicines*. Tokyo, Yakuji Nippon, 1993.
16. *Medicinal plants in China*. Manila, World Health Organization, 1989 (WHO Regional Publications, Western Pacific Series, No. 2).
17. *Quality control methods for medicinal plant materials*. Geneva, World Health Organization, 1998.
18. *Deutsches Arzneibuch 1996. Vol. 2. Methoden der Biologie*. Stuttgart, Deutscher Apotheker Verlag, 1996.
19. *European pharmacopoeia*, 3rd ed. Strasbourg, Council of Europe, 1997.
20. *Guidelines for predicting dietary intake of pesticide residues*, 2nd rev. ed. Geneva, World Health Organization, 1997 (unpublished document WHO/FSF/FOS/97.7; available from Food Safety, WHO, 1211 Geneva 27, Switzerland).
21. Taylor SJ, McDowell IJ. Determination of curcuminoid pigments in turmeric (*Curcuma domestica* Val) by reversed-phase high-performance liquid chromatography. *Chromatographia*, 1992, 34:73–77.
22. International Organization for Standardization. Turmeric—Determination of colouring power—Spectrophotometric method. *ISO 5566*, 1982.
23. König WA et al. Enantiomeric composition of the chiral constituents of essential oils. Part 2: Sesquiterpene hydrocarbon. *Journal of high resolution chromatography*, 1994, 17:315–320.
24. Zhao DY, Yang MK. Separation and determination of curcuminoids in *Curcuma longa* L. and its preparation by HPLC. *Yao hsueh hsueh pao*, 1986, 21:382–385.
25. Bruneton J. *Pharmacognosy, phytochemistry, medicinal plants*. Paris, Lavoisier, 1995.

26. German Commission E Monograph, Curcumae longae rhizoma. *Bundesanzeiger,* 1985, 223:30 November.
27. Thamlikitkul V et al. Randomized double blind study of *Curcuma domestica* Val. for dyspepsia. *Journal of the Medical Association of Thailand,* 1989, 72:613–620.
28. Intanonta A et al. *Treatment of abdominal pain with Curcuma longa L.* (Report submitted to Primary Health Care Office, Ministry of Public Health, Thailand, 1986.)
29. Prucksunand C et al. Effect of the long turmeric (*Curcuma longa* L.) on healing peptic ulcer: A preliminary report of 10 case studies. *Thai journal of pharmacology,* 1986, 8:139–151.
30. Masuda T et al. Anti-oxidative and anti-inflammatory curcumin-related phenolics from rhizomes of *Curcuma domestica. Phytochemistry,* 1993, 32:1557–1560.
31. Arora RB et al. Anti-inflammatory studies on *Curcuma longa* (turmeric). *Indian journal of medical research,* 1971, 59:1289–1295.
32. Yegnanarayan R, Saraf AP, Balwani JH. Comparison of antiinflammatory activity of various extracts of *Curcuma longa* (Linn). *Indian journal of medical research,* 1976, 64:601–608.
33. Permpiphat U et al. Pharmacological study of *Curcuma longa.* In: *Proceedings of the Symposium of the Department of Medical Science, Mahidol University, Bangkok, Thailand, Dec 3–4, 1990.*
34. Gupta SS, Chandra D, Mishra N. Anti-inflammatory and antihyaluronidase activity of volatile oil of *Curcuma longa* (Haldi). *Indian journal of physiology and pharmacology,* 1972, 16:254.
35. Chandra D, Gupta SS. Anti-inflammatory and antiarthritic activity of volatile oil of *Curcuma longa. Indian journal of medical research,* 1972, 60:138–142.
36. Tripathi RM, Gupta SS, Chandra D. Anti-trypsin and antihyaluronidase activity of volatile oil of *Curcuma longa* (Haldi). *Indian journal of pharmacology,* 1973, 5:260–261.
37. Ghatak N, Basu N. Sodium curcuminate as an effective antiinflammatory agent. *Indian journal of experimental biology,* 1972, 10:235–236.
38. Srimal RC, Dhawan BN. Pharmacology of diferuloyl methane (curcumin), a non-steroidal anti-inflammatory agent. *Journal of pharmacy and pharmacology,* 1973, 25:447–452.
39. Mukhopadhyay A et al. Antiinflammatory and irritant activities of curcumin analogs in rats. *Agents and actions,* 1982, 12:508–515.
40. Rao TS, Basu N, Siddiqui HH. Anti-inflammatory activity of curcumin analogs. *Indian journal of medical research,* 1982, 75:574–578.
41. Ammon HP, Wahl MA. Pharmacology of *Curcuma longa. Planta medica,* 1991, 57:1–7.
42. Kunchandy E, Rao MN. Oxygen radical scavenging activity of curcumin. *International journal of pharmacognosy,* 1990, 58:237–240.
43. Kinoshita G, Nakamura F, Maruyama T. Immunological studies on polysaccharide fractions from crude drugs. *Shoyakugaku zasshi,* 1986, 40:325–332.
44. Sakai K et al. Effects of extracts of Zingiberaceae herbs on gastric secretion in rabbits. *Chemical and pharmaceutical bulletin,* 1989, 37:215–217.
45. Muderji B, Zaidi SH, Singh GB. Spices and gastric function. Part I. Effect of *Curcuma longa* on the gastric secretion in rabbits. *Journal of scientific and industrial research,* 1981, 20:25–28.
46. Rafatullah S et al. Evaluation of turmeric (*Curcuma longa*) for gastric and duodenal antiulcer activity in rats. *Journal of ethnopharmacology,* 1990, 29:25–34.
47. Bhatia A, Singh GB, Khanna NM. Effect of curcumin, its alkali salts and *Curcuma longa* oil on histamine-induced gastric ulceration. *Indian journal of experimental biology,* 1964, 2:158–160.
48. Sinha M et al. Study of the mechanism of action of curcumin: an antiulcer agent. *Indian journal of pharmacy,* 1975, 7:98–99.

49. Prasad DN et al. Studies on ulcerogenic activity of curcumin. *Indian journal of physiology and pharmacology*, 1976, 20:92–93.
50. Gupta B et al. Mechanisms of curcumin induced gastric ulcers in rats. *Indian journal of medical research*, 1980, 71:806–814.
51. Srimal RC, Dhawan BN. In: Arora BA, ed. *Development of Unani drugs from herbal sources and the role of elements in their mechanism of action*. New Delhi, Hamdard National Foundation Monograph, 1985.
52. Deodhar SD, Sethi R, Srimal RC. Preliminary study on anti-rheumatic activity of curcumin (diferuloyl methane). *Indian journal of medical research*, 1980, 71:632–634.
53. Satoskar RR, Shah Shenoy SG. Evaluation of antiinflammatory property of curcumin (diferuloyl methane) in patient with postoperative inflammation. *International journal of clinical pharmacology, therapy and toxicology*, 1986, 24:651–654.
54. Rockwell P, Raw I. A mutagenic screening of various herbs, spices and food additives. *Nutrition and cancer*, 1979, 1:10–15.
55. Yamamoto H, Mizutani T, Nomura H. Studies on the mutagenicity of crude drug extracts. I. *Yakugaku zasshi*, 1982, 102:596–601.
56. Nagabhushan M, Bhide SV. Nonmutagenicity of curcumin and its antimutagenic action versus chili and capsaicin. *Nutrition and cancer*, 1986, 8:201–210.
57. Garg SK. Effect of *Curcuma longa* (rhizomes) on fertility in experimental animals. *Planta medica*, 1974, 26:225–227.
58. Vijayalaxmi. Genetic effects of tumeric and curcumin in mice and rats. *Mutation research*, 1980, 79:125–132.
59. Farnsworth NF, Bunyapraphatsara N, eds. *Thai medicinal plants, recommended for a primary health care system*. Bangkok, Prachachon, 1992.
60. Seetharam KA, Pasricha JS. Condiments and contact dermatitis of the finger-tips. *Indian journal of dermatology, venereology and leprology*, 1987, 53:325–328.

Radix Echinaceae

Definition

Radix Echinaceae consists of the fresh or dried roots of *Echinacea angustifolia* D.C. var. *angustifolia* or its variety *strigosa* McGregor, or *E. pallida* (Nutt.) Nutt. (Asteraceae) (*1–3*).

Synonyms

Echinacea angustifolia D.C. var. angustifolia

Brauneria angustifolia Heller, *Echinacea pallida* var. *angustifolia* (D.C.) Cronq. (*4, 5*).

Echinacea pallida (Nutt.) Nutt.

Echinacea angustifolia Hook, *Rudbeckia pallida* Nutt., *Brauneria pallida* Britt., *Echinacea pallida* f. *albida* Steyerm (*4, 5*).

E. *angustifolia* and *E. pallida* were regarded as varieties of the same species or even identical plants. However, in a revision of the genus *Echinacea* in 1968, McGregor (*4*) classified them as two distinct species with *E. angustifolia* further divided into two varieties (*4, 5*). A considerable amount of commercial "*E. angustifolia*" cultivated in Europe was, in fact, *E. pallida*. Data on *E. angustifolia* published prior to 1987 and based on material of commerce from Europe should be reviewed with caution (*5*).

Current commercial preparations are derived primarily from *E. angustifolia* and *E. pallida* roots; the preparation of a monograph on *E. purpurea* root awaits further data.

Asteraceae are also known as Compositae.

Selected vernacular names

Echinacea angustifolia D.C. var. angustifolia

American coneflower, black sampson, cock up head, coneflower, echinacea root, Igelkopf, Indian head, Kansas snakeroot, Kegelblume, narrow-leaved purple coneflower root, purple coneflower, Sonnenhut, racine d'echinacea (*5–10*).

Echinacea pallida (Nutt.) Nutt.

Blasser Igelkopf, blasse Kegelblume, blasser Sonnenhut, pale coneflower root, pale purple coneflower root, pallida root (*8, 10*).

Description

Echinacea species are hardy, herbaceous perennials with either simple or branched stems. The terminal single flowering heads have fertile disc florets that terminate in spines (paleae). These are surrounded by infertile drooping or spreading ray flowers that have 2 or 3 teeth at each end. The leaf shape varies from lanceolate to ovate, its margin may be dentate and the leaf may be pubescent or smooth. Roots are either single taproot or fibrous in form (*6–11*).

Echinacea angustifolia D.C. var. angustifolia

Stems simple or occasionally branched, 10–50 cm high, smooth or hirsute below, hirsute or tuberculate-hispid above; leaves oblong-lanceolate to elliptical, entire, dark green tuberculate-hirsute to tuberculate-hispid; basal leaves short- to long-petiolate, 5–27 cm long, 1–4 cm broad, lower cauline leaves petiolate, 4–15 cm long, 0.5–3.8 cm broad, upper cauline leaves sessile, acute; heads 1.5–3 cm high, 1.5–2.5 cm broad exclusive of ligules, phyllaries in three or four series, lanceolate, acute, entire, 6–11 mm long, 2–3 mm wide, tuberculate-hirsute or tuberculate-hispid; rays spreading, 2–3.8 cm long, 5–8 mm wide, white, pinkish or purplish; disc corollas 6–8.5 mm long, lobes 1.2–2 mm long; achenes 4–5 mm long, pappus a toothed crown; pollen grains yellow, 19–26 μm in diameter; haploid chromosome number $n = 11$ (*4*).

Echinacea pallida (Nutt.) Nutt.

Stems simple, rarely branched, 40–90 cm high, sparsely hirsute below, more densely so above; leaves oblong-lanceolate to long-elliptical, entire, dark green, hirsute on both surfaces, triple-veined; basal leaves 10–35 cm long, 1–4 cm broad, the cauline leaves 10–25 cm long, 1–2.5 cm broad, acute, petiolate below to sessile above; phyllaries lanceolate to narrowly oblong, 8–17 mm long, 2–4 mm broad, hirsute, ciliate, three or four series gradually passing into the echinaceous pales; rays reflexed, 4–9 cm long, 5–8 mm broad, purplish, pink, or white; pales 1–1.3 cm long, body 8–10 mm long, awn 2.5–3.5 mm long; disc floret 8–10 mm long, lobes 2–3 mm long, achenes 3.7–5 mm long, glabrous, pappus a toothed crown, teeth about even, longest 1 mm; pollen grains white, 24–28.5 μm in diameter; haploid chromosome number $n = 22$ (*4*).

Plant material of interest: fresh or dried roots
General appearance
Echinacea angustifolia D.C. var. *angustifolia*

Cylindrical or slightly tapering and sometimes spirally twisted, passing imperceptibly into a rhizome in the upper part; rhizome up to about 15 mm in diameter, roots 4–10 mm in diameter; outer surface pale brown to yellowish brown; rhizomes crowned with remains of the aerial stem and sometimes showing surface annulations; roots longitudinally wrinkled and deeply furrowed; fracture short when dry but becoming tough and pliable on exposure to air (*12*).

Echinacea pallida (Nutt.) Nutt.

Similar in appearance to *E. angustifolia* (*5–7*).

Organoleptic properties

Odour, mild, aromatic; taste, sweet initially but quickly becoming bitter followed by a tingling sensation on the tongue (*12*).

Microscopic characteristics

The roots of the two species are very similar. The transverse section shows a thin outer bark separated by a distinct cambium line from a wide xylem; a small circular pith in the rhizome. Cork composed of several rows of thin-walled cells containing yellowish brown pigment; cortex parenchymatous; rhizome with occasional small groups of thick-walled, lignified fibres in the pericycle; phloem and xylem composed of very narrow strands of vascular tissue separated by wide, non-lignified medullary rays; xylem vessels lignified, 25–75 µm in diameter, usually reticulate thickening but occasionally with spiral or annular thickening; stone cells, occurring singly or in small groups, varying considerably in size and shape from rounded to rectangular to elongated and fibre-like, up to 300 µm long and 20–40 µm wide, with intercellular spaces containing a dense black deposit; schizogenous oleoresin canals; spherocrystalline masses of inulin occur throughout the parenchymatous tissue. In *E. angustifolia* oleoresin canals, 80–150 µm in diameter and containing yellowish orange oleoresin, are present only outside the central cylinder, but in *E. pallida* they are present both inside and outside. In *E. angustifolia* the narrow, 300–800 µm long, lignified fibres are in scattered groups usually surrounded by phytomelanin deposits, while in *E. pallida* they are present only in the periphery of the cortex and they are mostly single, wider, and shorter, 100–300 µm, and phytomelanin is often absent (*9, 12*).

Powdered plant material

E. angustifolia

Powdered rhizome and roots are brown with a slight aromatic odour and initially a sweet taste, quickly becoming bitter and leaving a tingling sensation on the tongue. Thin-walled polygonal cork cells with red-brown contents; lignified reticulately thickened vessels; abundant stone cells of various shapes; fragments of oleoresin canals with reddish brown contents; abundant thin-walled parenchyma with spherocrystalline masses of inulin (*12*).

E. pallida

Descriptions of powdered *E. pallida* are currently unavailable.

Geographical distribution

Echinacea species are native to the Atlantic drainage area of the United States of America and Canada, but not Mexico. Their distribution centres are in Arkansas, Kansas, Missouri, and Oklahoma in the United States of America (*4*). *E. pallida* was cultivated in Europe for a number of years and was mistaken for *E. angustifolia* (*9*).

General identity tests

Macroscopic and microscopic examinations (*5–7, 9, 12*). Chemical finger-prints of lipophilic constituents, echinacosides, and other caffeic acid derivatives in methanol extracts can be obtained by thin-layer chromatography and high-performance liquid chromatography (*5, 13, 14*).

Purity tests
Microbiology

The test for *Salmonella* spp. in Radix Echinaceae products should be negative. The maximum acceptable limits of other microorganisms are as follows (*15–17*). For preparation of decoction: aerobic bacteria—not more than 10^7/g; fungi—not more than 10^5/g; *Escherichia coli*—not more than 10^2/g. Preparations for internal use: aerobic bacteria—not more than 10^5/g or ml; fungi—not more than 10^4/g or ml; enterobacteria and certain Gram-negative bacteria—not more than 10^3/g or ml; *Escherichia coli*—0/g or ml.

Foreign organic matter

Not more than 3% (*2, 3, 12*). Does not contain roots of *Parthenium integrifolium* L., commonly known as "American feverfew", which have been found to be adulterants of or substitutes for Radix Echinaceae (*5, 6, 9, 13*).

Total ash

Not more than 9% (*12*).

Acid-insoluble ash

Not more than 3% (*12*).

Water-soluble extractive

Not less than 15% (*12*).

Moisture

Not more than 10% (*3*).

Pesticide residues

To be established in accordance with national requirements. Normally, the maximum residue limit of aldrin and dieldrin in Radix Echinaceae is not more than 0.05 mg/kg (*17*). For other pesticides, see WHO guidelines on quality control methods for medicinal plants (*15*) and guidelines for predicting dietary intake of pesticide residues (*18*).

Heavy metals

Recommended lead and cadmium levels are no more than 10 and 0.3 mg/kg, respectively, in the final dosage form of the plant material (*15*).

Radioactive residues

For analysis of strontium-90, iodine-131, caesium-134, caesium-137, and plutonium-239, see WHO guidelines on quality control methods for medicinal plants (*15*).

Other purity tests

Chemical tests and tests of dilute ethanol-soluble extractive to be established in accordance with national requirements.

Chemical assays

Essential oil (0.2–2%) and echinacoside (0.4–1.7%) in both *E. angustifolia* and *E. pallida* roots (*5*).

Quantitative analysis of echinacoside, cynarin, chicoric acid, chlorogenic acid derivatives, and other constituents by high-performance liquid chromatography (*5, 19*).

Major chemical constituents

A number of chemical entities have been identified and reported to be biologically active, including a volatile oil, alkamides, polyalkenes, polyalkynes, caffeic acid derivatives, and polysaccharides (*5–7, 9–11*).

The volatile oil contains, among other compounds, pentadeca-(1,8-Z)-diene (44%), 1-pentadecene, ketoalkynes and ketoalkenes.

More than 20 alkamides, mostly isobutylamides of C_{11}–C_{16} straight-chain fatty acids with olefinic or acetylenic bonds, or both, are found in the roots; the highest concentration is in *E. angustifolia*, followed by *E. purpurea*, and the lowest is in *E. pallida*. The main alkamide is a mixture of isomeric dodeca-2,4,8,10-tetraenoic acid isobutylamides.

Caffeic acid ester derivatives present include echinacoside, cynarin, and chicoric acid. Cynarin is present only in *E. angustifolia*, thus distinguishing it from the closely related *E. pallida*.

Polysaccharide constituents are of two types: a heteroxylan of relative molecular mass about 35 000 and an arabinorhamnogalactan of relative molecular mass about 45 000.

Other constituents include trace amounts of pyrrolizidine alkaloids (tussilagine (0.006%) and isotussilagine). At these concentrations, the alkaloids are considered to be non-toxic (*7, 20*), and since they lack the 1,2-unsaturated necine ring of alkaloids such as senecionine (structure in box) from *Senecio* species, they are considered to have no hepatotoxic potential (*5*).

Structures of representative constituents are presented below.

(2E,4E,8Z,10E)- and (2E,4E,8Z,10Z)-dodeca-2,4,8,10-tetraenoic acid isobutylamides

chicoric acid

or enantiomer [(+)-isomer]
echinolone

cynarin (1,5-dicaffeylquinic acid)

echinacoside

Necine ring pyrrolizidine alkaloids :

tussilagine   isotussilagine

1,2-saturated

senecionine

1,2-unsaturated

Dosage forms

Powdered roots, and galenics and preparations thereof for internal use (*9*).

Medicinal uses
Uses supported by clinical data
Preparations of Radix Echinaceae are administered orally in supportive therapy for colds and infections of the respiratory and urinary tract (*1, 5–7, 9, 11, 21–23*). Beneficial effects in the treatment of these infections are generally thought to be brought about by stimulation of the immune response (*5, 6, 9, 10*).

Uses described in pharmacopoeias and in traditional systems of medicine
None.

Uses described in folk medicine, not supported by experimental or clinical data
Treatment of yeast infections, side-effects of radiation therapy, rheumatoid arthritis, and food poisoning (*1, 5, 6, 9, 24*).

Pharmacology
Experimental pharmacology
Current claims for the effectiveness of Radix Echinaceae as a stimulator of the immune system are based on over 350 scientific studies in the past 50 years. Numerous *in vitro* and *in vivo* studies have documented the activation of an immune response after treatment with Radix Echinaceae extracts. The immunostimulant effect is brought about by three mechanisms: activation of phagocytosis and stimulation of fibroblasts; increasing respiratory activity; and causing increased mobility of the leukocytes (*5, 9, 11*). Chemically standardized extracts, derived from roots and aerial parts from the three *Echinacea* species, have been assessed for their phagocytotic potential. All ethanolic root extracts increased phagocytosis *in vitro* (*25*). Inhibition of hyaluronidase activity, stimulation of the activity of the adrenal cortex, stimulation of the production of properdin (a serum protein which can neutralize bacteria and viruses), and stimulation of interferon production have also been reported after *Echinacea* treatments (*26*). The pharmacological activity of *Echinacea* spp. has been attributed to five component fractions in addition to the essential oil, namely the alkylamides, caffeic acid derivatives, polyalkynes, polyalkenes and polysaccharides (*6*). The lipophilic amides, alkamides and caffeic acid derivatives appear to contribute to the immunostimulant activity of the alcoholic *Echinacea* extracts by stimulating phagocytosis of polymorphonuclear neutrophil granulocytes (*5, 23, 27*). High molecular weight polysaccharides, including heteroxylan, which activates phagocytosis, and arabinogalactan, which promotes the release of tumour necrosis factor and the production of interleukin-1 and interferon beta (*24, 26*), have also been implicated in the activity of the aqueous extracts and the powdered drug when taken orally. The overall immunostimulant activity of

the alcoholic and aqueous *Echinacea* extracts appears to depend on the combined effects of several constituents (*5, 9, 27*).

Echinacea extracts inhibit streptococcal and tissue hyaluronidase (*28*). Inhibition of tissue and bacterial hyaluronidase is thought to localize the infection and prevent the spread of causative agents to other parts of the body. In addition to the direct antihyaluronidase activity, an indirect effect on the hyaluronic acid–hyaluronidase system has been reported (*29, 30*). Stimulation of new tissue production by increasing the activity of fibroblasts, and stimulation of both blood- and tissue-produced phagocytosis, appear to be involved in this mechanism (*29*).

Echinacea extracts have anti-inflammatory activity. An alkylamide fraction from *Echinacea* roots markedly inhibited activity *in vitro* in the 5-lipoxygenase model (porcine leukocytes) (*31*). Topical application of a crude polysaccharide extract from *E. angustifolia* has been reported to reduce inflammation in the rat paw oedema model (*32, 33*).

Clinical pharmacology

One placebo-controlled clinical study of 160 patients with infections of the upper respiratory tract has been performed (*34*). Significant improvement was observed after patients were treated with an aqueous-alcoholic tincture (1:5) at 90 drops/day (900 mg roots). The duration of the illness decreased from 13 to 9.8 days for bacterial infections, and from 12.9 to 9.1 days for viral infections (*34*).

Contraindications
External use

Allergy to plants in the Asteraceae.

Internal use

Should not be used in serious conditions such as tuberculosis, leukosis, collagenosis, multiple sclerosis, AIDS, HIV infection and autoimmune disorders. *Echinacea* preparations should not be administered to people with a known allergy to any plant of the Asteraceae (*1*). Parenteral administration is rarely indicated owing to potential adverse side-effects (see Adverse reactions).

Warnings

None.

Precautions
General

Internal use should not exceed a period of 8 successive weeks (*1*).

Carcinogenesis, mutagenesis, impairment of fertility

Mutagenicity and carcinogenicity tests were negative (5, 9, 35). Doses up to a polysaccharide concentration of 500 µg/ml caused no increase in sister chromatid exchange or structural chromosome aberrations (35).

Pregnancy: teratogenic effects

There are no reliable studies on this subject. Therefore, administration of Radix Echinaceae during pregnancy is not generally recommended (1).

Nursing mothers

There are no reliable studies on this subject. Therefore, nursing mothers should not take Radix Echinaceae without consulting a physician (1).

Paediatric use

Oral administration of *Echinacea* preparations is not recommended for children, except on the advice of a physician.

Other precautions

No information was available concerning drug interactions, drug and laboratory test interactions, and non-teratogenic effects on pregnancy.

Adverse reactions

External use

Allergic reactions.

Internal use

Allergic reactions, shivering, fever, and headache.

Posology

E. angustifolia root

Unless otherwise prescribed, hot water (about 150 ml) is poured over about 0.5 teaspoon (about 1 g) of powdered plant material, allowed to steep for 10 minutes, passed through a strainer, and taken orally three times a day between meals (7).

Liquid extract (1:5, 45% ethanol), 0.5–1 ml three times daily (7). Tincture (1:5, 45% ethanol), 2–5 ml three times daily (7).

E. pallida root

Unless otherwise prescribed: daily dose, tincture (1:5 with 50% ethanol by volume) from original dry extract (50% ethanol), corresponding to 900 mg of root (9).

References

1. German Commission E Monograph, Echinaceae angustifoliae radix; Echinaceae pallidae radix. *Bundesanzeiger*, 1992, 162:29 August.
2. *National formulary* IX. Washington, DC, American Pharmaceutical Association, 1950.
3. *Deutsches Arzneibuch 1996*. Stuttgart, Deutscher Apotheker Verlag, 1996.
4. McGregor RL. The taxonomy of the genus *Echinacea* (Compositae). *University of Kansas science bulletin*, 1968, 48:113–142.
5. Bauer R, Wagner H. *Echinacea* species as potential immunostimulatory drugs. In: Wagner H, Farnsworth NR, eds. *Economic and medicinal plants research, Vol. 5*. London, Academic Press, 1991:253–321.
6. Awang DVC, Kindack DG. Herbal medicine, *Echinacea. Canadian pharmaceutical journal*, 1991, 124:512–516.
7. Bradley PR, ed. *British herbal compendium, Vol. 1*. Bournemouth, British Herbal Medicine Association, 1992.
8. Hänsel R et al., eds. *Hagers Handbuch der pharmazeutischen Praxis*, 5th ed., Vol. 6. Berlin, Springer, 1994
9. Bisset NG. *Max Wichtl's herbal drugs & phytopharmaceuticals*. Boca Raton, FL, CRC Press, 1994.
10. Foster S. *Echinacea, the purple coneflowers*. Austin, TX, The American Botanical Council, 1991 (Botanical Series, 301).
11. Bruneton J. *Pharmacognosy, phytochemistry, medicinal plants*. Paris, Lavoisier, 1995.
12. *British herbal pharmacopoeia*. London, British Herbal Medicine Association, 1990.
13. Bauer R, Khan IA, Wagner H. Echinacea-Drogen, Standardisierung mittels HPLC und DC. *Deutsche Apotheker Zeitung*, 1986, 126:1065–1070.
14. Bauer R, Khan IA, Wagner H. *Echinacea*: Nachweis einer Verfälschung von *Echinacea purpurea* (L.) Moench. mit *Parthenium integrifolium* L. *Deutsche Apotheker Zeitung*, 1987, 127:1325–1330.
15. *Quality control methods for medicinal plant materials*. Geneva, World Health Organization, 1998.
16. *Deutsches Arzneibuch 1996, Vol. 2. Methoden der Biologie*. Stuttgart, Deutscher Apotheker Verlag, 1996.
17. *European Pharmacopoeia*, 3rd ed. Strasbourg, Council of Europe, 1997.
18. *Guidelines for predicting dietary intake of pesticide residues*, 2nd rev. ed. Geneva, World Health Organization, 1997 (unpublished document WHO/FSF/FOS/97.7; available from Food Safety, WHO, 1211 Geneva 27, Switzerland).
19. Bauer R, Remiger P, Wagner H. *Echinacea*—Vergleichende DC- und HPLC-Analyse der Herba-Drogen von *Echinacea purpurea, E. pallida* und *E. angustifolia* (3. Mitt.). *Deutsche Apotheker Zeitung*, 1988, 128:174–180.
20. Röder E, Wiedenfeld H, Hille T, Britz-Kirstgen R. Pyrrolizidine in *Echinacea angustifolia* DC and *Echinacea purpurea* M. Isolation and analysis. *Deutsche Apotheker Zeitung*, 1984, 124:2316–2317.
21. Iwu MM. *Handbook of African medicinal plants*. Boca Raton, FL, CRC Press, 1993.
22. Schöneberger D. The influence of immune-stimulating effects of pressed juice from *Echinacea purpurea* on the course and severity of colds. *Forum immunologie*, 1992, 8:2–12.
23. Melchart D et al. Immunomodulation with *Echinacea*: a systematic review of controlled clinical trials. *Phytomedicine*, 1994, 1:245–254.
24. Viehmann P. Results of treatment with an Echinacea-based ointment. *Erfahrungsheilkunde*, 1978, 27:353–358.
25. Bauer R et al. Immunological *in vivo* examinations of *Echinacea* extracts. *Arzneimittel-Forschung*, 1988, 38:276–281.
26. Haas H. *Arzneipflanzenkunde*. Mannheim, BI Wissenschaftsverlag, 1991:134–135.

27. Bauer R, Wagner H. *Echinacea. Handbuch für Apotheker und andere Naturwissenschaftler.* Stuttgart, Wissenschaftliche Verlagsgesellschaft, 1990.
28. Büsing KH. Hyaluronidase inhibition by Echinacin. *Arzneimittel-Forschung*, 1952, 2:467–469.
29. Koch FE, Haase H. A modification of the spreading test in animal assays. *Arzneimittel-Forschung*, 1952, 2:464–467.
30. Koch FE, Uebel H. The influence of *Echinacea purpurea* upon the hypohyseal-adrenal system. *Arzneimittel-Forschung*, 1953, 3:133–137.
31. Wagner H et al. *In vitro* inhibition of arachidonate metabolism by some alkamides and prenylated phenols. *Planta medica*, 1988, 55:566–567.
32. Tubaro A et al. Anti-inflammatory activity of a polysaccharidic fraction of *Echinacea angustifolia*. *Journal of pharmacy and pharmacology*, 1987, 39:567–569.
33. Tragni E et al. Anti-inflammatory activity of *Echinacea angustifolia* fractions separated on the basis of molecular weight. *Pharmaceutical research communications*, 1988, 20(Suppl. V):87–90.
34. Bräunig B, Knick E. Therapeutische Erfahrungen mit Echinaceae pallidae bei grippalen Infekten. Ergebnisse einer plazebokontrollierten Doppelblindstudie. *Naturheilpraxis*, 1993, 46:72–75.
35. Kraus C, Abel G, Schimmer O. Untersuchung einiger Pyrrolizidinalkaloide auf chromosomenschädigende Wirkung in menschlichen Lymphocyten *in vitro*. *Planta medica*, 1985, 51:89–91.

Herba Echinaceae Purpureae

Definition

Herba Echinaceae Purpureae consists of the fresh or dried aerial parts of *Echinacea purpurea* (L.) Moench harvested in full bloom (Asteraceae) (*1*).

Synonyms

Brauneria purpurea (L.) Britt., *Echinacea intermedia* Lindl., *E. purpurea* (L.) Moench f., *E. purpurea* (L.) Moench var. *arkansana* Steyerm., *E. speciosa* Paxt., *Rudbeckia purpurea* L., *R. hispida* Hoffm., *R. serotina* Sweet (*2, 3*).

Asteraceae are also known as Compositae.

Selected vernacular names

Coneflower, purple coneflower herb, purpurfarbener Igelkopf, purpurfarbene Kegelblume, purpurfarbener Sonnenhut, red sunflower, roter Sonnenhut (*4–8*).

Description

A hardy, herbaceous perennial. Stems erect, stout, branched, hirsute or glabrous, 60–180 cm high; basal leaves ovate to ovate-lanceolate, acute, coarsely or sharply serrate, petioles up to 25 cm long, blades to 20 cm long and 15 cm wide, blade abruptly narrowing to base, often cordate, decurrent on petiole, 3–5 veined; cauline leaves petiolate below, sessile above, 7–20 cm long, 1.5–8 cm broad, coarsely serrate to entire, rough to the touch on both surfaces; phyllaries linear-lanceolate, attenuate, entire, pubescent on outer surface, ciliate, passing into the chaff; heads 1.5–3 cm long and 5–10 mm broad, purplish; pales 9–13 mm long, awn half as long as body; disc corollas 4.5–5.5 mm long, lobes 1 mm long; achene 4–4.5 mm long, pappus a low crown of equal teeth; pollen grains yellow, 19–21 μm in diameter; haploid chromosome number $n = 11$ (*2*).

Plant material of interest: fresh or dried aerial parts

General appearance

The macroscopic characteristics of Herba Echinaceae Purpureae are as described above under Description. An abbreviated description is currently unavailable.

Organoleptic properties
Mild, aromatic odour; initially sweet taste that quickly becomes bitter.

Microscopic characteristics
A description of the microscopic characteristics of a cross-section of the aerial parts of the plant is currently unavailable.

Powdered plant material
A description of the powdered plant material is currently unavailable.

Geographical distribution
Echinacea purpurea is native to the Atlantic drainage area of the United States of America and Canada, but not Mexico. Its distribution centres are in Arkansas, Kansas, Missouri, and Oklahoma in the United States of America (*2*). *Echinacea purpurea* has been introduced as a cultivated medicinal plant in parts of north and eastern Africa and in Europe (*9*).

General identity tests
Macroscopic examination (*2*) and thin-layer chromatography and high-performance liquid chromatography (*4, 10–13*) of the lipophilic constituents and chicoric acid in methanol extracts.

Purity tests
Microbiology
The test for *Salmonella* spp. in Herba Echinaceae Purpureae should be negative. The maximum acceptable limits of other microorganisms are as follows (*14–16*). For preparation of decoction: aerobic bacteria—not more than 10^7/g; fungi—not more than 10^5/g; Escherichia *coli*—not more than 10^2/g. Preparations for internal use: aerobic bacteria—not more than 10^5/g or ml; fungi—not more than 10^4/g or ml; enterobacteria and certain Gram-negative bacteria—not more than 10^3/g or ml; Escherichia *coli*—0/g or ml. Preparations for external use: aerobic bacteria—not more than 10^2/g or ml; fungi—not more than 10^2/g or ml; enterobacteria and certain Gram-negative bacteria—not more than 10^1/g or ml.

Pesticide residues
To be established in accordance with national requirements. Normally, the maximum residue limit of aldrin and dieldrin in Herba Echinaceae Purpureae is not more than 0.05 mg/kg (*16*). For other pesticides, see WHO guidelines on quality control methods for medicinal plants (*14*) and guidelines for predicting dietary intake of pesticide residues (*17*).

Heavy metals

Recommended lead and cadmium levels are no more than 10 and 0.3 mg/kg, respectively, in the final dosage form of the plant material (*14*).

Radioactive residues

For analysis of strontium-90, iodine-131, caesium-134, caesium-137, and plutonium-239, see WHO guidelines on quality control methods for medicinal plants (*14*).

Other purity tests

Chemical tests and tests for acid-insoluble ash, dilute ethanol-soluble extractive, foreign organic matter, moisture, total ash, and water-soluble extractive to be established in accordance with national requirements.

Chemical assays

For essential oil (0.08–0.32%); chicoric acid (1.2–3.1%) (*4*). Quantitative analysis of echinacoside, chicoric acid, isobutylamides, and other constituents by high-performance liquid chromatography (*4*). Quantitative analysis of alkamides and caffeic acid derivatives by thin-layer chromatography and high-performance liquid chromatography (*4, 12*).

Major chemical constituents

A number of chemical entities have been identified, including alkamides, polyalkenes, polyalkynes, caffeic acid derivatives, and polysaccharides (*3, 5–9*).

The volatile oil contains, among other compounds, borneol, bornyl acetate, pentadeca-8-(Z)-en-2-one, germacrene D, caryophyllene, and caryophyllene epoxide.

Isobutylamides of C_{11}–C_{16} straight-chain fatty acids with olefinic or acetylenic bonds (or both) are found in the aerial parts of Herba Echinaceae Purpureae, with the isomeric dodeca-(2E,4E,8Z,10E/Z)-tetraenoic acid isobutylamides.

The caffeic acid ester derivative chicoric acid is the major active compound of this class found in the aerial parts of *Echinacea purpurea*, with a concentration range of 1.2–3.1%. Chicoric acid methyl ester and other derivatives are also present.

Polysaccharide constituents from Herba Echinaceae Purpureae are of two types: a heteroxylan of average relative molecular mass about 35 000 (e.g. PS-I), and an arabinorhamnogalactan of average relative molecular mass about 45 000 (e.g. PS-II).

Other constituents include trace amounts of pyrrolizidine alkaloids (tussilagine (0.006%) and isotussilagine). At these concentrations, the alkaloids are considered to be non-toxic (*8*). Furthermore, because these alkaloids lack the 1,2-unsaturated necine ring of alkaloids such as senecionine (structure in box) from *Senecio* species, they are considered to be non-hepatotoxic (*3*).

Structures of representative constituents are presented below.

chicoric acid

Necine ring pyrrolizidine alkaloids :

tussilagine   isotussilagine   senecionine

1,2-saturated   1,2-unsaturated

Dosage forms

Powdered aerial part, pressed juice and galenic preparations thereof for internal and external use (*1, 3*).

Medicinal uses

Uses supported by clinical data

Herba Echinaceae Purpureae is administered orally in supportive therapy for colds and infections of the respiratory and urinary tract (*1, 3, 5, 7, 8, 18*). Beneficial effects in the treatment of these infections are generally thought to be brought about by stimulation of the immune response (*3, 5, 7*). External uses include promotion of wound healing and treatment of inflammatory skin conditions (*1, 3, 5, 7, 8, 9, 19*).

Uses described in pharmacopoeias and in traditional systems of medicine

None.

Uses described in folk medicine, not supported by experimental or clinical data

Other medical uses claimed for Herba Echinaceae Purpureae include treatment of yeast infections, side-effects of radiation therapy, rheumatoid arthritis, blood poisoning, and food poisoning (*1, 5, 7, 9*).

Pharmacology
Experimental pharmacology

Current claims of the effectiveness of *Echinacea purpurea* as a stimulator of the immune system are based on numerous scientific studies. The immunostimulant effect is brought about by three mechanisms: activation of phagocytosis and stimulation of fibroblasts; increasing respiratory activity; and increased mobility of the leukocytes (*3, 5, 8*). Phagocytic activity of standardized extracts of the aerial parts of *E. purpurea* has been determined. A lyophylisate of the expressed juice of Herba Echinaceae Purpureae significantly increased the percentage of phagocytizing human granulocytes and stimulated the phagocytosis of yeast particles *in vitro* (*20, 21*). Inhibition of hyaluronidase activity, stimulation of the activity of the adrenal cortex, stimulation of the production of properdin (a serum protein which can neutralize bacteria and viruses), and stimulation of interferon production have also been reported after *Echinacea* treatments (*22*). The pharmacological activity of *Echinacea* spp. has been attributed to five component fractions in addition to the essential oil, namely the alkylamides, caffeic acid derivatives, polyalkynes, polyalkenes, and polysaccharides (*7*). The lipophilic amides, alkamides, and caffeic acid derivatives appear to contribute to the immunostimulant activity of the alcoholic *Echinacea* extracts by stimulating phagocytosis of polymorphonuclear neutrophil granulocytes (*3, 23, 24*). High molecular weight polysaccharides, including heteroxylan, which activates phagocytosis, and arabinogalactan, which promotes the release of tumour necrosis factor and the production of interleukin-1 and interferon beta (*19, 22*), have also been implicated in the activity of the aqueous extracts and the powdered drug when taken orally. The overall immunostimulant activity of the alcoholic and aqueous *Echinacea* extracts appears to depend on the combined effects of several constituents (*3, 5, 23*).

Topical applications of *Echinacea* extracts have been traditionally used to promote wound healing. The first published work on the mechanism of this action was by Büsing (*25*), who investigated the effect of *Echinacea* spp. on streptococcal and tissue hyaluronidase. Inhibition of tissue and bacterial hyaluronidase is thought to localize the infection and prevent the spread of causative agents to other parts of the body. In addition to the direct antihyaluronidase activity, an indirect effect on the hyaluronic acid–hyaluronidase system has been reported (*26*). Stimulation of new tissue production by increasing fibroblast activity, and stimulation of both blood- and tissue-produced phagocytosis, appear to be involved in this mechanism (*26*). The polysaccharide fraction (echinacin B) appears to promote wound healing by forming a hyaluronic acid–polysaccharide complex that indirectly leads to the inhibition of hyaluronidase (27).

In *in vitro* experiments, an ethanol extract (65% by volume) of Herba Echinaceae Purpureae inhibited the contraction of collagen by mouse fibroblasts, measured by the collagen lattice diameter (28).

Mouse macrophages pretreated with polysaccharides that were isolated from the supernatant of Herba Echinaceae Purpureae cell culture increased production of tumour necrosis factor alpha, interleukin-1, and interferon beta-2 and increased cytotoxicity against tumour cells and microorganisms (*Leishmania enreittii*) (29–31).

Purified polysaccharides isolated from large-scale cell cultures of *E. purpurea* enhanced the spontaneous motility of human polymorphonuclear leukocytes under soft agar and increased the ability of these cells to kill *Staphylococcus aureus*. Human monocytes were activated to secrete tumour necrosis factor alpha, interleukin-1, and interleukin-6 while the expression of class II human leukocyte antigens was unaffected (32).

For purified caffeic acid derivatives, antiviral activities have been demonstrated (33). Incubation of vesicular stomatitis virus (VSV) with 125 µg/ml of chicoric acid for 4 hours reduced the number of viral particles in mouse L-929 murine cells by more than 50% (34).

Clinical pharmacology

Recently 26 controlled clinical trials (18 randomized, 11 double-blind) were systematically reviewed in Germany (24), Nineteen trials studied the prophylaxis or curative treatment of infections, four trials studied the reduction of side-effects of chemotherapy, and three investigated the modulation of specific immune parameters. The review concluded that *Echinacea*-containing preparations are efficacious immunomodulators (24). However, it also concluded that there was insufficient evidence for clear therapeutic recommendations as to which preparation or dosage to use for a specific indication (24).

A large-scale longitudinal trial (4598 patients) studied the effects of an ointment containing a lyophylisate of the expressed juice of Herba Echinaceae Purpureae. The ointment was used to treat inflammatory skin conditions, wounds, eczema, burns, herpes simplex, and varicose ulcerations of the legs (19). Therapeutic benefit from the ointment was observed in 85.5% of the cases. The treatment periods ranged from 7.1 to 15.5 days (19).

Contraindications

External use

Allergy to the plant.

Internal use

Should not be used in serious conditions such as tuberculosis, leukosis, collagenosis, multiple sclerosis, AIDS, HIV infection, and autoimmune disorders.

Echinacea preparations should not be administered to people with a known allergy to any plant of the Asteraceae (*1*).

Warnings

No information available.

Precautions

General

Internal or external use should not exceed a period of 8 successive weeks (*1*).

Carcinogenesis, mutagenesis, impairment of fertility

Mutagenicity and carcinogenicity test results were negative (*3, 5, 35*). Doses up to a polysaccharide concentration of 500 mg/ml caused no increase in sister chromatid exchange or structural chromosome aberrations (*35*).

Pregnancy: teratogenic effects

There are no reliable studies on this subject. Therefore, administration of the drug during pregnancy is not recommended (*1*).

Nursing mothers

There are no reliable studies on this subject. Nursing mothers should not take the drug without consulting a physician (*1*).

Paediatric use

Oral administration of *Echinacea* preparations is not recommended for small children, except on the advice of a physician. Herba Echinaceae Purpureae may be used for external treatment of small superficial wounds.

Other precautions

No information available concerning drug interactions, drug and laboratory test interactions, or non-teratogenic effects on pregnancy.

Adverse reactions

Occasionally allergic reactions may occur owing to allergy to plants in the Asteraceae (Compositae).

Posology

Oral daily dosage of Herba Echinaceae Purpureae, 6–9 ml expressed juice (*1*) for no longer than 8 successive weeks (*1*). External use of semisolid preparations containing at least 15% pressed juice (*1*) for no longer than 8 successive weeks (*1*). Information on dosages for children is not available (*7*).

References

1. German Commission E Monograph, Echinaceae purpureae radix. *Bundesanzeiger*, 1992, 162:29 August.
2. McGregor RL. The taxonomy of the genus *Echinacea* (Compositae). *University of Kansas science bulletin*, 1968, 48:113–142.
3. Bauer R, Wagner H. *Echinacea* species as potential immunostimulatory drugs. In: Wagner H, Farnsworth NR, eds. *Economic and medicinal plants research*. Vol. 5. London, Academic Press, 1991:253–321.
4. Hänsel R et al., eds. *Hagers Handbuch der pharmazeutischen Praxis, Vol. 6*, 5th ed. Berlin, Springer, 1994.
5. Bisset NG. *Max Wichtl's herbal drugs & phytopharmaceuticals*. Boca Raton, FL, CRC Press, 1994.
6. Farnsworth NR, ed. *NAPRALERT database*. Chicago, University of Illinois at Chicago, IL, March 15, 1995 production (an on-line database available directly through the University of Illinois at Chicago or through the Scientific and Technical Network (STN) of Chemical Abstracts Services).
7. Awang DVC, Kindack DG. Herbal medicine, *Echinacea*. *Canadian pharmaceutical journal*, 1991, 124:512–516.
8. Bruneton J. *Pharmacognosy, phytochemistry, medicinal plants*. Paris, Lavoisier, 1995.
9. Iwu MM. *Handbook of African medicinal plants*. Boca Raton, FL, CRC Press, 1993.
10. Bauer R, Khan IA, Wagner H. Echinacea-Drogen Standardisierung mittels HPLC und DC. *Deutsche Apotheker Zeitung*, 1986, 126:1065–1070.
11. Bauer R, Khan IA, Wagner H. *Echinacea*: Nachweis einer Verfälschung von *Echinacea purpurea* (l.) Moench. mit *Parthenium integrifolium* L. *Deutsche Apotheker Zeitung*, 1987, 127:1325–1330.
12. Bauer R, Remiger P, Wagner H. Echinacea—Vergleichende DC- und HPLC-Analyse der Herba-drogen von *Echinacea purpurea*, *E. pallida* und *E. angustifolia* (3. Mitt.). *Deutsche Apotheker Zeitung*, 1988, 128:174–180.
13. Bauer R, Wagner H. Echinacea—Der Sonnenhut—Stand der Forschung. *Zeitschrift für Phytotherapie*, 1988, 9:151.
14. *Quality control methods for medicinal plant materials*. Geneva, World Health Organization, 1998.
15. *Deutsches Arzneibuch 1996. Vol. 2. Methoden der Biologie*. Stuttgart, Deutscher Apotheker Verlag, 1996.
16. *European pharmacopoeia*, 3rd ed. Strasbourg, Council of Europe, 1997.
17. *Guidelines for predicting dietary intake of pesticide residues*, 2nd rev. ed. Geneva, World Health Organization, 1997 (unpublished document WHO/FSF/FOS/97.7; available from Food Safety, WHO, 1211 Geneva 27, Switzerland).
18. Schöneberger D. The influence of immune-stimulating effects of pressed juice from *Echinacea purpurea* on the course and severity of colds. *Forum immunologie*, 1992, 8:2–12.
19. Viehmann P. Results of treatment with an Echinacea-based ointment. *Erfahrungsheilkunde*, 1978, 27:353–358.
20. Stotzem CD, Hungerland U, Mengs U. Influence of *Echinacea purpurea* on the phagocytosis of human granulocytes. *Medical science research*, 1992, 20:719–720.
21. Bittner E. *Die Wirkung von Echinacin auf die Funktion des Retikuloendothelialen Systems* [Dissertation]. Freiburg, University of Freiburg, 1969.
22. Haas H. *Arzneipflanzenkunde*. Mannheim, BI Wissenschaftsverlag, 1991:134–135.
23. Bauer R, Wagner H. *Echinacea. Handbuch für Apotheker und andere Naturwissenschaftler*. Stuttgart, Wissenschaftliche Verlagsgesellschaft, 1990.
24. Melchart D et al. Immunomodulation with *Echinacea*—a systematic review of controlled clinical trials. *Phytomedicine*, 1994, 1:245–254.

25. Büsing KH. Hyaluronidase inhibition by Echinacin. *Arzneimittel-Forschung*, 1952, 2:467–469.
26. Koch FE, Haase H. A modification of the spreading test in animal assays. *Arzneimittel-Forschung*, 1952, 2:464–467.
27. Bonadeo I, Bottazzi G, Lavazza M. Essenze-Profumi-Piante. *Officin–Aromi-Saponi-Cosmetici-Aerosol*, 1971, 53:281–295.
28. Zoutewelle G, van Wijk R. Effects of *Echinacea purpurea* extracts on fibroblast populated collagen lattice contraction. *Phytotherapy research*, 1990, 4:77–81.
29. Steinmüller C et al. Polysaccharides isolated from plant cell cultures of *Echinacea purpurea* enhance the resistance of immunosuppressed mice against systemic infections with *Candida albicans* and *Listeria monocytogenes*. *International journal for immunopharmacology*, 1993, 15:605–614.
30. Stempel M et al. Macrophage activation and induction of macrophage cytotoxicity by purified polysaccharide fractions from the plant *Echinacea purpurea*. *Infection and immunity*, 1984:845–849.
31. Luettig B et al. Macrophage activation by polysaccharide arabinogalactan isolated from plant cell cultures of *Echinacea purpurea*. *Journal of the National Cancer Institute*, 1989, 81:669–675.
32. Roesler J et al. Application of purified polysaccharides from cell cultures of the plant *Echinacea purpurea* to test subjects mediates activation of the phagocyte system. *International journal for immunopharmacology*, 1991, 13:931–941.
33. Cheminat A et al. Caffeoyl conjugates from *Echinacea* species: structures and biological activity. *Phytochemistry*, 1988, 27:2787–2794.
34. Müller-Jakic B et al. *In vitro* inhibition of cyclooxygenase and 5-lipoxygenase by alkamides from *Echinacea* and *Achillea* species. *Planta medica*, 1993:37–42.
35. Kraus C, Abel G, Schimmer O. Untersuchung einiger Pyrrolizidinalkaloide auf chromosomenschädigende Wirkung in menschlichen Lymphocyten *in vitro*. *Planta medica*, 1985, 51:89–91.

Herba Ephedrae

Definition

Herba Ephedrae consists of the dried stem or aerial part of *Ephedra sinica* Stapf or other ephedrine-containing *Ephedra* species (Ephedraceae) (*1–5*).

Synonyms

None.

Selected vernacular names

Amsania, budshur, chewa, Chinese ephedra, ephédra, horsetail, hum, huma, joint fir, khama, ma hoàng, ma huang, máhuáng, mao, maoh, maou, mao-kon, môc tac ma hoàng, mu-tsei-ma-huang, phok, san-ma-huang, shrubby, soma, song tuê ma hoàng, trung aa hoàng, tsao-ma-huang, tutgantha (*4–10*).

Description

Erect or prostrate, green, almost leafless shrub, 20–90 cm high. Branches erect, short, glaucous green, somewhat flat, 1.0–1.5 mm in diameter, with small sparse longitudinal striae, fasciated at the nodes; nodes reddish brown; internode 2.5–5.5 cm long × 2 mm in diameter. Small triangular leaves opposite, reduced to scales, barely 2 mm. Flowers in summer, unisexual, dioecious; male flowers pedunculate or nearly sessile, grouped in catkins composed of 4 to 8 pairs of flowers with about 8 anthers; female flowers biflorous, pedunculate with 3 or 4 pairs of bracts, the naked ovule surrounded by an urn-shaped perianth sheath, fruiting with often fleshy red succulent bracts, 2-seeded (*4, 7, 11*).

Plant material of interest: stem or aerial part

General appearance

Macroscopically, Herba Ephedrae occurs as thin cylindrical or ellipsoidal cylinder, 1–2 mm in diameter; 3.5–5.5 cm in length of internode; light green to yellow-green; numerous parallel vertical furrows on the surface; scaly leaves at the node portion; leaves, 2–4 mm in length, light brown to brown in colour, usually opposite at every node, adhering at the base to form a tubular sheath around the stem. Under a magnifying glass, the transverse section of the stem appears as circle and ellipse, the outer portion greyish green to yellow-green in colour, and the centre filled with a red-purple substance or hollow. When fractured at an internode, the outer part is fibrous and easily split vertically (*1*).

Organoleptic properties
Odour, slight; taste, slightly bitter and astringent, giving a slight sensation of numbness on the tongue (*1*).

Microscopic characteristics
The epidermal cells of the stem are covered with a moderately thick granular cuticle; the cells are polygonal or subrectangular, axially elongated, having straight anticlinal walls. The stomata are few and are of the ranunculaceous type with lignified appendages. The epidermis of the scaly leaf is covered with smooth (upper) or warty (lower) cuticle and consists of subrectangular to polygonal cells, having straight or sometimes slightly beaded anticlinal walls; few stomata are present resembling those of stem. The epidermis of the apical and marginal regions of the scaly leaf shows short papillae-like outgrowths. Chlorenchymatous palisade-like cells form the outer zone of the cortex; rounded ordinary parenchymatous cells form the inner zone of the cortex. Cortical parenchyma and pith cells contain an amorphous reddish brown substance. Non-lignified or lignified hypodermal and pericyclic fibres, which have thick walls, bear slit-like pits and blunt, slightly tapering, occasionally forked ends. The vessels of the secondary xylem of the stem are lignified with bordered pits, having rounded or oval apertures. The vessel segments have much inclined end walls, bearing foraminate perforation plates. The tracheids and fibrous tracheids of secondary xylem of the stem are lignified with bordered pits having oval or slit-like apertures. The fibres of the scaly leaf are lignified, usually irregular or nearly straight, having moderately thick walls and blunt or sometimes forked ends. Few, small, rounded, simple and compound starch granules with indistinct hilum are present in cortical parenchyma, pith, and medullary ray cells. Few, small prisms of calcium oxalate are present in the cortical parenchyma (*4*).

Powdered plant material
Powdered Herba Ephedrae is greyish green. Numerous thick fragments of cutinized outer walls of epidermis vary from colourless to varying shades of brown or red; numerous fragments of sclerenchyma fibres with extremely thickened, non-lignified to lignified walls, narrow, frequently indistinct lumina and sharp pointed ends; fragments of vascular tissue showing tracheids with bordered pores and occasional spiral and pitted tracheae; numerous chlorenchyma cells; starch grains simple, spheroidal to occasionally ovate, averaging up to 1.2 μm but occasionally up to 20 μm; fragments of epidermis with rectangular cells and granular contents, some with sunken elliptical stomata; fragments of

146

lignified or non-lignified pith parenchyma, some of the cells showing mucilage sacs; papillae; granules of calcium oxalate (*4, 6*).

Geographical distribution

Ephedra species are found in Afghanistan, Central America, China, India, regions of the Mediterranean, Mongolia, and North America (*4, 6–12*).

General identity tests

Macroscopic and microscopic examinations and microchemical tests for the presence of alkaloids with Mayer's reagent (*1–5, 7*).

Purity tests
Microbiology

The test for *Salmonella* spp. in Herba Ephedrae products should be negative. The maximum acceptable limits for other microorganisms are as follows (*13–15*). For preparation of decoction: aerobic bacteria—not more than 10^7/g; fungi—not more than 10^5/g; *Escherichia coli*—not more than 10^2/g. Preparations for internal use: aerobic bacteria—not more than 10^5/g or ml; fungi—not more than 10^4/g or ml; enterobacteria and certain Gram-negative bacteria—not more than 10^3/g or ml; *Escherichia coli*—0/g or ml.

Foreign organic matter

Woody stems, not more than 5% (*1*). Does not contain stems of Equisetaceae or Gramineae plants, nor any other foreign matter (*1*).

Total ash

Not more than 9% (3).

Acid-insoluble ash

Not more than 2% (*1*).

Moisture

Not more than 9% (3).

Pesticide residues

To be established in accordance with national requirements. Normally, the maximum residue limit of aldrin and dieldrin for Herba Ephedrae is not more than 0.05 mg/kg (*15*). For other pesticides, see WHO guidelines on quality control methods for medicinal plants (*13*) and guidelines for predicting dietary intake of pesticide residues (*16*).

Heavy metals

Recommended lead and cadmium levels are no more than 10 and 0.3 mg/kg, respectively, in the final dosage form of the plant material (*13*).

Radioactive residues

For analysis of strontium-90, iodine-131, caesium-134, caesium-137, and plutonium-239, see WHO guidelines on quality control methods for medicinal plants (*13*).

Other purity tests

Chemical, dilute ethanol-soluble extractive, and water-soluble extractive tests to be established in accordance with national requirements.

Chemical assays

Contains not less than 0.7% total alkaloids, calculated as ephedrine by high-performance liquid chromatography in the Japanese pharmacopoeia; or not less than 0.8% of total alkaloids, calculated as ephedrine in the Chinese pharmacopoeia (*1, 2*).

Thin-layer (*17*), gas–liquid (*18*) or high-performance liquid (*19*) chromatographic analysis for ephedrine and related alkaloids are available.

Major chemical constituents

The major active principle found in Herba Ephedrae is (−)-ephedrine in concentrations of 40–90% of the total alkaloid fraction, accompanied by (+)-pseudoephedrine. Other trace alkaloids in the alkaloid complex include (−)-norephedrine, (+)-norpseudoephedrine, (−)-methylephedrine and (+)-methylpseudoephedrine. The total alkaloid content can exceed 2% depending on the species (*20*). Not all *Ephedra* species contain ephedrine or alkaloids.

(−)-ephedrine   (−)-methylephedrine   (−)-norephedrine

(+)-pseudoephedrine   (+)-methylpseudoephedrine   (+)-norpseudoephedrine

Dosage forms
Powdered plant material; extracts and other galenicals. Store in well closed, light-resistant containers.

Medicinal uses
Uses supported by clinical data
Herba Ephedrae preparations are used in the treatment of nasal congestion due to hay fever, allergic rhinitis, acute coryza, common cold, and sinusitis. The drug is further used as a bronchodilator in the treatment of bronchial asthma (4, 8, 10, 21–23).

Uses described in pharmacopoeias and in traditional systems of medicine
Herba Ephedrae has been used for the treatment of urticaria, enuresis, narcolepsy, myasthenia gravis, and chronic postural hypotension (4, 8, 22, 23).

Uses described in folk medicine, not supported by experimental or clinical data
Other medical uses claimed for Herba Ephedrae preparations include its use as an analgesic, an antiviral agent, an antitussive and expectorant, an antibacterial, and an immune stimulant (10, 24, 25).

Clinical pharmacology
Two of the main active constituents of Herba Ephedrae, ephedrine and pseudoephedrine, are potent sympathomimetic drugs that stimulate α-, β_1- and β_2- adrenoceptors (22, 23). Pseudoephedrine's activity is similar to ephedrine, but its hypertensive effects and stimulation of the central nervous system are somewhat weaker. Part of ephedrine's peripheral action is due to the release of norepinephrine, but the drug also directly affects receptors. Tachyphylaxis develops to its peripheral actions, and rapidly repeated doses become less effective owing to the depletion of norepinephrine stores (22).

Cardiovascular actions
Like epinephrine (adrenaline), ephedrine excites the sympathetic nervous system, causing vasoconstriction and cardiac stimulation. Ephedrine differs from epinephrine in that it is orally active, has a much longer duration of action, and has more pronounced activity in the central nervous system, but is much less potent (22, 23). The drug stimulates the heart rate, as well as cardiac output, and increases peripheral resistance, thereby producing a lasting rise in blood pressure. The cardiovascular effects of ephedrine persist up to ten times as long as

149

those of epinephrine (22). Ephedrine elevates both the systolic and diastolic pressures and pulse pressure. Renal and splanchnic blood flows are decreased, while coronary, cerebral, and muscle blood flows are increased (22, 23).

Bronchodilator and nasal decongestant

Ephedrine, like epinephrine, relaxes bronchial muscles and is a potent bronchodilator owing to its activation of the β-adrenoceptors in the lungs (22, 23). Bronchial muscle relaxation is less pronounced but more sustained with ephedrine than with epinephrine. As a consequence, ephedrine should be used only in patients with mild cases of acute asthma and in chronic cases that require maintenance medication. Ephedrine, like other sympathomimetics with α-receptor activity, causes vasoconstriction and blanching when applied topically to nasal and pharyngeal mucosal surfaces (22, 23). Continued, prolonged use of these preparations (>3 days) may cause rebound congestion and chronic rhinitis (26). Both ephedrine and pseudoephedrine are useful orally as nasal decongestants in cases of allergic rhinitis, but they may not be very effective for the treatment of nasal congestion due to colds.

Central nervous system

Mydriasis occurs after local application of ephedrine (3–5%) to the eye, but the effect lasts for only a few hours (22). Ephedrine is of little value as a mydriatic in the presence of inflammation. The activity of the smooth muscles of the uterus is usually reduced by ephedrine; consequently, the drug has been used to relieve the pain of dysmenorrhoea (22).

Ephedrine is a potent stimulator of the central nervous system. The effects of the drug may last for several hours after oral administration (23). Thus, preparations containing Herba Ephedrae have been promoted for use in weight reduction and thermogenesis (fat burning) (27, 28). The safety and effectiveness of these preparations is currently an issue of debate and requires further investigation (29).

Ephedrine stimulates the α-adrenoceptors of the smooth muscle cells of the bladder base, which increases the resistance to the outflow of urine (23). Thus Herba Ephedrae has been used in the treatment of urinary incontinence and nocturnal enuresis.

Contraindications

Herba Ephedrae should not be administered to patients with coronary thrombosis, diabetes, glaucoma, heart disease, hypertension, thyroid disease, impaired circulation of the cerebrum, phaeochromocytoma, or enlarged prostate (10, 21, 23). Co-administration of Herba Ephedrae preparations with monoamine oxidase inhibitors is contraindicated as the combination may cause severe, possibly fatal, hypertension (23).

150

Warnings

Dosage should be reduced or treatment discontinued if nervousness, tremor, sleeplessness, loss of appetite or nausea occurs. Not for children under 6 years of age. Keep out of the reach of children (30). Continued, prolonged use may cause dependency.

Precautions

General

Insomnia may occur with continued use of Herba Ephedrae preparations (23).

Drug interactions

In combination with cardiac glycosides or halothane, may cause heart rhythm disturbances (21); with guanethidine, may cause an enhancement of sympathomimetic effect (21); with monoamine oxidase inhibitors, can cause severe, possibly fatal, hypertension (26); with ergot alkaloid derivatives or oxytocin, may increase risk of high blood pressure (21).

Carcinogenesis, mutagenesis, impairment of fertility

Extracts of *Ephedra sinica* are not mutagenic in the *Salmonella*/microsome reversion assay (31).

Pregnancy: teratogenic effects

Ephedra sinica did not have any teratogenic effects *in vivo* (32).

Pregnancy: nonteratogenic effects

Ephedra sinica is not abortifacient in rats (32). Clinical studies in humans are not available; therefore, use of the drug during pregnancy is not generally recommended.

Nursing mothers

There are no reliable studies on this subject. Therefore, nursing mothers should not take Herba Ephedrae without consulting a physician.

Paediatric use

Herba Ephedrae should not be administered to children under 6 years of age.

Other precautions

No information available concerning drug and laboratory test interactions.

Adverse reactions

In large doses Herba Ephedrae products can cause nervousness, headaches, insomnia, dizziness, palpitations, skin flushing and tingling, and vomiting (21).

The principal adverse effects of ephedrine and Herba Ephedrae are stimulation of the central nervous system, nausea, tremors, tachycardia, and urine retention (*24*). Continued, prolonged use (>3 days) of topical preparations containing Herba Ephedrae, for the treatment of nasal congestion, may cause rebound congestion and chronic rhinitis (*26*). Continued prolonged use of oral preparations may cause dependency (*21*).

Posology

Crude plant material: 1–6 g for decoction daily (*8, 21*). Liquid extract (1:1 in 45% alcohol): 1–3 ml daily (*21*). Tincture (1:4 in 45% alcohol): 6–8 ml daily (*21*).

References

1. *The pharmacopoeia of Japan XII*. Tokyo, The Society of Japanese Pharmacopoeia, 1991.
2. *Pharmacopoeia of the People's Republic of China* (English ed.). Guangzhou, Guangdong Science and Technology Press, 1992.
3. *Deutsches Arzneibuch 1996*. Stuttgart, Deutscher Apotheker Verlag, 1996.
4. *African pharmacopoeia*, 1st ed. Lagos, Organization of African Unity, Scientific, Technical & Research Commission, 1985.
5. *Vietnam materia medica*. Hanoi, Ministry of Health, 1972.
6. Hsu HY. *Oriental materia medica, a concise guide*. Long Beach, CA, Oriental Healing Arts Institute, 1986.
7. Youngken HW. *Textbook of pharmacognosy*, 6th ed. Philadelphia, Blakiston, 1950.
8. *Medicinal plants in China*. Manila, World Health Organization, 1989 (WHO Regional Publications, Western Pacific Series, No. 2).
9. *The Indian pharmaceutical codex. Vol. I. Indigenous drugs*. New Delhi, Council of Scientific & Industrial Research, 1953.
10. Farnsworth NR, ed. *NAPRALERT database*. Chicago, University of Illinois at Chicago, IL, March 15, 1995 production (an on-line database available directly through the University of Illinois at Chicago or through the Scientific and Technical Network (STN) of Chemical Abstracts Services).
11. Tyler VE, Brady LR, Robbers JE, eds. *Pharmacognosy*, 9th ed. Philadelphia, Lea & Febiger, 1988.
12. Morton JF. *Major medicinal plants: botany, culture and use*. Springfield, IL, Charles C Thomas, 1977.
13. *Quality control methods for medicinal plant materials*. Geneva, World Health Organization, 1998.
14. *Deutsches Arzneibuch 1996. Vol. 2. Methoden der Biologie*. Stuttgart, Deutscher Apotheker Verlag, 1996.
15. *European pharmacopoeia*, 3rd ed. Strasbourg, Council of Europe, 1997.
16. *Guidelines for predicting dietary intake of pesticide residues*, 2nd rev. ed. Geneva, World Health Organization, 1997 (unpublished document WHO/FSF/FOS/97.7; available from Food Safety, WHO, 1211 Geneva 27, Switzerland).
17. Zhang JS, Tian Z, Lou ZC. Detection and identification of the alkaloids in Herba *Ephedra* (Ma huang) by chemical tests and HPTLC. *Yaowu fenxi zazhi*, 1992, 12:38–41.
18. Cui JF et al. Analysis of alkaloids in Chinese *Ephedra* species by gas chromatographic methods. *Phytochemical analysis*, 1991, 2:116–119.

19. Zhang JS, Tian Z, Lou ZC. Simultaneous determination of six alkaloids in Ephedra Herba by high performance liquid chromatography. *Planta medica*, 1988, 54:69–70.
20. Bruneton J. *Pharmacognosy, phytochemistry, medicinal plants*. Paris, Lavoisier, 1995.
21. German Commission E Monograph, Ephedrae herba. *Bundesanzeiger*, 1991, 11:17 January.
22. *Goodman and Gilman's the pharmacological basis of therapeutics*, 6th ed. New York, MacMillan, 1985:169–170.
23. Goodman LS et al. *Goodman and Gilman's the pharmacological basis of therapeutics*, 8th ed. New York, MacMillan, 1993:213–214.
24. Kim TH, Yang KS, Hwang EZ, Park SB. Effect of Ephedrae Herba on the immune response in mice. *Korean journal of pharmacognosy*, 1991, 22:183–191.
25. Konno C et al. Ephedroxane, anti-inflammatory principal of *Ephedra* herbs. *Phytochemistry*, 1979, 18:697–698.
26. *Handbook of non-prescription drugs*, 8th ed. Washington, DC, American Pharmaceutical Association, 1986.
27. Daley PA et al. Ephedrine, caffeine and aspirin: safety and efficacy for the treatment of human obesity. *International journal of obesity*, 1993, 17(Suppl. 1):S73–S78.
28. Pardoe AU, Gorecki DKJ, Jones D. Ephedrine alkaloid patterns in herbal products based on Ma Huang (*Ephedra sinica*). *International journal of obesity*, 1993, 17(Suppl. 1):S82.
29. Adverse events with *Ephedra* and other botanical dietary supplements. *FDA medical bulletin*, 1994, 24:3.
30. Policy Statement on *Ephedra sinica* (Ma huang). Austin, TX, American Herbal Products Association 1994.
31. Morimoto I et al. Mutagenicity screening of crude drugs with *Bacillus subtilis* rec-assay and *Salmonella*/microsome reversion assay. *Mutation research*, 1982, 97:81–102.
32. Lee EB. Teratogenicity of the extracts of crude drugs. *Korean journal of pharmacognosy*, 1982, 13:116–121.

Folium Ginkgo

Definition

Folium Ginkgo consists of the dried whole leaf of *Ginkgo biloba* L. (Ginkgoaceae).

Synonyms

Pterophyllus salisburiensis Nelson, *Salisburia adiantifolia* Smith, *Salisburia macrophylla* C. Koch (*1–4*).

Selected vernacular names

Eun-haeng, gin-nan, ginkgo, ginkgo balm, ginkgo leaves, ginkyo, ginan, icho, ityo, kew tree, maidenhair tree, pei-wen, temple balm, yin guo, yinhsing (*1–5*).

Description

A monotypic dioecious plant that is the only living representative of the Ginkgoales. It has a grey bark, reaches a height of 35 m and a diameter of 3–4 m (sometimes up to 7 m), and has fan-like leaves that are deciduous, alternate, lengthily petiolate, bilobate, base wedge-shaped, 6–9 cm broad (sometimes up to 15–20 cm), turning yellow in autumn. Venation dichotomously branching, seemingly parallel. Staminate and ovulate strobili borne on separate trees; staminate strobili consisting of naked pairs of anthers in catkin-like clusters; ovulate strobili in the form of long, slender, fused stalks bearing a single naked ovule which is fertilized by motile sperm cells, developing into 2 seeds. Seeds yellow when mature, foul-smelling, drupe-like, the middle layer of integument becoming hard or stone-like, the outer layer fleshy (*3, 4*).

Plant material of interest: dried leaf

The kernel (nut, seed) is used in Chinese medicine (*6, 7*).

General appearance

The leaves are green, grey-yellow, brown or blackish; the upper side of a leaf may be somewhat darker than the underside. The leaves are fan-shaped, long-petioled and have two lobes with forked veins radiating from the petiole end (*2, 4, 8*).

Organoleptic properties
Ginkgo leaves have a weak characteristic odour (*2, 4, 8*).

Microscopic characteristics
Young leaves have abundant trichomes that become confined to the petiole base as the leaf ages. While the leaves have no midrib, dichotomous venation with regular, numerous branching parallel veins arises from two vascular strands within the petiole. Stomata occur almost exclusively on the lower surface of the leaf. The epidermis of the upper and underside of the leaf consists of undulated, irregular, mostly long extended cells. In the cross-section, the epidermal cells appear nearly isodiametric and from above appear to be slightly undulated, with the upper cells appearing larger. The outer walls of the epidermal cells are covered with a more or less thin layer of cuticle. In the area of vascular bundles there are remarkable long extended narrow cells with slightly undulated walls. Numerous druses of calcium oxalate occur near the vascular bundles (*2, 4*).

Powdered plant material
The colour of the powder agrees with that of the leaves. The powder shows fragments of the epidermis with wavelike indentations irregular in form with generally elongated cells; large stomal openings of the anisocytic type; markedly elongated, narrow cells with only weakly undulated walls in the vascular areas and without marked indentations. The equifacial mesophyll comprises excretory vesicles, secretory cells, and idioblasts, as well as intermittent calcium oxalate druses, in the region of the vascular fascicles (*2, 8*).

Geographical distribution
Native to China, but grown as an ornamental shade tree in Australia, south-east Asia, Europe, Japan, and the United States of America (*1–3, 6*). It is commercially cultivated in France and the United States of America (*2*).

General identity tests
Macroscopic and microscopic examinations (*2, 8*). Thin-layer chromatographic analysis for the presence of the characteristic flavonoids, ginkgolides, and bilobalide (*9*); high-performance liquid chromatographic analysis for flavonoids (*10*), ginkgolides, and bilobalide (*2*); and gas–liquid chromatographic evaluation of ginkgolides and bilobalide (*11*).

Purity tests
Microbiology
The test for *Salmonella* spp. in Folium Ginkgo should be negative. The maximum acceptable limits of other microorganisms are as follows (*12–14*). For preparation of decoction: aerobic bacteria—not more than 10^7/g; fungi—not

more than 10^5/g; *Escherichia coli*—not more than 10^2/g. Preparations for internal use: aerobic bacteria—not more than 10^5/g or ml; fungi—not more than 10^4/g or ml; enterobacteria and certain Gram-negative bacteria—not more than 10^3/g or ml; *Escherichia coli*—0/g or ml.

Foreign organic matter

Not more than 5% of twigs and not more than 2% of other foreign matter (*15*).

Total ash

Not more than 11% (*15*).

Pesticide residues

To be established in accordance with national requirements. Normally, the maximum residue limit of aldrin and dieldrin in Folium Ginkgo is not more than 0.05 mg/kg (*14*). For other pesticides, see WHO guidelines on quality control methods for medicinal plants (*12*), and guidelines for predicting dietary intake of pesticide residues (*16*).

Heavy metals

Recommended lead and cadmium levels are not more than 10 and 0.3 mg/kg, respectively, in the final dosage form of the plant material (*12*).

Radioactive residues

For analysis of strontium-90, iodine-131, caesium-134, caesium-137, and plutonium-239, see WHO guidelines on quality control methods for medicinal plants (*12*).

Other purity tests

Acid-insoluble ash, acid-insoluble extractive, chemical, and moisture tests to be established in accordance with national requirements.

Chemical assays

Flavonoids not less than 0.5% calculated as flavonol glycosides or 0.2–0.4% calculated as aglycones (*17*); also contains ginkgolides (0.06–0.23%) and bilobalide (up to 0.26%) (*2*, *17*).

Qualitative and quantitative determination of flavonoid glycosides is carried out after hydrolysis to the aglycones kaempferol, quercetin, and isorhamnetin. The qualitative presence or absence of biflavones (*17*) is determined by high-performance liquid chromatography; and qualitative and quantitative determination of the diterpene ginkgolides and sesquiterpene bilobalide by high-performance liquid chromatography (*2*, *18*) or gas–liquid chromatography (*11*).

Certain commercial products used for clinical and experimental biological studies, e.g. EGb 761 and LI 1370, do not contain biflavones.

Major chemical constituents

Folium Ginkgo contains a wide variety of phytochemicals, including alkanes, lipids, sterols, benzenoids, carotenoids, phenylpropanoids, carbohydrates, flavonoids, and terpenoids (*18, 19*). The major constituents are flavonoids of which mono-, di-, and tri-glycosides and coumaric acid esters that are based on the flavonols kaempferol and quercetin dominate. Lesser quantities of glycosides are derived from isorhamnetin, myricetin, and 3′-methylmyricetin. Non-glycosidic biflavonoids, catechins, and proanthocyanidins are also present (*15*). Characteristic constituents of this plant material are the unique diterpene lactones ginkgolides A, B, C, J, and M and the sesquiterpene lactone bilobalide (*17*). Representative structures of the major and characteristic constituents are presented below.

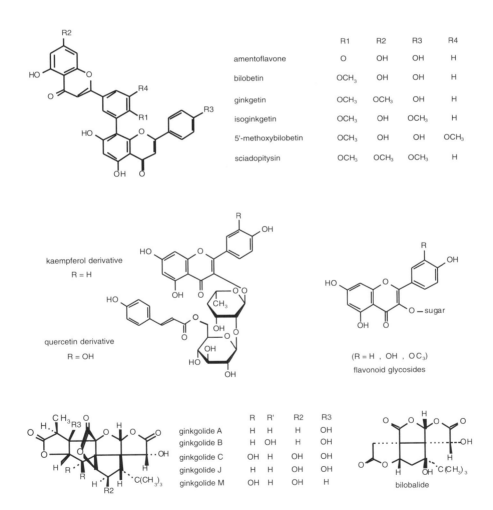

	R1	R2	R3	R4
amentoflavone	O	OH	OH	H
bilobetin	OCH₃	OH	OH	H
ginkgetin	OCH₃	OCH₃	OH	H
isoginkgetin	OCH₃	OH	OCH₃	H
5′-methoxybilobetin	OCH₃	OH	OH	OCH₃
sciadopitysin	OCH₃	OCH₃	OCH₃	H

	R	R'	R2	R3
ginkgolide A	H	H	H	OH
ginkgolide B	H	OH	H	OH
ginkgolide C	OH	H	OH	OH
ginkgolide J	H	H	OH	OH
ginkgolide M	OH	H	OH	H

157

Dosage forms

Standardized extracts (dry extracts from dried leaves, extracted with acetone and water, drug:extract ratio 35–67:1) contain 22–27% flavone glycosides and 5–7% terpene lactones, of which approximately 2.8–3.4% consists of ginkgolides A, B, and C and 2.6–3.2% bilobalide. The level of ginkgolic acids is below 5 mg/kg. Coated tablets and solution for oral administration are prepared from standardized purified extracts (*20, 21*).

Medicinal uses

Uses supported by clinical data

Extracts as described above (Dosage forms) have been used for symptomatic treatment of mild to moderate cerebrovascular insufficiency (demential syndromes in primary degenerative dementia, vascular dementia, and mixed forms of both) with the following symptoms: memory deficit, disturbance in concentration, depressive emotional condition, dizziness, tinnitus, and headache (*1, 3, 20–22*). Such extracts are also used to improve pain-free walking distance in people with peripheral arterial occlusive disease such as intermittent claudication, Raynaud disease, acrocyanosis, and post-phlebitis syndrome, and to treat inner ear disorders such as tinnitus and vertigo of vascular and involutive origin (*20, 23–27*). Extracts and doses other than those described in Dosage forms and Posology are used for similar but milder indications (*28, 29*).

Uses described in pharmacopoeias and in traditional systems of medicine

None.

Uses described in folk medicine, not supported by experimental or clinical data

As a vermifuge, to induce labour, for the treatment of bronchitis, chronic rhinitis, chilblains, arthritis, and oedema (*3, 5*).

Pharmacology

Experimental pharmacology

Cerebrovascular insufficiency and peripheral vascular diseases

In vitro studies. A standardized extract of *Ginkgo biloba* (100 µg/ml) did not produce isometrically recordable contractions in isolated rabbit aorta but did potentiate the contractile effect of norepinephrine (*30*). Higher concentrations ($EC_{50} \approx 1.0$ mg/ml) produced a concentration-dependent contraction that could be antagonized by the α-adrenoceptor-blocking agent phentolamine (*30*). Both cocaine and desipramine, inhibitors of catecholamine re-uptake, potentiated the contractile effect of norepinephrine but inhibited the contractile effects of a standardized extract of G. *biloba* and tyramine (30). The results of these experiments indicate that the contractile action of G. *biloba* may be due to the release of catecholamines from endogenous tissue reserves, and this activity may explain some of the therapeutic effects of the drug in humans (e.g. improvement in cerebrovascular and peripheral vascular insufficiency) (1, 30). On the basis of experiments comparing the effects of an extract of G. *biloba*, phentolamine, propranolol, gallopamil, theophylline, and papaverine on the biphasic contractile response of norepinephrine in isolated rat aorta, researchers concluded that G. *biloba* had musculotropic action similar to that of papaverine (31). This activity was previously reported for the flavonoids quercetin, kaempferol, and isorhamnetin, isolated from the leaves of G. *biloba* (32). The flavonoids and papaverine both inhibit 3′,5′-cyclic-GMP phosphodiesterase, which in turn induces endothelium-dependent relaxation in isolated rabbit aorta by potentiating the effects of endothelium-derived relaxing factors (1).

In vitro studies have demonstrated that G. *biloba* extracts scavenge free radicals (33–37). *Ginkgo biloba* extracts have been reported to reduce free radical-lipid peroxidation induced by NADPH-Fe^{3+} systems in rat microsomes (33), and to protect human liver microsomes from lipid peroxidation caused by ciclosporin A (34). The extract also inhibits the generation of reactive oxygen radicals in human leukocytes treated with phorbol myristate acetate (35). The antioxidant action of G. *biloba* extract may prolong the half-life of endothelium-derived relaxing factor by scavenging superoxide anions (36, 37). Both the flavonoid and terpenoid constituents of G. *biloba* appear to aid the free-radical scavenging activity of the drug (37).

Ginkgo biloba extract protected against brain tissue hypoxic damage *in vitro*. The ginkgolides and bilobalide were responsible for the antihypoxic activity of the extract (38, 39). Ginkgolides A and B have been shown to protect rat hippocampal neurons against ischaemic damage, which may be due to their ability to act as antagonists to receptors for platelet-activating factor (PAF) (40–42).

In vivo studies. Oral administration of G. *biloba* extract protected rats against induced cerebral ischaemia (43–45). Intravenous perfusion of a G. *biloba* extract prevented the development of multiple cerebral infarction in dogs injected with fragments of an autologous clot into a common carotid artery (46). These data suggest that G. *biloba* extract, administered after clot formation, may have some beneficial effects on acute cerebral infarction or ischaemia caused by embolism (1). Other experiments demonstrated that animals treated with G. *biloba* extract survived under hypoxic conditions longer than did untreated controls (47, 48). Longer survival was due not only to significant improvements in cerebral blood flow, but also to an increase in the level of glucose and ATP (44, 48–50). Other studies have shown that a G. *biloba* extract devoid of ginkgolides but containing bilobalide had protective activity when administered intraperitoneally to mice with induced hypobaric hypoxia (51, 52). Intravenous infusion of G. *biloba* extract significantly increased pial arteriolar diameter in cats (53) and improved cerebral blood flow in rats (*53*). The active constituents of *G. biloba* responsible for increasing cerebral blood flow appeared to be the non-flavonoid compounds (*54*); ginkgolide B may be responsible for this action owing to its PAF-antagonist activity (*55, 56*). Furthermore, intravenous administration of a standardized *G. biloba* extract and ginkgolide B to rats showed that the extract, but not ginkgolide B, decreased the brain's use of glucose (*57*).

The constituents of *G. biloba* responsible for its anti-ischaemic activity remain undefined. The flavonoids, ginkgolides, and bilobalide have all been suggested, but it is possible that other constituents may be responsible.

An extract of *G. biloba* was effective in the *in vivo* treatment of cerebral oedema, a condition of excessive hydration of neural tissues owing to damage by neurotoxic agents (such as triethyltin) or trauma (*58–60*). Bilobalide appeared to play a significant role in the antioedema effect (*61, 62*). Oral or subcutaneous administration of an extract of *G. biloba* to rats with acute and chronic phases of adriamycin-induced paw inflammation partially reversed the increase in brain water, sodium, and calcium and the decrease in brain potassium associated with sodium arachidonate-induced cerebral infarction (*63*).

Mice treated with a standardized extract of *G. biloba* (100 mg/kg, orally for 4–8 weeks) showed improved memory and learning during appetitive operant conditioning (*64*).

Vestibular and auditory effects

Ginkgo biloba extract improved the sum of action potentials in the cochlea and acoustic nerve in cases of acoustically produced sound trauma in guinea-pigs (*1, 65*). The mechanism reduced the metabolic damage to the cochlea. Oral or parenteral administration of a standardized *G. biloba* extract to mice (2 mg/kg) improved the ultrastructure qualities of vestibular sensory epithelia when the tissue was fixed by vascular perfusion (*66*). Improvement was due to the effects of the drug on capillary permeability and general microcirculation (*1, 66*).

Positive effects on vestibular compensation were observed after administration of *G. biloba* extract (50 mg/kg intraperitoneally) to rats and cats that had undergone unilateral vestibular neurectomy (*67, 68*).

Antagonism of platelet-activating factor (PAF)

The ginkgolides, and in particular ginkgolide B, are known antagonists of PAF (*69–73*). PAF is a potent inducer of platelet aggregation, neutrophil degranulation, and oxygen radical production leading to increased microvascular permeability and bronchoconstriction. Intravenous injections of PAF induced transient thrombocytopenia in guinea-pigs, which was accompanied by non-histamine-dependent bronchospasm (*69, 70*). Ginkgolide B has been shown to be a potent inhibitor of PAF-induced thrombocytopenia and bronchoconstriction (*71, 72*). PAF or ovalbumin-induced bronchoconstriction in sensitized guinea-pigs was inhibited by an intravenous injection of ginkgolide B (1–3 mg/kg) 5 minutes prior to challenge (*73*).

Clinical pharmacology

Cerebral insufficiency

Cerebral insufficiency is an inexact term to describe a collection of symptoms associated with dementia (*21*, *22*). In dementia owing to degeneration with neuronal loss and impaired neurotransmission, decline of intellectual function is associated with disturbances in the supply of oxygen and glucose. In clinical studies *G. biloba* effectively managed symptoms of cerebral insufficiency including difficulty in concentration and memory, absent-mindedness, confusion, lack of energy, tiredness, decreased physical performance, depressive mood, anxiety, dizziness, tinnitus, and headache (*20–22*). Several mechanisms of action of *G. biloba* have been described: effects on blood circulation such as the vasoregulating activity of arteries, capillaries, veins (increased blood flow); rheological effects (decreased viscosity, by PAF-receptor antagonism); metabolic changes such as increased tolerance to anoxia; beneficial influence on neurotransmitter disturbances; and prevention of damage to membranes by free radicals (*22*). Treatment of humans with *G. biloba* extract has been shown to improve global and local cerebral blood flow and microcirculation (*74–76*), to protect against hypoxia (*77*), to improve blood rheology, including inhibition of platelet aggregation (*74*, *78–81*), to improve tissue metabolism (*82*), and to reduce capillary permeability (*83*).

A critical review of 40 published clinical trials (up to the end of 1990) using an orally administered *G. biloba* extract in the treatment of cerebral insufficiency concluded that only eight of the studies were well performed (*21*, *22*). Almost all trials reported at least a partially positive response at dosages of 120–160 mg a day (standardized extract) and treatment for at least 4–6 weeks (*21*, *22*). In a comparison of *G. biloba* with published trials using co-dergocrine (dihydroergotoxine), a mixture of ergoloid mesilates used for the same purpose, both *G. biloba* extract and co-dergocrine showed similar efficacy. A direct comparison of 120 mg of *G. biloba* standardized extract and 4.5 mg co-dergocrine showed similar improvements in both groups after 6 weeks (*84*).

A meta-analysis of 11 placebo-controlled, randomized double-blind studies in elderly patients given *G. biloba* extract (150 mg orally per day) for cerebral insufficiency concluded that eight studies were well performed (*85*). Significant differences were found for all analysed single symptoms, indicating the superiority of the drug in comparison with the placebo. Analysis of the total score of clinical symptoms indicated that seven studies confirmed the effectiveness of *G. biloba* extract, while one study was inconclusive (*85*).

Peripheral arterial occlusive disease

The effectiveness of *G. biloba* extract in the treatment of intermittent claudication (peripheral arterial occlusive disease Fontaine stage II), as compared with a placebo, was demonstrated in placebo-controlled, double-blind clinical trials by a statistically significant increase in walking distance (*1*, *23*, *24*). Sixty patients with peripheral arterial occlusive disease in Fontaine stage IIb who were treated with the drug (120–160 mg for 24 weeks) and underwent physical training also clearly increased their walking distance (*25*).

Out of 15 controlled trials (up to the end of 1990) only two (*23*, *24*) were of acceptable quality (*22–24*). The results of both studies were positive and showed an increase in walking distance in patients with intermittent claudication after 6 months (*23*), and an improvement of pain at rest in patients treated with 200 mg of *G. biloba* extract for 8 weeks (*24*).

After meta-analysis of five placebo-controlled clinical trials (up to the end of 1991) of *G. biloba* extract in patients with peripheral arterial disease, investigators concluded that the extract exerted a highly significant therapeutic effect (*26*).

Vertigo and tinnitus

Ginkgo biloba extracts have been used clinically in the treatment of inner ear disorders such as hearing loss, vertigo, and tinnitus. In a placebo-controlled, double-blind study of 68 patients with vertiginous syndrome of recent onset, treatment with *G. biloba* extract (120–160 mg daily, for 4–12 weeks) produced a statistically significant improvement as compared with the placebo group (*27*).

The results of clinical studies on the treatment of tinnitus have been contradictory. At least six clinical studies have assessed the effectiveness of *G. biloba* extract for the treatment of tinnitus. Three studies reported positive results (*86*, *87*, *88*). One multicentre, randomized, double-blind, 13-month study of 103 patients with tinnitus showed that all patients improved, irrespective of the prognostic factor, when treated with *G. biloba* extract (160 mg/day for 3 months) (*86*). Three other clinical trials reported negative outcomes (*89–91*). Statistical analysis of an open study (80 patients) without placebo, coupled with a double-blind, placebo-controlled part (21 patients), demonstrated that a concentrated *G. biloba* extract (29.2 mg/day for 2 weeks) had no effect on tinnitus (*91*).

Contraindications

Hypersensitivity to *G. biloba* preparations (*20*).

Warnings

No information available.

Precautions

Carcinogenesis, mutagenesis, impairment of fertility

Investigations with *G. biloba* extracts have shown no effects that were mutagenic, carcinogenic, or toxic to reproduction (*20*).

Pregnancy: non-teratogenic effects

The safety of Folium Ginkgo for use during pregnancy has not been established.

Nursing mothers

Excretion of Folium Ginkgo into breast milk and its effects on the newborn have not been established.

Other precautions

No information is available concerning general precautions or drug interactions, drug and laboratory test interactions, teratogenic effects on pregnancy, or paediatric use.

Adverse reactions

Headaches, gastrointestinal disturbances, and allergic skin reactions are possible adverse effects (*20*).

Posology

Dried extract (as described in Dosage forms), 120–240 mg daily in 2 or 3 divided doses (*2*); 40 mg extract is equivalent to 1.4–2.7 g leaves (*20*). Fluid extract (1 : 1), 0.5 ml 3 times a day (*1, 2*).

References

1. DeFeudis FV. *Ginkgo biloba extract (egb 761): pharmacological activities and clinical applications.* Paris, Elsevier, Editions Scientifiques, 1991:1187.
2. Hänsel R et al., eds. *Hagers Handbuch der pharmazeutischen Praxis*, Vol. 6, 5th ed. Berlin, Springer-Verlag, 1994.
3. Squires R. *Ginkgo biloba. Australian traditional medicine society* (ATOMS), 1995:9–14.
4. Huh H, Staba EJ. The botany and chemistry of *Ginkgo biloba* L. *Journal of herbs, spices and medicinal plants*, 1992, 1:91–124.
5. Farnsworth NR, ed. *NAPRALERT database.* University of Illinois at Chicago, IL, August 8, 1995 production (an on-line database available directly through the University of Illinois at Chicago or through the Scientific and Technical Network (STN) of Chemical Abstracts Services).
6. Keys JD. *Chinese herbs, their botany, chemistry and pharmacodynamics.* Rutland, VT, CE Tuttle, 1976:30–31.
7. *Pharmacopoeia of the People's Republic of China* (English ed.). Guangzhou, Guangdong Science and Technology Press, 1992:64.
8. Melzheimer V. *Ginkgo biloba* L. aus Sicht der systematischen und angewandten Botanik. *Pharmazie in unserer Zeit*, 1992, 21:206–214.
9. Van Beek TA, Lelyveld GP. Thin layer chromatography of bilobalide and ginkgolides A, B, C and J on sodium acetate impregnated silica gel. *Phytochemical analysis*, 1993, 4:109–114.
10. Hasler A, Meier B, Sticher O. Identification and determination of the flavonoids from *Ginkgo biloba* by HPLC. *Journal of chromatography*, 1992, 605:41–48.
11. Hasler A, Meier B. Determination of terpenes from *Ginkgo biloba* by GLC. *Pharmacy and pharmacology letters*, 1992, 2:187–190.

12. *Quality control methods for medicinal plant materials.* Geneva, World Health Organization, 1998.
13. *Deutsches Arzneibuch 1996. Vol. 2. Methoden der Biologie.* Stuttgart, Deutscher Apotheker Verlag, 1996.
14. *European pharmacopoeia,* 3rd ed. Strasbourg, Council of Europe, 1997.
15. Sticher O. Biochemical, pharmaceutical and medical perspectives of *Ginkgo* preparations. In: *New Drug Development from Herbal Medicines in Neuropsychopharmacology. Symposium of the XIXth CINP Congress, Washington, DC, June 27–July 1, 1994.*
16. *Guidelines for predicting dietary intake of pesticide residues,* 2nd rev. ed. Geneva, World Health Organization, 1997 (unpublished document WHO/FSF/FOS/97.7; available from Food Safety, WHO, 1211 Geneva 27, Switzerland).
17. Sticher O. Quality of *Ginkgo* preparations. *Planta medica,* 1993, 59:2–11.
18. Van Beek TA et al. Determination of ginkgolides and bilobalide in *Ginkgo biloba* leaves and phytochemicals. *Journal of chromatography,* 1991, 543:375–387.
19. Hasler A et al. Complex flavonol glycosides from the leaves of *Ginkgo biloba. Phytochemistry,* 1992, 31:1391.
20. German Commission E monograph, Trockenextrakt (35–67:1) aus *Ginkgo-biloba-*Blättern Extrakt mit Aceton-Wasser. *Bundesanzeiger,* 1994, 46:7361–7362.
21. Kleijnen J, Knipschild P. *Ginkgo biloba. Lancet,* 1992, 340:1136–1139.
22. Kleijnen J, Knipschild P. *Ginkgo biloba* for cerebral insufficiency. *British journal of clinical pharmacology,* 1992, 34:352–358.
23. Bauer U. Six month double-blind randomized clinical trial of *Ginkgo biloba* extract versus placebo in two parallel groups in patients suffering from peripheral arterial insufficiency. *Arzneimittel-Forschung,* 1984, 34:716–720.
24. Saudreau F, Serise JM, Pillet J. Efficacité de l'extrait de *Ginkgo biloba* dans le traitement des artériopathies obliterantes chroniques des membres inferieurs au stade III de la classification de Fontaine. *Journal malade vasculare,* 1989, 14:177–182.
25. Blume J et al. Placebokontrollierte Doppelblindstudie zur Wirksamkeit von *Ginkgo biloba*-Spezialextrakt EGb 761 bei austrainierten Patienten mit Claudicatio intermittens. *VASA,* 1996, 2:1–11.
26. Schneider B. *Ginkgo biloba* Extrakt bei peripheren arteriellen Verschlußkrankheiten. *Arzneimittel-Forschung,* 1992, 42:428–436.
27. Haguenauer JP et al. Traitement des troubles de l'equilibre par l'extrait de *Ginkgo biloba. Presse medicale,* 1986, 15:1569–1572.
28. Coeur et circulation, 02.97.0 Troubles de l'artériosclérose. *IKS monthly bulletin,* 1994, 6:532–533.
29. Kade F, Miller W. Dose-dependent effects of *Ginkgo biloba* extraction on cerebral, mental and physical efficiency: a placebo controlled double blind study. *British journal of clinical research,* 1993, 4:97–103.
30. Auguet M, DeFeudis FV, Clostre F. Effects of *Ginkgo biloba* on arterial smooth muscle responses to vasoactive stimuli. *General pharmacology,* 1982, 13:169–171, 225–230.
31. Auguet M, Clostre F. Effects of an extract of *Ginkgo biloba* and diverse substances on the phasic and tonic components of the contraction of an isolated rabbit aorta. *General pharmacology,* 1983, 14:277–280.
32. Peter H, Fisel J, Weisser W. Zur Pharmakologie der Wirkstoffe aus *Ginkgo biloba. Arzneimittel-Forschung,* 1966, 16:719–725.
33. Pincemail J et al. In: Farkas L, Gabor M, Kallay F, eds. *Flavonoids and bioflavonoids.* Szeged, Hungary, 1985:423.
34. Barth SA et al. Influences of *Ginkgo biloba* on cyclosporin induced lipid peroxidation in human liver microsomes in comparison to vitamin E, glutathione and N-acetylcysteine. *Biochemical pharmacology,* 1991, 41:1521–1526.
35. Pincemail J et al. *Ginkgo biloba* extract inhibits oxygen species production generated

by phorbol myristate acetate stimulated human leukocytes. *Experientia*, 1987, 43:181–184.

36. Pincemail J, Dupuis M, Nasr C. Superoxide anion scavenging effect and superoxide dismutase activity of *Ginkgo biloba* extract. *Experientia*, 1989, 45:708–712.
37. Robak J, Gryglewski RJ. Flavonoids are scavengers of superoxide anions. *Biochemical pharmacology*, 1988, 37:837–841.
38. Oberpichler H et al. Effects of *Ginkgo biloba* constituents related to protection against brain damage caused by hypoxia. *Pharmacological research communications*, 1988, 20:349–352.
39. Krieglstein J. Neuroprotective effects of *Ginkgo biloba* constituents. *European journal of pharmaceutical sciences*, 1995, 3:39–48.
40. Braquet P. The ginkgolides: potent platelet-activating factor antagonists isolated from *Ginkgo biloba* L.: chemistry, pharmacology and clinical application. *Drugs of the future*, 1987, 12:643–648.
41. Oberpichler H. PAF-antagonist ginkgolide B reduces postischemic neuronal damage in rat brain hippocampus. *Journal of cerebral blood flow and metabolism*, 1990, 10:133–135.
42. Prehn JHM, Krieglstein J. Platelet-activating factor antagonists reduce excitotoxic damage in cultured neurons from embryonic chick telencephalon and protect the rat hippocampus and neocortex from ischemic injury *in vivo*. *Journal of neuroscience research*, 1993, 34:179–188.
43. Larssen RG, Dupeyron JP, Boulu RG. Modèles d'ischémie cérébrale expérimentale par microsphères chez le rat. Étude de l'effet de deux extraits de *Ginkgo biloba* et du naftidrofuryl. *Thérapie*, 1978, 33:651–660.
44. Rapin JR, Le Poncin-Lafitte M. Consommation cérébrale du glucose. Effet de l'extrait de *Ginkgo biloba*. *Presse médica*, 1986, 15:1494–1497.
45. Le Poncin-Lafitte MC, Rapin J, Rapin JR. Effects of *Ginkgo biloba* on changes induced by quantitative cerebral microembolization in rats. *Archives of international pharmacodynamics*, 1980, 243:236–244.
46. Cahn J. Effects of *Ginkgo biloba* extract (GBE) on the acute phase of cerebral ischaemia due to embolisms. In: Agnoli A et al., eds. *Effects of Ginkgo biloba extract on organic cerebral impairment*. London, John Libbey, 1985:43–49.
47. Chatterjee SS. Effects of *Ginkgo biloba* extract on cerebral metabolic processes. In: Agnoli A et al., eds. *Effects of Ginkgo biloba extract on organic cerebral impairment*. London, John Libby, 1985:5–14.
48. Karcher L, Zagermann P, Krieglstein J. Effect of an extract of *Ginkgo biloba* on rat brain energy metabolism in hypoxia. *Naunyn-Schmiedeberg's archives of pharmacology*, 1984, 327:31–35.
49. Le Poncin-Lafitte M et al. Ischémie cérébrale après ligature non simultanèe des artères carotides chez le rat: effet de l'extrait de *Ginkgo biloba*. *Semaine hopitale Paris*, 1982, 58:403–406.
50. Iliff LD, Auer LM. The effect of intravenous infusion of Tebonin (*Ginkgo biloba*) on pial arteries in cats. *Journal of neurosurgical science*, 1982, 27:227–231.
51. Duverger D. Anoxie hypobare chez la souris avec les différents extraits de *Ginkgo biloba*. Le Plessis Robinson, France, Institut Henri-Beaufour, 1989 (Report no. 1116/89/DD/HK).
52. Duverger D. Anoxie hypobare chez la souris avec l'un des constituants de l'EGB:le HE 134. Le Plessis Robinson, France, Institut Henri-Beaufour, 1990 (Report no. 1182/90/DD/HK).
53. Krieglstein J, Beck T, Seibert A. Influence of an extract of *Ginkgo biloba* on cerebral blood flow and metabolism. *Life sciences*, 1986, 39:2327–2334.
54. Beck T et al. Comparative study on the effects of two extract fractions of *Ginkgo biloba* on local cerebral blood flow and on brain energy metabolism in the rat under

hypoxia. In: Krieglstein J, ed. *Pharmacology of cerebral ischemia.* Amsterdam, Elsevier, 1986:345–350.

55. Krieglstein J, Oberpichler H. *Ginkgo biloba* und Hirnleistungsstörungen. *Pharmazeutische Zeitung,* 1989, 13:2279–2289.

56. Oberpichler H et al. Effects of *Ginkgo biloba* constituents related to protection against brain damage caused by hypoxia. *Pharmacology research communications,* 1988, 20:349–352.

57. Lamor Y et al. Effects of ginkgolide B and *Ginkgo biloba* extract on local cerebral glucose utilization in the awake adult rat. *Drug development research,* 1991, 23:219–225.

58. Chatterjee SS, Gabard B. Effect of an extract of *Ginkgo biloba* on experimental neurotoxicity. *Archives of pharmacology,* 1984, 325(Suppl.), Abstr. 327.

59. Otani M et al. Effect of an extract of *Ginkgo biloba* on triethyltin-induced cerebral oedema. *Acta neuropathology,* 1986, 69:54–65.

60. Borzeix MG. Effects of *Ginkgo biloba* extract on two types of cerebral oedema. In: Agnoli A et al., eds. *Effects of Ginkgo biloba extract on organic cerebral impairment.* London, John Libbey, 1985:51–56.

61. Chatterjee SS, Gabard BL, Jaggy HEW. Pharmaceutical compositions containing bilobalide for the treatment of neuropathies. US Patent no. 4,571,407 (Feb 18, 1986).

62. Sancesario G, Kreutzberg GW. Stimulation of astrocytes affects cytotoxic brain oedema. *Acta neuropathology,* 1986, 72:3–14.

63. DeFeudis FV et al. *Some in vitro and in vivo actions of an extract of Ginkgo biloba (GBE 761).* In: Agnoli A et al., eds. *Effects of Ginkgo biloba extract on organic cerebral impairment.* London, John Libbey, 1985:17–29.

64. Winter E. Effects of an extract of *Ginkgo biloba* on learning and memory in mice. *Pharmacology, biochemistry and behavior,* 1991, 38:109–114.

65. Stange VG et al. Adaptationsverhalten peripherer und zentraler akustischer Reizantworten des Meerschweinchens unter dem Einfluss verschiedener Fraktionen eines Extraktes aus *Ginkgo biloba. Arzneimittel-Forschung,* 1976, 26:367–374.

66. Raymond J. Effets de l'extrait de *Ginkgo biloba* sur la préservation morphologique des épithéliums sensoriels vestibulaires chez la souris. *Presse médicale,* 1986, 15:1484–1487.

67. Denise P, Bustany P. The effect of *Ginkgo biloba* (EGb 761) on central compensation of a total unilateral peripheral vestibular deficit in the rat. In: Lacour M et al., eds. *Vestibular compensation: facts, theories and clinical perspectives.* Paris, Elsevier, 1989:201–208.

68. Lacour M, Ez-Zaher L, Raymond J. Plasticity mechanisms in vestibular compensation in the cat are improved by an extract of *Ginkgo biloba* (EGb 761). *Pharmacology, biochemistry and behavior,* 1991, 40:367–379.

69. Vargaftig BB et al. Platelet-activating factor induces a platelet-dependent bronchoconstriction unrelated to the formation of prostaglandin derivatives. *European journal of pharmacology,* 1982, 65:185–192.

70. Vargaftig BB, Benveniste J. Platelet-activating factor today. *Trends in pharmacological sciences,* 1983, 4:341–343.

71. Desquand S et al. Interference of BN 52021 (ginkgolide B) with the broncho-pulmonary effects of PAF-acether in the guinea-pig. *European journal of pharmacology,* 1986, 127:83–95.

72. Desquand S, Vargaftig BB. Interference of the PAF-acether antagonist BN 52021 in bronchopulmonary anaphylaxis. Can a case be made for a role for PAF-acether in bronchopulmonary anaphylaxis in the guinea-pig? In: Braquet P, ed. *Ginkgolides, Vol. 1.* Barcelona, JR Prous, 1988:271–281.

73. Braquet P et al. Involvement of platelet activating factor in respiratory anaphylaxis, demonstrated by PAF-acether inhibitor BN 52021. *Lancet,* 1985, **i**:1501.

74. Költringer P et al. Die Mikrozirkulation und Viskoelastizität des Vollblutes unter

Ginkgo biloba extrakt. Eine plazebokontrollierte, randomisierte Doppelblind-Studie. *Perfusion*, 1989, 1:28–30.

75. Költringer P et al. Mikrozirkulation unter parenteraler *Ginkgo biloba* Extrakt-Therapie. *Wiener Medizinische Wochenschrift*, 1989, 101:198–200.
76. Jung F et al. Effect of *Ginkgo biloba* on fluidity of blood and peripheral microcirculation in volunteers. *Arzneimittel-Forschung*, 1990, 40:589–593.
77. Schaffler K, Reeh PW. Doppelblindstudie zur hypoxieprotektiven Wirkung eines standardisierten *Ginkgo-biloba*-Präparates nach Mehrfachverabreichung an gesunden Probanden. *Arzneimittel-Forschung*, 1985, 35:1283–1286.
78. Hofferberth B. Simultanerfassung elektrophysiologischer, psychometrischer und rheologischer Parameter bei Patienten mit hirnorganischem Psychosyndrom und erhöhtem Gefässrisiko—Eine Placebo-kontrollierte Doppelblindstudie mit *Ginkgo biloba*-Extrakt EGB 761. In: Stodtmeister R, Pillunat LE, eds. *Mikrozirkulation in Gehirn und Sinnesorganen*. Stuttgart, Ferdinand Enke, 1991:64–74.
79. Witte S. Therapeutical aspects of *Ginkgo biloba* flavone glucosides in the context of increased blood viscosity. *Clinical hemorheology*, 1989, 9:323–326.
80. Artmann GM, Schikarski C. *Ginkgo biloba* extract (EGb 761) protects red blood cells from oxidative damage. *Clinical hemorheology*, 1993, 13:529–539.
81. Ernst E, Marshall M. Der Effekt von *Ginkgo-biloba*-Spezialextrakt EGb 761 auf die Leukozytenfilterabilität—Eine Pilotstudie. *Perfusion*, 1992, 8:241–244.
82. Rudofsky G. Wirkung von *Ginkgo-biloba*-extrakt bei arterieller Verschlusskrankheit. *Fortschritte der Medizin*, 1987, 105:397–400.
83. Lagrue G, et al. Oedèmes cycliques idiopathiques. Rôle de l'hyperperméabilité capillaire et correction par l'extrait de *Ginkgo biloba*. *Presse médicale*, 1986, 15:1550–1553.
84. Gerhardt G, Rogalla K, Jaeger J. Medikamentöse Therapie von Hirnleistungsstörungen. Randomisierte Vergleichsstudie mit Dihydroergotoxin und *Ginkgo biloba*-Extrakt. *Fortschritte der Medizin*, 1990, 108:384–388.
85. Hopfenmüller W. Nachweis der therapeutischen Wirksamkeit eines *Ginkgo biloba* Spezialextraktes. *Arzneimittel-Forschung*, 1994, 44:1005–1013.
86. Meyer B. Etude multicentrique randomisée a double insu face au placebo du traitement des acouphènes par l'extrait de *Ginkgo biloba*. *Presse médicale*, 1986, 15:1562–1564.
87. Sprenger FH. Gute Therapieergebnisse mit *Ginkgo biloba*. *Ärztliche Praxis*, 1986, 12:938–940.
88. Witt U. Low power laser und *Ginkgo*-Extrakte als Kombinationstherapie. Hamburg, Germany (unpublished document; available through *NAPRALERT*, see reference 5).
89. Coles RRA. Trial of an extract of *Ginkgo biloba* (EGB) for tinnitus and hearing loss. *Clinical otolaryngology*, 1988, 13:501–504.
90. Fucci JM et al. *Effects of Ginkgo biloba extract on tinnitus: a double blind study*. St. Petersberg, FL, Association for Research in Otolaryngology, 1991.
91. Holgers KM, Axelson A, Pringle I. *Ginkgo biloba* extract for the treatment of tinnitus. *Audiology*, 1994, 33:85–92.

Radix Ginseng

Definition

Radix Ginseng is the dried root of *Panax ginseng* C.A. Meyer (Araliaceae) (*1–5*).[1]

Synonyms

Panax schinseng Nees (*2*).

Other *Panax* species, including *P. quinquefolius* L. (American ginseng), *P. notoginseng* Burk. (San-chi ginseng), *P. pseudoginseng* Wall. ssp. *japonicus* Hara = *P. japonicus* C.A. Meyer (Japanese chikutsu ginseng) and *P. notoginseng* ssp. *himalaicus* (Himalayan ginseng) have also been referred to as "ginseng" and used medically (*6, 7*). However, scientific documentation of these species is insufficient to justify the preparation of a monograph at this time.

Selected vernacular names

Chosen ninjin, ginseng, Ginsengwurzel, hakusan, hakushan, higeninjin, hongshen, hungseng, hungshen, hunseng, jenseng, jenshen, jinpi, kao-li-seng, korean ginseng, minjin, nhan sam, ninjin, ninzin, niuhuan, Oriental ginseng, otane ninjin, renshen, san-pi, shanshen, sheng-sai-seng, shenshaishanshen, shengshaishen, t'ang-seng, tyosenninzin, yakuyo ninjin, yakuyo ninzin, yeh-shan-seng, yuan-seng, yuanshen (*1, 2, 4–10*).

Description

A perennial herb with characteristic branched roots extending from the middle of the main root in the form of a human figure. Stem erect, simple, and not branching. Leaves verticillate, compound, digitate, leaflets 5, with the 3 terminal leaflets larger than the lateral ones, elliptical or slightly obovate, 4–15 cm long by 2–6.5 cm wide; apex acuminate; base cuneate; margin serrulate or finely bidentate. In general, 1 leaf in the first year with 1 leaflet added annually until the sixth year. Inflorescence a small terminal umbel, hemispherical in early summer. Flowers polygamous, pink. Calyx vaguely 5-toothed. Petals 5, stamens 5. Fruit a small berry, nearly drupaceous, and red when ripe in autumn (*8*).

---

[1] Steamed *Panax ginseng* root is listed in the Japanese pharmacopoeia as "Red Ginseng (Ginseng Radix Rubra)" (*2*).

Plant material of interest: dried root
General appearance
The main root is fusiform or cylindrical, 2.5–20 cm long by 0.5–3.0 cm in diameter; externally greyish yellow; upper part or entire root exhibiting sparse, shallow, interrupted, and coarse transverse striations and distinct longitudinal wrinkles; lower part bearing 2–5 branching lateral roots and numerous slender rootlets with inconspicuous minute tubercles. Rhizomes 1–4 cm long by 0.3–1.5 cm in diameter, mostly constricted and curved, bearing adventitious roots and sparse depressed circular stem scars. Texture relatively hard, fracture yellowish white, cambium ring brownish yellow, starchy (1–5).

Organoleptic properties
Colour, greyish white to amber-yellow; odour, characteristic; taste, slightly sweet at first, followed by a slight bitterness (1, 2).

Microscopic characteristics
The transverse section shows cork consisting of several rows of cells; cortex narrow; phloem showing clefts in the outer part, and parenchymatous cells densely arranged and scattered with resin canals containing yellow secretions in the inner part; cambium in a ring; xylem rays broad, vessels singly scattered or grouped in an interrupted radial arrangement, and occasionally accompanied by non-lignified fibres; parenchyma cells containing abundant starch grains and a few clusters of calcium oxalate (1, 3–5).

Powdered plant material
Yellowish white; fragments of resin canals containing yellow secretions; clusters of calcium oxalate (20–68 µm in diameter), few, with acute angles; cork cells subsquare or polygonal, with thin and sinuous walls; reticulate and scalariform vessels 10–56 µm in diameter; starch granules fairly abundant, simple, subspheroidal, semicircular, or irregular polygonal (4–30 µm in diameter), singly or in groups of two to four (1–5).

Geographical distribution
Mountain regions of China (Manchuria), the Democratic People's Republic of Korea, Japan, the Republic of Korea, and the Russian Federation (eastern Siberia) (7, 8). It is commercially produced mainly by cultivation (6).

General identity tests
Macroscopic and microscopic examinations, microchemical tests, and thin-layer chromatographic analysis (1–5).

Purity tests
Microbiology
The test for *Salmonella* spp. in Radix Ginseng products should be negative. The maximum acceptable limits of other microorganisms are as follows (*11–13*). For preparation of decoction: aerobic bacteria—not more than 10^7/g; fungi—not more than 10^5/g; *Escherichia coli*—not more than 10^2/g. Preparations for internal use: aerobic bacteria—not more than 10^5/g or ml; fungi—not more than 10^4/g or ml; enterobacteria and certain Gram-negative bacteria—not more than 10^3/g or ml; *Escherichia coli*—0/g or ml.

Foreign organic matter
Not more than 2% (*2, 3*).

Total ash
Not more than 4.2% (*2*).

Acid-insoluble ash
Not more than 1% (*4*).

Sulfated ash
Not more than 12% (*5*).

Alcohol-soluble extractive
Not less than 14.0% (*2*).

Pesticide residues
To be established in accordance with national requirements. Normally, the maximum residue limit of aldrin and dieldrin for Radix Ginseng is not more than 0.05 mg/kg (*13*). For other pesticides, see WHO guidelines on quality control methods for medicinal plants (*11*) and guidelines for predicting dietary intake of pesticide residues (*14*).

Heavy metals
Recommended lead and cadmium levels are no more than 10 and 0.3 mg/kg, respectively, in the final dosage form of the plant material (*11*).

Radioactive residues
For analysis of strontium-90, iodine-131, caesium-134, caesium-137, and plutonium-239, see WHO guidelines on quality control methods for medicinal plants (*11*).

Other purity tests

Chemical and water-soluble extractive tests to be established in accordance with national requirements.

Chemical assays

Microchemical, thin-layer chromatographic, and spectrophotometric methods are used for the qualitative and quantitative analysis of ginsenosides (*1–5*). High-performance liquid chromatography (*15–17*) and liquid chromatography–mass spectrometry (*18*) methods are also available.

Characteristic saponins known as ginsenosides, not less than 1.5% calculated as ginsenoside Rg_1 (D-glucopyranosyl-6β-glucopyranosyl-20S-protopanaxatriol, relative molecular mass 800) (3, 5).

Major chemical constituents

The major chemical constituents are triterpene saponins. More than 30 are based on the dammarane structure, and one (ginsenoside Ro) is derived from oleanolic acid (*6, 7, 17, 19*). The dammarane saponins are derivatives of either protopanaxadiol or protopanaxatriol. Members of the former group include ginsenosides Ra_{1-3}, Rb_{1-3}, Rc, Rc_2, Rd, Rd_2, and Rh_2; (20S)-ginsenoside Rg_3; and malonyl ginsenosides Rb_1, Rb_2, Rc, and Rd. Examples of protopanaxatriol saponins are ginsenosides Re_2, Re_3, Rf, Rg_1, Rg_2, and Rh_1; 20-gluco-ginsenoside Rf; and (20R)-ginsenosides Rg_2 and Rh_1. Those considered most important are ginsenosides Rb_1, Rb_2, Rc, Rd, Rf, Rg_1, and Rg_2; Rb_1, Rb_2, and Rg_1 are the most abundant. Representative structures are presented below.

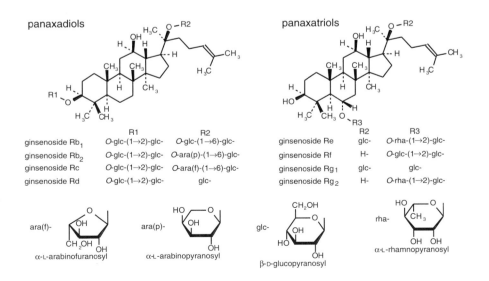

	R1	R2
ginsenoside Rb_1	O-glc-(1→2)-glc-	O-glc-(1→6)-glc-
ginsenoside Rb_2	O-glc-(1→2)-glc-	O-ara(p)-(1→6)-glc-
ginsenoside Rc	O-glc-(1→2)-glc-	O-ara(f)-(1→6)-glc-
ginsenoside Rd	O-glc-(1→2)-glc-	glc-

	R2	R3
ginsenoside Re	glc-	O-rha-(1→2)-glc-
ginsenoside Rf	H-	O-glc-(1→2)-glc-
ginsenoside Rg_1	glc-	glc-
ginsenoside Rg_2	H-	O-rha-(1→2)-glc-

ara(f)-   α-L-arabinofuranosyl

ara(p)-   α-L-arabinopyranosyl

glc-   β-D-glucopyranosyl

rha-   α-L-rhamnopyranosyl

Dosage forms

Crude plant material, capsules and tablets of powdered drugs, extracts, tonic drinks, wines, and lozenges. Store in a cool, dry place in well-sealed containers (*20*).

Medicinal uses

Uses supported by clinical data

Radix Ginseng is used as a prophylactic and restorative agent for enhancement of mental and physical capacities, in cases of weakness, exhaustion, tiredness, and loss of concentration, and during convalescence (*21–29*).

Uses described in pharmacopoeias and in traditional systems of medicine

Radix Ginseng has been used clinically in the treatment of diabetes (*1*), but further clinical studies are needed. The drug is also used in the treatment of impotence, prevention of hepatotoxicity, and gastrointestinal disorders such as gastritis and ulcers (*1*, *7*).

Uses described in folk medicine, not supported by experimental or clinical data

Treatment of liver disease, coughs, fever, tuberculosis, rheumatism, vomiting of pregnancy, hypothermia, dyspnoea, and nervous disorders (*7*).

Pharmacology

Experimental pharmacology

The suggested mode of action of Radix Ginseng is twofold. First, the drug has an "adaptogenic" effect (*30*), which produces a non-specific increase in the body's own defences against exogenous stress factors and noxious chemicals (*31*). Secondly, the drug promotes an overall improvement in physical and mental performance (*30–33*).

Treatment of cultured mammalian cells, isolated organs, and animal models (primarily mice and rats) with Radix Ginseng before or during exposure to physical, chemical, or psychological stress increased the ability of the respective model systems to resist the damaging effects of various stressors (*31*). These results were demonstrated in cases of radiation poisoning (*34–36*), viral infection and tumour load (*37*, *38*), alcohol or carbon tetrachloride poisoning (*39–41*), oxygen deprivation and hypobaric pressure (*42*, *43*), light or temperature stress, emotional stress, and electrical shock or restricted movement (*44*, *45*, *46*). The mechanism by which the drug exerts its activity is most likely through the hypothalamus–pituitary–adrenal axis (*47–49*) and through its immunostimulant effect (*50*).

Intraperitoneal administration to rats of ginseng saponin fractions or the ginsenosides Rb_1, Rb_2, Rc, Rd, and Re elevated serum levels of adrenocorticotropic hormone (ACTH) and corticosterone (51, 52). Pretreatment with dexamethasone, which blocks hypothalamus and pituitary functions, prevented ginseng saponin-mediated release of ACTH and corticosterone, and thereby demonstrated that the increase in serum corticosterone by ginseng occurs indirectly through release of ACTH from the pituitary (51, 52).

The immunomodulatory activity of ginseng appears to be at least partly responsible for its adaptogenic effect (50, 53, 54). Alcohol extracts of Radix Ginseng stimulated phagocytosis *in vitro*, were mitogenic in cultured human lymphocytes, stimulated the production of interferon, and enhanced the activity of natural killer cells (55, 56). Intraperitoneal administration of an extract of the drug to mice stimulated cell-mediated immunity against Semliki Forest virus, elevated antibody levels against sheep red blood cells and natural killer cells (57), and stimulated the production of interferon (58).

Improvement in physical and mental performance has been observed in mice and rats after oral or intraperitoneal administration of the drug (59–63). Oral administration of ginseng saponin fractions to mice increased endurance and prolonged swimming time in swimming tests (63). However, two studies concluded that ginseng had no positive effects on the physical performance in mice and rats (64, 65). The adaptogenic effects of Radix Ginseng are generally attributed to the ginsenosides (66, 67). The ginsenosides have been shown to alter mechanisms of fuel homeostasis during prolonged exercise, by increasing the capacity of skeletal muscle to oxidize free fatty acids in preference to glucose for cellular energy production (59). Other constituents of Radix Ginseng, such as vanillic and salicylic acid, have also been reported to have "antifatigue" activity in rats (68). Furthermore, the antioxidant activity of ginseng was associated with both the ginsenosides and the flavonoid constituents (31, 69). The ginsenosides protected pulmonary vascular endothelium against free-radical-induced injury (69).

Mice given ginseng extract or ginsenosides Rb_1 and Rg_2 orally during passive avoidance response tests showed an improvement in learning ability which was negatively influenced by stress (30), and rats showed improved retention of learned behaviour (70). Ginsenosides Rg_1 and Rb_1 are the active nootropic constituents of the drug (66), and improve memory and learning in normal as well as cognition-impaired animals. The mode of action involves an increase in the synthesis and release of acetylcholine, and a decrease of brain serotonin levels (66). In cerebral and coronary blood vessels, extracts of Radix Ginseng produced vasodilatation, which improved brain and coronary blood flow (71). The vasodilatory activity of the ginsenosides appears to be primarily due to relaxation of vascular smooth muscles. The ginsenosides block the constricting effects of norepinephrine in isolated aorta strips, and inhibit the uptake of $^{45}Ca^{2+}$ in the membrane and sarcolemma of rabbit heart tissue. Inhibition of Ca^{2+} uptake in the muscle membrane contributes to the mechanism of vasodilatation (71).

A number of polypeptides and glycans isolated from Radix Ginseng, named GP and panaxans A–E, respectively, have demonstrated hypoglycaemic activity when given intraperitoneally to mice (72, 73). Two of the glycans, panaxans A and B, have been shown to stimulate hepatic glucose utilization by increasing the activity of glucose-6-phosphate 1-dehydrogenase, phosphorylase *a*, and phosphofructokinase (72). Panaxan A did not affect plasma insulin levels or insulin sensitivity, but panaxan B elevated the plasma insulin level by stimulating insulin secretion from pancreatic islets, and further enhanced insulin sensitivity by increasing insulin binding to receptors (72). The panaxans are not active after oral administration. Administration of GP (intravenously or subcutaneously) to mice or rats decreased blood glucose and liver glycogen levels (73). Radix Ginseng also contains a number of other constituents with hypoglycaemic activity (72, 74). Adenosine, isolated from a water extract of Radix Ginseng, enhanced lipogenesis and cyclic AMP accumulation of adipocytes, and some of the ginsenosides inhibited ACTH-induced lipolysis, suppressed insulin-stimulated lipogenesis, and stimulated the release of insulin from cultured islets (72).

Subcutaneous administration of a ginseng extract enhanced the mating behaviour of male rats (75). The drug further stimulated spermatogenesis in rat (76), and rabbit testes, and increased the motility and survival of rabbit sperm outside the body (75).

Intragastric or intradermal administration of an ethanol extract of the drug to rats decreased histamine-, pentagastrin-, carbachol- and vagal stimulation-induced gastric secretion, and inhibited gastric ulcers induced by stress or by pyloric ligation (77–79).

Liver-protectant activity of ginseng has been demonstrated *in vitro* and *in vivo* (80, 81). Intraperitoneal administration of Radix Ginseng extracts to normal and dexamethasone-treated rats did not influence the blood chemistry of normal rats, but it decreased aspartate aminotransferase and alanine aminotransferase levels in dexamethasone-treated animals, thereby demonstrating a liver-protectant effect (81). However, another study demonstrated that an intraperitoneal injection of a methanol extract of Radix Ginseng had no protective activity against carbon tetrachloride-induced hepatotoxicity in rats (82).

Clinical pharmacology

Antifatigue activity

The results of clinical studies measuring increased performance and antifatigue effects of ginseng extracts are conflicting and, in general, most studies suffer from poor methodology, lack of proper controls, and no standardization of the ginseng extracts used. The influence of chronic Radix Ginseng administration (2 g/day orally for 4 weeks) on substrate utilization, hormone production, endurance, metabolism, and perception of effort during consecutive days of exhaustive exercise in 11 naval cadets was reported. No significant differences were observed between the control group and the group receiving the ginseng supplementation (*83*). Another clinical trial with eight participants reported no significant difference between placebo and ginseng administration during exhaustive exercise after 7 days of treatment (*84*). A randomized, double-blind, cross-over study sought the effects of ginseng on circulatory, respiratory, and metabolic functions during maximal exercise in 50 men (21–47 years old) (*24*). Total tolerated workload and maximal oxygen uptake were significantly higher following ginseng administration than with placebo. At the same workload, oxygen consumption, plasma lactate levels, ventilation, carbon dioxide production, and heart rate during exercise were all lower in the ginseng treatment group. The results indicated that the ginseng preparations effectively increased the work capacity of the participants by improving oxygen utilization (*24*). A placebo-controlled, cross-over study determined the effects of ginseng on the physical fitness of 43 male triathletes (*25*). The participants received 200 mg of a ginseng preparation twice daily for two consecutive training periods of 10 weeks. No significant changes were observed during the first 10-week period, but ginseng appeared to prevent the loss of physical fitness (as measured by oxygen uptake and oxygen pulse) during the second 10-week period (*25*). Two further studies with athletes given 100 mg of a standardized ginseng extract twice daily for 9 weeks reported significant improvement in aerobic capacity and reduction in blood lactate and heart rates (*26, 27*), but placebos or controls were not used in either of the two studies. Further extension of these studies using placebo-controlled, double-blind trials demonstrated significant improvement in the ginseng group as compared with the placebo group (*28*). Similar results were reported in another study on athletes, and the differences between the ginseng and placebo groups lasted for approximately 3 weeks after the last ginseng dose (*29*). The effects of 1200 mg of Radix Ginseng in a placebo-controlled, double-blind cross-over study in fatigued night nurses were assessed and the results were compared with placebo and with effects on nurses engaged in daytime work (*22*). Ginseng restored ratings on tests of mood, competence, and general performance, and the study concluded that ginseng had anti-fatigue activity (*22*).

Aqueous and standardized ginseng extracts were tested in a placebo-controlled, double-blind study for immunomodulatory actions (*85*). Sixty healthy volunteers were divided into three groups of 20 each and were given either a placebo or 100 mg of aqueous ginseng extract or 100 mg of standardized ginseng extract, every 12 hours for 8 weeks. Blood samples drawn from the volunteers revealed an increase in chemotaxis of polymorphonuclear leukocytes, the phagocytic index, and the total number of T3 and T4 lymphocytes after 4 and 8 weeks of ginseng therapy, as compared with the placebo group. The group receiving the standardized extract also increased their T4:T8 ratio and the activity of natural killer cells. The conclusion of this study was that ginseng extract stimulated the immune system in humans, and that the standardized extract was more effective than the aqueous extract (*85*).

Psychomotor activity

A double-blind, placebo-controlled clinical study assessed the effect of standardized ginseng extract (100 mg twice daily for 12 weeks) on psychomotor performance in 16 healthy individuals (23). Various tests of pyschomotor performance found a favourable effect on attention, processing, integrated sensory–motor function, and auditory reaction time. The study concluded that the drug was superior to the placebo in improving certain psychomotor functions in healthy subjects (23).

Antidiabetic activity

Radix Ginseng has been shown in clinical studies to have beneficial effects in both insulin-dependent and non-insulin-dependent diabetic patients (86, 87). Oral administration of ginseng tablets (200 mg daily for 8 weeks) to 36 non-insulin-dependent patients elevated mood, improved physical performance, reduced fasting blood glucose and serum aminoterminal propeptide of type III procollagen concentrations, and lowered glycated haemoglobin (87).

Impotence

Ginseng extracts improved sperm production in men and may have some usefulness in treating impotence (32). The ginsenosides, which appear to be the active components, are thought to depress blood prolactin levels, thereby increasing libido (32). In one clinical study, 90 patients with erectile dysfunction were treated with ginseng saponins (600 mg orally per day). Treatment improved rigidity, tumescence, and libido, but not the frequency of coitus (88).

Contraindications

None (21, 50, 89, 90).

Warnings

No information available.

Precautions

General

Diabetic patients should consult a physician prior to taking Radix Ginseng, as ginseng intake may slightly reduce blood glucose levels (86, 87).

Drug interactions

There are two reports of an interaction between Radix Ginseng and phenelzine, a monoamine oxidase inhibitor (91, 92). The clinical significance of this interaction has not been evaluated.

Drug and laboratory test interactions

None reported.

Carcinogenesis, mutagenesis, impairment of fertility

Radix Ginseng is not carcinogenic or mutagenic *in vitro*, and does not have any effect on fertility (*90*).

Pregnancy: teratogenic effects

Radix Ginseng is not teratogenic *in vivo* (*90*).

Pregnancy: non-teratogenic effects

The safety of Radix Ginseng for use in pregnancy has not been established.

Nursing mothers

Excretion of Radix Ginseng compounds into breast milk and its effects on the newborn have not been established.

Paediatric use

The safety and efficacy of Radix Ginseng use in children have not been established.

Adverse reactions

Various researchers who studied Radix Ginseng extracts using conventional toxicological methods in five different animal models reported no acute or chronic toxicity of the extract (*89, 90, 93*).

On the basis of Radix Ginseng's long use, and the relative infrequency of significant demonstrable side-effects, it has been concluded that the use of Radix Ginseng is not associated with serious adverse effects if taken at the recommended dose (*90, 93*). However, in Siegel's open study of 133 patients ingesting large quantities, ginseng was reported to result in hypertension, nervousness, irritability, diarrhoea, skin eruptions, and insomnia, which were collectively called ginseng abuse syndrome (GAS) (*94*). Critical analysis of this report has shown that there were no controls or analyses to determine the type of ginseng being ingested or the constituents of the preparation taken, and that some of the amounts ingested were clearly excessive (as much as 15 g per day, where the recommended daily dose is 0.5–2 g) (*50, 90, 95*). When the dose was decreased to 1.7 g/day the symptoms of the "syndrome" were rare. Thus the only conclusion that can be validly extracted from the Siegel study is that the excessive and uncontrolled intake of ginseng products should be avoided (*90*). One case of ginseng-associated cerebral arteritis has been reported in a patient consuming a high dose of an ethanol extract of ginseng root (approximately 6 g in one dose) (*96*). However, again the type and quantity of ginseng extract were not reported. Two cases of mydriasis and disturbance in accommodation, as well as dizziness have been reported after ingestion of large doses (3–9 g) of an unspecified type of ginseng preparation (*97*).

Estrogenic-like side-effects have been reported in both premenopausal and postmenopausal women following the use of ginseng. Seven cases of mastalgia (*98–100*) and one case of vaginal bleeding in a postmenopausal woman (*101*) were reported after ingestion of unspecified ginseng products. An increased libido in premenopausal women has also been reported (*100*). Specific studies on the possible hormonal side-effects of ginseng have been carried out with a standardized ginseng extract (*102–104*). Under physiological conditions, there is no interaction of the ginseng extract with either cytosolic estrogen receptors isolated from mature rat uterus or progesterone receptors from human myometrium (*102*). Furthermore, clinical studies have demonstrated that a standardized ginseng extract does not cause a change in male and female hormonal status (*103, 104*).

Posology

Unless otherwise prescribed, daily dose (taken in the morning): dried root 0.5–2 g by decoction; doses of other preparations should be calculated accordingly (*21, 23, 89*).

References

1. *Pharmacopoeia of the People's Republic of China* (English ed.). Guangzhou, Guangdong Science and Technology Press, 1992.
2. *The pharmacopoeia of Japan XII*. Tokyo, The Society of Japanese Pharmacopoeia, 1991.
3. *Pharmacopée française*. Paris, Adrapharm, 1996.
4. *Deutsches Arzneibuch 1996*. Stuttgart, Deutscher Apotheker Verlag, 1996.
5. *Pharmacopoeia helvetica VII*. Berne, Département fédéral de l'intérieur, 1994.
6. Shibata S et al. Chemistry and pharmacology of *Panax*. In: Wagner H, Farnsworth NR, Hikino H, eds. *Economic and medicinal plants research, Vol. 1*. London, Academic Press, 1985.
7. Bruneton J. *Pharmacognosy, phytochemistry, medicinal plants*. Paris, Lavoisier, 1995.
8. *Medicinal plants in China*. Manila, World Health Organization, 1989 (WHO Regional Publications, Western Pacific Series, No. 2).
9. Hsu HY. *Oriental materia medica, a concise guide*. Long Beach, CA, Oriental Healing Arts Institute, 1986.
10. Farnsworth NR, ed. *NAPRALERT database*. Chicago, University of Illinois at Chicago, IL, August 8, 1995 production (an on-line database available directly through the University of Illinois at Chicago or through the Scientific and Technical Network (STN) of Chemical Abstracts Services).
11. *Quality control methods for medicinal plant materials*. Geneva, World Health Organization, 1998.
12. *Deutsches Arzneibuch 1996. Vol. 2. Methoden der Biologie*. Stuttgart, Deutscher Apotheker Verlag, 1996.
13. *European pharmacopoeia*, 3rd ed. Strasbourg, Council of Europe, 1997.
14. *Guidelines for predicting dietary intake of pesticide residues*, 2nd rev. ed. Geneva,

World Health Organization, 1997 (unpublished document WHO/FSF/FOS/97.7; available from Food Safety, WHO, 1211 Geneva 27, Switzerland).

15. Sticher O, Soldati F. HPLC separation and quantitative determination of ginsenosides from *Panax ginseng, Panax quinquefolium* and from ginseng drug preparations. 1. *Planta medica,* 1979, 36:30–42.

16. Sticher O, Soldati F. HPLC separation and quantitative determination of ginsenosides from *Panax ginseng, Panax quinquefolium* and from ginseng drug preparations. 2. *Planta medica,* 1979, 39:348–357.

17. Cui JF. Identification and quantification of ginsenosides in various commercial ginseng preparations. *European journal of pharmaceutical sciences,* 1995, 3:77–85.

18. van Breemen RB et al. Electrospray liquid chromatography/mass spectrometry of ginsenosides. *Analytical chemistry,* 1995, 67:3985–3989.

19. Sprecher E. Ginseng: miracle drug or phytopharmacon? *Deutsche Apotheker Zeitung,* 1987, 9:52–61.

20. *British herbal pharmacopoeia.* London, British Herbal Medicine Association, 1990.

21. German Commission E Monograph, Ginseng radix. *Bundesanzeiger,* 1991, 11:17 January.

22. Hallstrom C, Fulder S, Carruthers M. Effect of ginseng on the performance of nurses on night duty. *Comparative medicine East and West,* 1982, 6:277–282.

23. D'Angelo L et al. Double-blind, placebo-controlled clinical study on the effect of a standardized ginseng extract on psychomotor performance in healthy volunteers. *Journal of ethnopharmacology,* 1986, 16:15–22.

24. Pieralisi G, Ripari P, Vecchiet L. Effects of a standardized ginseng extract combined with dimethylaminoethanol bitartrate, vitamins, minerals, and trace elements on physical performance during exercise. *Clinical therapeutics,* 1991, 13:373–382.

25. Van Schepdael P. Les effets du ginseng G115 sur la capacité physique de sportifs d'endurance. *Acta therapeutica,* 1993, 19:337–347.

26. Forgo I, Kirchdorfer AM. The effect of different ginsenoside concentrations on physical work capacity. *Notabene medici,* 1982, 12:721–727.

27. Forgo I, Kirchdorfer AM. On the question of influencing the performance of top sportsmen by means of biologically active substances. *Ärztliche Praxis,* 1981, 33:1784–1786.

28. Forgo I. Effect of drugs on physical performance and hormone system of sportsmen. *Münchener Medizinische Wochenschrift,* 1983, 125:822–824.

29. Forgo I, Schimert G. The duration of effect of the standardized ginseng extract in healthy competitive athletes. *Notabene medici,* 1985, 15:636–640.

30. Wagner H, Norr H, Winterhoff H. Plant adaptogens. *Phytomedicine,* 1994, 1:63–76.

31. Sonnenborn U, Proppert Y. Ginseng (*Panax ginseng* C.A. Meyer). *British journal of phytotherapy,* 1991, 2:3–14.

32. Owen RT. Ginseng: A pharmacological profile. *Drugs of today,* 1981, 17:343–351.

33. Phillipson JD, Anderson LA. Ginseng-quality, safety and efficacy? *Pharmaceutical journal,* 1984, 232:161–165.

34. Takeda A, Yonezawa M, Katoh N. Restoration of radiation injury by ginseng. I. Responses of X-irradiated mice to ginseng extracts. *Journal of radiation research,* 1981, 22:323–335.

35. Yonezawa M, Katoh N, Takeda A. Restoration of radiation injury by ginseng. IV. Stimulation of recoveries in CFUs and megakaryocyte counts related to the prevention of occult blood appearance in X-irradiated mice. *Journal of radiation research,* 1985, 26:436–442.

36. Zhang JS et al. Modification of radiation response in mice by fractionated extracts of *Panax ginseng. Radiation research,* 1987, 112:156–163.

37. Qian BC et al. Effects of ginseng polysaccharides on tumor and immunological function in tumor-bearing mice. *Yao hsueh hsueh pao,* 1987, 8:277–280.

38. Yun TK, Yun YS, Han IW. An experimental study on tumor inhibitory effect of red ginseng in mice and rats exposed to various chemical carcinogens. In: *Proceedings of the third International Ginseng Symposium.* Seoul, Korean Ginseng Research Institute, 1980:87–113.

39. Choi CW, Lee SI, Huk K. Effect of ginseng on hepatic alcohol metabolizing enzyme system activity in chronic alcohol-treated mouse. *Korean journal of pharmacognosy*, 1984, 20:13–21.

40. Hikino H et al. Antihepatotoxic actions of ginsenosides from *Panax ginseng* roots. *Planta medica*, 1985, 51:62–64.

41. Nakagawa S et al. Cytoprotective activity of components of garlic, ginseng and ciwujia on hepatocyte injury induced by carbon tetrachloride *in vitro*. *Hiroshima journal of medical science*, 1985, 34:303–309.

42. Chen X et al. Protective effects of ginsenosides on anoxia/reoxygenation of cultured rat monocytes and on reperfusion injuries against lipid peroxidation. *Biomedica biochimica acta*, 1987, 46:646–649.

43. Lu G, Cheng XJ, Yuan WX. Protective action of ginseng root saponins on hypobaric hypoxia in animals. *Yao hsueh hsueh pao*, 1988, 9:391–394.

44. Banerjee U, Izquierdo JA. Anti-stress and antifatigue properties of *Panax ginseng*: Comparison with piracetam. *Acta physiologica et therapeutica Latinoamericana*, 1982, 32:277–285.

45. Cheng XJ et al. Protective effects of ginsenosides on anoxia/reoxygenation of cultured rat myocytes and on reperfusion injuries against lipid peroxidation. *Biomedica biochimica acta*, 1987, 46:646–649.

46. Saito H. Neuropharmacological studies on *Panax ginseng*. In: Chang HM et al., eds. *Advances in Chinese medicinal materials research*. Singapore, World Scientific Publishing, 1974:509–518.

47. Filaretov AA et al. Effect of adaptogens on the activity of the pituitary-adrenocortical system in rats. *Bulletin of experimental biology and medicine*, 1986, 101:627–629.

48. Lu G, Cheng XJ, Yuan WX. Effects of the ginseng root saponins on serum corticosterone and brain neurotransmitters of mice under hypobaric and hypoxic environment. *Yao hsueh hsueh pao*, 1988, 9:489–492.

49. Ng TB, Li WW, Yeung HW. Effects of ginsenosides, lectins, and *Momordica charantia* insulin-like peptides on corticosterone production by isolated rat adrenal cells. *Journal of ethnopharmacology*, 1987, 21:21–29.

50. Sonnenborn U. Ginseng-Nebenwirkungen: Fakten oder Vermutungen? *Medizinische Monatsschrift für Pharmazeuten*, 1989, 12:46–53.

51. Hiai S et al. Stimulation of pituitary-adrenocortical system by ginseng saponin. *Endocrinology Japan*, 1979, 26:661.

52. Hiai S, Sasaki S, Oura H. Effects of Ginseng saponin on rat adrenal cyclic AMP. *Planta medica*, 1979, 37:15–19.

53. Singh VK, Agarwal SS, Gupta BM. Immunomodulatory activity of *Panax ginseng* extract. *Planta medica*, 1984, 50:462–465.

54. Sonnenborn U. Ginseng—neuere Untersuchungen immunologischer, und endokrinologischer Aktivitäten einer alten Arzneipflanze. *Deutsche Apotheker Zeitung*, 1987, 125:2052–2055.

55. Fulder S. The growth of cultured human fibroblasts treated with hydrocortisone and extracts of the medicinal plant *Panax ginseng*. *Experimental gerontology*, 1977, 12:125–131.

56. Gupta S et al. A new mitogen and interferon inducer. *Clinical research*, 1980, 28:504A.

57. Singh VK, Agarwal SS, Gupta BM. Immunomodulatory effects of *Panax ginseng* extract. *Planta medica*, 1984, 50:459.

58. Jie YH, Cammisuli S, Baggiolini M. Immunomodulatory effects of *Panax ginseng* C. A. Meyer in the mouse. *Agents and actions*, 1984, 15:386–391.

59. Avakian EV et al. Effect of *Panax ginseng* on energy metabolism during exercise in rats. *Planta medica*, 1984, 50:151–154.
60. Brekhman II, Dardymov IV. Pharmacological investigation of glycosides from ginseng and *Eleutherococcus*. *Journal of natural products*, 1969, 32:46–51.
61. Hassan Samira MM et al. Effect of the standardized ginseng extract G 115 on the metabolism and electrical activity of the rabbit's brain. *Journal of international medical research*, 1985, 13:342–348.
62. Petkov V. Effect of ginseng on the brain biogenic monoamines and 3′,5′-AMP system. Experiments on rats. *Arzneimittel-Forschung*, 1978, 28:338–339.
63. Bombardelli E, Cristoni A, Lietti A. The effect of acute and chronic ginseng saponins treatment on adrenals function: biochemistry and pharmacological aspects. In: *Proceedings of the third International Ginseng Symposium*. Seoul, Korean Ginseng Research Institute, 1980:9–16.
64. Lewis WH, Zenger VE, Lynch RG. No adaptogen response of mice to ginseng and *Eleutherococcus* infusions. *Journal of ethnopharmacology*, 1983, 8:209–214.
65. Martinez B, Staba EJ. The physiological effects of *Aralia, Panax* and *Eleutherococcus* on exercised rats. *Japanese journal of pharmacology*, 1984, 35:79–85.
66. Liu CX, Xiao PG. Recent advances in ginseng research in China. *Journal of ethnopharmacology*, 1992, 36:27–38.
67. Yang ZW. Renshen. In: Chang HM, But PPH, eds., *Pharmacology and applications of Chinese materia medica*, Vol. 1. Singapore, World Scientific Publishing, 1986:17–31.
68. Han BH, Han YN, Park MH. Chemical and biochemical studies on antioxidant components of ginseng. In: Chang HM, Tso WW, Koo A. *Advances in Chinese medicinal materials research*. World Scientific Publishing, Singapore, 1985:485–498.
69. Kim H et al. Ginsenosides protect pulmonary vascular endothelium against radical-induced injury. *Biochemical and biophysical research communications*, 1992, 189, 670–676.
70. Petkov VD et al. Memory effects of standardized extracts of *Panax ginseng* (G115), *Ginkgo biloba* (GK501) and their combination Gincosan (PHL00701). *Planta medica*, 1993, 59:106–114.
71. Huang KC. Herbs with multiple actions. In: *The pharmacology of Chinese herbs*. Boca Raton, FL, CRC Press, 1993:21–48.
72. Marles R, Farnsworth NR. Antidiabetic plants and their active constituents. *Phytomedicine*, 1995, 2:137–189.
73. Wang BX et al. Studies on the mechanism of ginseng polypeptide induced hypoglycemia. *Yao hsueh hsueh pao*, 1989, 25:727–731.
74. Davydov VV, Molokovsky A, Limarenko AY, Efficacy of ginseng drugs in experimental insulin-dependent diabetes and toxic hepatitis. *Patologichezkaia Fiziologiia I Eksperimentalkaia Terapiia*, 1990, 5:49–52.
75. Kim C. Influence of ginseng on mating behavior in male rats. *American journal of Chinese medicine*, 1976, 4:163–168.
76. Yamamoto M. Stimulatory effect of *Panax ginseng* principals on DNA and protein synthesis in rat testes. *Arzneimittel-Forschung*, 1977, 27:1404–1405.
77. Suzuki Y et al. Effects of tissue cultured ginseng on the function of the stomach and small intestine. *Yakugaku zasshi*, 1991, 111:765–769.
78. Suzuki Y et al. Effects of tissue cultured ginseng on gastric secretion and pepsin activity. *Yakugaku zasshi*, 1991, 111:770–774.
79. Matsuda H, Kubo M. Pharmacological study on *Panax ginseng* C.A. Meyer. II. Effect of red ginseng on the experimental gastric ulcer. *Yakugaku zasshi*, 1984, 104:449–453.
80. Hikino H. Antihepatotoxic activity of crude drugs. *Yakugaku zasshi*, 1985, 105:109–118.
81. Lin JH et al. Effects of ginseng on the blood chemistry profile of dexamethasone-treated male rats. *American journal of Chinese medicine*, 1995, 23:167–172.

82. Kumazawa N et al. Protective effects of various methanol extracts of crude drugs on experimental hepatic injury induced by carbon tetrachloride in rats. *Yakugaku zasshi*, 1990, 110:950–957.
83. Knapik JJ, Wright JE, Welch MJ. The influence of *Panax ginseng* on indices of substrate utilization during repeated, exhaustive exercise in man. *Federation proceedings*, 1983, 42:336.
84. Morris AC, Jacobs I, Kligerman TM. No ergogenic effect of ginseng extract after ingestion. *Medical science of sports exercise*, 1994, 26:S6.
85. Scaglione F et al. Immunomodulatory effects of two extracts of *Panax ginseng* C.A. Meyer. *Drugs, experimental and clinical research*, 1990, 26:537–542.
86. Kwan HJ, Wan JK. Clinical study of treatment of diabetes with powder of the steamed insam (ginseng) produced in Kaesong, Korea. *Technical information*, 1994, 6:33–35.
87. Sotaniemi EA, Haapakoski E, Rautio A. Ginseng therapy in non-insulin-dependent diabetic patients. *Diabetes care*, 1995, 18:1373–1375.
88. Choi HK, Seong DW. Effectiveness for erectile dysfunction after the administration of Korean red ginseng. *Korean journal of ginseng science*, 1995, 19:17–21.
89. Bradley PR, ed. *British herbal compendium*, Vol. 1. Guildford UK, British Herbal Medicine Association, 1992:115–118.
90. Sonnenborn U, Hänsel R. *Panax ginseng*. In: De Smet PAGM et al., eds. *Adverse reactions of herbal drugs*. Springer-Verlag, Berlin, 1992:179–192.
91. Jones BD, Runikis AM. Interaction of ginseng with phenelzine. *Journal of clinical psychopharmacology*, 1987, 7:201–202.
92. Shader RI, Greenblatt DJ. Phenelzine and the dream machine-ramblings and reflections. *Journal of clinical psychopharmacology*, 1985, 5:67.
93. Soldati F. Toxicological studies on ginseng. *Proceedings of the fourth International Ginseng Symposium*. Daejeon, Republic of Korea, Korean Ginseng and Tobacco Research Institute, 1984.
94. Siegel RK. Ginseng abuse syndrome: problems with the panacea. *Journal of the American Medical Association*, 1979, 241:1614–1615.
95. Tyler V. Performance and immune deficiencies. In: *Herbs of choice*. New York, Pharmaceutical Products Press, 1994:155–157.
96. Ryu SJ, Chien YY. Ginseng-associated cerebral arteritis. *Neurology*, 1995, 45:829–830.
97. Lou BY et al. Eye symptoms due to ginseng poisoning. *Yen ko hsueh pao*, 1989, 5:96–97.
98. Palmer BV, Montgomery AC, Monteiro JC. Gin Seng and mastalgia. *British medical journal*, 1978, 279:1284.
99. Koriech OM. Ginseng and mastalgia. *British medical journal*, 1978, 297:1556.
100. Punnonen R, Lukola A. Oestrogen-like effect of ginseng. *British medical journal*, 1980, 281:1110.
101. Hopkins MP, Androff L, Benninghoff AS. Ginseng face cream and unexplained vaginal bleeding. *American journal of obstetrics and gynecology*, 1988, 159:1121–1122.
102. Buchi K, Jenny E. On the interference of the standardized ginseng extract G115 and pure ginsenosides with agonists of the progesterone receptor of the human myometrium. *Phytopharm*, 1984:1–6.
103. Forgo I, Kayasseh L, Staub JJ. Effect of a standardized ginseng extract on general well-being, reaction capacity, pulmonary function and gonadal hormones. *Medizinische Welt*, 1981, 19:751–756.
104. Reinhold E. Der Einsatz von Ginseng in der Gynäkologie. *Natur- und Ganzheits Medizin*, 1990, 4:131–134.

Radix Glycyrrhizae

Definition

Radix Glycyrrhizae consists of the dried roots and rhizomes of *Glycyrrhiza glabra* L. and its varieties (*1–7*) or of *Glycyrrhiza uralensis* Fisch. (*6, 7*) (Fabaceae).[1]

Synonyms

Liquiritae officinalis Moench is a synonym of *Glycyrrhiza glabra* L. (*1*).

Selected vernacular names

Glycyrrhiza glabra L. *and its varieties*

Adimaduram, akarmanis, asloosoos, aslussos, athimaduram, athimaduramu, athimathuram, bekh-e-mahak, bois doux, cha em thet, estamee, gancao, glycyrrhiza, herbe aux tanneurs, hsi-pan-ya-kan-tsao, irk al hiel, irk al hilou, irksos, jakyakgamcho-tang, jashtimadhu, jethimadh, jethimadha, kanpo, kanzo, kan-ts'ao, kum cho, Lakritzenwurzel, licorice, licorice root, liquiritiae radix, liquorice, liquorice root, madhuyashti, madhuyashti rasayama, mulathee, muleti, mulhatti, neekhiyu, Persian licorice, racine de reglisse, racine douce, reglisse, reglisse officinalis, rhizoma glycyrrhizae, Russian licorice, Russian liquorice, Russisches Süssholz, si-pei, sinkiang licorice, Spanish licorice, Spanish liquorice, Spanisches Süssholz, Süssholzwurzel, sweet root, sweetwood, ud al sus, velmi, walmee, welmii, xi-bei, yashti, yashtimadhu, yashtimadhukam, yashtomadhu (*1–15*).

Glycyrrhiza uralensis Fisch.

Chinese licorice, Chinese liquorice, gancao, kan-ts'ao, kanzo, kanzoh, licorice root, liquiritiae radix, north-eastern Chinese licorice, saihokukanzoh, tohoku kanzo, tongpei licorice, tung-pei-kan-tsao, Ural liquorice, uraru-kanzo (*14–17*).

---

[1] *Glycyrrhiza inflata* Bat. is listed in the Chinese pharmacopoeia (*6*). However, literature references to botanical, chemical, and biological studies on this species are rare. Therefore, it has not been included in this monograph.

Description
Glycyrrhiza glabra L. and its varieties

A perennial plant, up to more than 1 m in height, erect, with highly developed stoloniferous roots. Leaves compound, 9–17 alternate imparipinnate leaflets, oblong to elliptical-lanceolate, acute or obtuse; racemes loose, shorter than the leaves or a little longer. Flowers 1 cm long. Flat pods oblong to linear, 1–3 cm long by 6 mm wide, more or less densely echinate glandular, many-seeded or abbreviated, 2- or 3-seeded (*1, 11*).

Glycyrrhiza uralensis Fisch.

A perennial glandular herb, 30–100 cm high. Stem erect, with short whitish hairs and echinate glandular hairs; the lower part of the stem is woody. Leaves alternate, imparipinnate; leaflets 7–17, ovate-elliptical, 2–5.5 cm long by 1–3 cm wide; apex obtuse-rounded; base rounded; both surfaces covered with glandular hairs and short hairs. Stipules lanceolate. Inflorescence an axillary cluster. Flowers purplish, papilionaceous; calyx villous. Fruit a flat pod, oblong, sometimes falcate, 6–9 mm wide, densely covered with brownish echinate glandular hairs. Seeds 2–8. The root is cylindrical, fibrous, flexible, 20–22 cm long and 15 mm in diameter, with or without cork, cork reddish, furrowed, light yellow inside (*16*).

Plant material of interest: dried root and rhizome
General appearance
Glycyrrhiza glabra L. and its varieties

The commercial variety, *G. glabra* var. *typica* Regel & Herd, known as Spanish liquorice, consists generally of roots and rhizomes in nearly cylindrical pieces, up to 1 m long and 5–20 mm in diameter; externally, the bark is brownish grey to dark brown, longitudinally wrinkled, occasionally bearing small dark buds in rhizomes or small circular or transverse rootlet-scars in roots. The peeled root is yellow, smooth, fibrous, finely striated; fracture, fibrous in the bark and splintery in the wood; internally, bright yellow. A distinct cambium ring separates the yellowish grey bark from the finely radiate yellow wood; central pith, only in rhizomes (*1, 2, 7*).

The commercial variety, *G. glabra* var. *glandulifera* (Wald et Kit) Regel & Herd, known as Russian liquorice, consists mainly of roots, in cylindrical pieces somewhat tapering and sometimes longitudinally split; 15–40 cm long, 1–5 cm in diameter. The enlarged crown of the root may attain up to 10 cm in diameter; externally, the unpeeled root purplish brown, somewhat scaly, with stem scars at the top; the peeled root yellowish, coarsely striated; fracture as for Spanish type; internally, yellow, radiating (*1*).

Glycyrrhiza uralensis Fisch.

The roots and rhizomes are cylindrical, fibrous, flexible, 20–100 cm long, 0.6–3.5 cm in diameter, with or without cork. Externally reddish brown or greyish brown, longitudinally wrinkled, furrowed, lenticellate, and with sparse rootlet scars. Texture compact, fracture slightly fibrous, yellowish white, starchy; cambium ring distinct, rays radiate, some with clefts. Rhizomes cylindrical, externally with bud scars, pith present in the centre of fracture (*6*, *7*, *16*, *17*).

Organoleptic properties

Odour slight and characteristic (*1*, *6*, *7*); taste, very sweet (*1*, *6*, *7*, *13*, *15*, *17*).

Microscopic characteristics

In transverse section the cork is thick, brown or purplish brown, formed of several layers of flattened polygonal thin-walled cells; cortex of phelloderm in root somewhat narrow, yellow fibres of parenchyma cells contain isolated prisms of calcium oxalate; phloem, wide, yellow, traversed by numerous wavy parenchymatous medullary rays, 1–8 cells wide and consisting of numerous radial groups of fibres, each surrounded by a crystal sheath of parenchyma cells. Each cell usually contains a prism of calcium oxalate and layers of parenchyma alternating with sieve tissue, the latter occasionally obliterated, appearing as refractive irregular structures; phloem fibres, very long, with very narrow lumen and strongly thickened stratified walls which are cellulosic in the inner part of the phloem and slightly lignified in the outer; xylem, yellow, distinctly radiate; xylem rays, consisting of small pale yellow parenchyma, groups of fibres similar to those of the phloem but more lignified, and surrounded by crystal-sheath, tracheids, and large wide lumen vessels, 80–200 µm in diameter, with thick yellow reticulate walls or with numerous oval bordered pits with slit-shaped openings. Other parenchyma cells contain small round or oval starch granules. Pith, only in rhizome, dark yellow, parenchymatous. Root, with 4-arch primary xylem, no pith and shows 4 broad primary medullary rays, radiating from the centre at right angles to one another. In peeled liquorice, the cork, cortex, and sometimes part of the phloem are absent (*1*).

Powdered plant material

Light yellow in the peeled or brownish yellow or purplish brown in the unpeeled root. Characterized by the numerous fragments of the fibres accompanied by crystal-sheath, the fibres 8–25 µm, mostly 10–15 µm, in diameter; dark yellow fragments of vessels, 80–200 µm in diameter, containing solitary prismatic crystals of calcium oxalate, free or in cells 10–35 µm (mostly 15–25 µm) long; numerous simple oval, round or fusiform starch granules, free or in parenchyma cells, with no striation but occasionally showing hilum, 2–20 µm (mostly about 10 µm) in diameter; cork may be present (*1*, *2*, *7*).

Geographical distribution
Glycyrrhiza glabra
Native to central and south-western Asia and the Mediterranean region (*11, 12, 13*). It is cultivated in the Mediterranean basin of Africa, in southern Europe, and in India (*1, 11, 12, 13*).

Glycyrrhiza uralensis
Northern China, Mongolia, and Siberia (*16, 17*).

General identity tests
Macroscopic, microscopic, and microchemical examinations (*1–7*); and thin-layer chromatographic analysis for the presence of glycyrrhizin (*2–7*).

Purity tests
Microbiology
The test for *Salmonella* spp. in Radix Glycyrrhizae products should be negative. The maximum acceptable limits of other microorganisms are as follows (*18, 19, 20*). For preparation of decoction: aerobic bacteria—not more than 10^7/g; fungi—not more than 10^5/g; *Escherichia coli*—not more than 10^2/g. Preparations for internal use: aerobic bacteria—not more than 10^5/g or ml; fungi—not more than 10^4/g or ml; enterobacteria and certain Gram-negative bacteria—not more than 10^3/g or ml; *Escherichia coli*—0/g or ml.

Total ash
Not more than 7% (*6, 7*).

Acid-insoluble ash
Not more than 2% (*1–3, 6, 7*).

Sulfated ash
Not more than 10% (*2*).

Water-soluble extractive
Not less than 20% (*8*).

Dilute alcohol-soluble extractive
Not less than 25% (*7*).

Pesticide residues
To be established in accordance with national requirements. Normally, the maximum residue limit of aldrin and dieldrin for Radix Glycyrrhizae is not

more than 0.05 mg/kg (*20*). For other pesticides, see WHO guidelines on quality control methods for medicinal plants (*18*) guidelines for predicting dietary intake of pesticide residues (*21*).

Heavy metals

Recommended lead and cadmium levels are no more than 10 and 0.3 mg/kg, respectively, in the final dosage form of the plant material (*18*).

Radioactive residues

For analysis of strontium-90, iodine-131, caesium-134, caesium-137, and plutonium-239, see WHO guidelines on quality control methods for medicinal plants (*18*).

Other purity tests

Alcohol-soluble extractive, chemical, and foreign organic matter tests to be established in accordance with national requirements.

Chemical assays

Assay for glycyrrhizin (glycyrrhizic acid, glycyrrhizinic acid) content (at least 4%) by means of spectrophotometric (*1, 2*), thin-layer chromatographic–densitometric (*22, 23*) or high-performance liquid chromatographic (*24–26*) methods.

Major chemical constituents

The major constituents are triterpene saponins. Glycyrrhizin (glycyrrhizic acid, glycyrrhizinic acid) is the major component (2–9%); minor components occur in proportions that vary depending on the species and geographical location (*24–27*). Glycyrrhizin occurs as a mixture of potassium and calcium salts (*9*). It is a monodesmoside, which on hydrolysis releases two molecules of

isoliquiritigenin   R = H
isoliquiritin   R = β-D-glucopyranosyl

liquiritigenin   R = H
liquiritin   R = β-D-glucopyranosyl

glycyrrhizin or glycyrrhizic acid or glycyrrhizinic acid
aglycone = glycyrrhetic acid or glycyrrhetinic acid

D-glucuronic acid and the aglycone glycyrrhetic (glycyrrhetinic) acid (enoxolone) (*28*). Glycyrrhizin is generally regarded as the active principle of Radix Glycyrrhizae and is responsible for its sweetness, which is 50 times that of sucrose (*27*). Flavonoid constituents include liquiritigenin and isoliquiritigenin.

Dosage forms

Crude plant material, dried extract and liquid extract. Store in a well-closed container, protected from light and moisture (*1, 3*).

Medicinal uses

Uses supported by clinical data

None.

Uses described in pharmacopoeias and in traditional systems of medicine

As a demulcent in the treatment of sore throats, and as an expectorant in the treatment of coughs and bronchial catarrh. Also in the prophylaxis and treatment of gastric and duodenal ulcers, and dyspepsia (*1, 6, 8, 27–29*). As an anti-inflammatory agent in the treatment of allergic reactions (*27*), rheumatism and arthritis (*9*), to prevent liver toxicity, and to treat tuberculosis and adrenocorticoid insufficiency (*9, 30*).

Uses described in folk medicine, not supported by experimental or clinical data

As a laxative, emmenagogue, contraceptive, galactagogue, antiasthmatic drug, and antiviral agent (*15*). In the treatment of dental caries, kidney stones, heart disease (*15*), "consumption", epilepsy, loss of appetite, appendicitis, dizziness, tetanus, diphtheria, snake bite, and haemorrhoids (*11, 13*).

Pharmacology

Experimental pharmacology

The demulcent action of the drug is due primarily to glycyrrhizin (*27*). The antitussive and expectorant properties of the drug have also been attributed to glycyrrhizin, which accelerates tracheal mucus secretion (*27*).

The antiulcer activity of Radix Glycyrrhizae has been demonstrated both experimentally and clinically. Intraperitoneal, intraduodenal, or oral administration of aqueous or alcoholic extracts of Radix Glycyrrhizae reduced gastric secretions in rats, and it inhibited the formation of gastric ulcers induced by pyloric ligation, aspirin, and ibuprofen (*27, 31–32*). Glycyrrhizin and its aglycone (glycyrrhetic acid, enoxolone), two of the active constituents of Radix Glycyrrhizae, both have antiphlogistic activity and increase the rate of mucus secretion by the gastric mucosa (9). Deglycyrrhizinated liquorice (97% of glycyrrhizin is removed) effectively treated stress-induced ulcers in animal models (31–34). The mechanism of antiulcer activity involves acceleration of mucin excretion through increasing the synthesis of glycoprotein at the gastric mucosa, prolonging the life of the epithelial cells, and antipepsin activity (32).

The spasmolytic activity of Radix Glycyrrhizae has been demonstrated *in vivo* (guinea-pig, rabbit, and dog) (35–37), and appears to be due to the flavonoids liquiritigenin and isoliquiritigenin (38).

Glycyrrhizin reduces the toxic action of carbon tetrachloride- and galactosamine-induced cytotoxicity in cultured rat hepatocytes, through its antioxidant activity (9, 27). Glycyrrhizin inhibited histamine release from rat mast cells and prevented carbon tetrachloride-induced liver lesions and macrophage-mediated cytotoxicity (27). Intragastric administration of a flavonoid fraction isolated from Radix Glycyrrhizae to mice protected against carbon tetrachloride hepatotoxicity (39). Glycyrrhizin protected the liver apparently through its membrane stabilization effects (27).

The anti-inflammatory and antiallergic actions of the drug have been attributed to the corticosteroid-like activity of glycyrrhizin and glycyrrhetic acid (enoxolone). These compounds act indirectly by potentiating the activity of corticosteroids. *In vitro*, glycyrrhetic acid inhibits Δ^4 β-reductase, an enzyme that competitively inactivates steroid hormones, and 11β-hydroxysteroid dehydrogenase, the enzyme that deactivates cortisol (27). Glycyrrhizin given intraperitoneally suppressed contact dermatitis in mice, and was more effective than prednisolone, but no effects were observed after oral administration (9).

In vitro, the drug inhibits the growth of *Bacillus subtilis* (40), *Mycobacterium tuberculosis* (41), *Aspergillus spp.* (42), *Staphylococcus aureus*, *Mycobacterium smegmatis*, and *Candida albicans* (43).

Clinical pharmacology

Oral administration of Radix Glycyrrhizae to 15 patients with peptic ulcer reduced symptoms and improved healing in 75% of the cases (44). Glycyrrhetic acid (enoxolone), the active constituent, produced its antiulcer activity by inhibiting 15-hydroxyprostaglandin dehydrogenase and Δ^{13}-prostaglandin reductase (45). Inhibition of these two enzymes stimulated an increase in the concentration of prostaglandins E and $F_{2\alpha}$ in the stomach, which promoted the healing of peptic ulcers owing to a cytoprotective effect on the gastric mucosa (45). Carbenoxolone, a derivative of glycyrrhetic acid, has been used clinically for years in the treatment of gastric and duodenal ulcers (46).

Oral administration of deglycyrrhizinated liquorice (380 mg, 3 times daily) to 169 patients with chronic duodenal ulcers was as effective as antacid or cimetidine treatments (47). These results indicate that, in addition to glycyrrhetic acid, other unidentified constituents of Radix Glycyrrhizae contribute to its antiulcer activity.

Reports on the usefulness of liquorice extracts on body fluid homeostasis in patients with Addison disease are contradictory. One study found no positive effects (*48*), while three other studies noted an increase in weight gain and sodium retention (*49–51*).

Contraindications

Radix Glycyrrhizae is contraindicated in patients with hypertension, cholestatic disorders or cirrhosis of the liver, hypokalaemia, or chronic renal insufficiency, and during pregnancy (*9, 29*).

Warnings

Prolonged use of large doses (>50 g/day) of the drug for extended periods (>6 weeks) may increase water accumulation, causing swelling of the hands and feet. Sodium excretion is reduced and potassium excretion is increased. Blood pressure may rise.

Precautions

General

Radix Glycyrrhizae should not be taken concurrently with corticosteroid treatment. If sore throat or cough persists for more than 3 days, the patient should consult a physician.

Drug interactions

Because it increases potassium loss, Radix Glycyrrhizae should not be administered for prolonged use with thiazide and loop diuretics or cardiac glycosides (*29*). Because it reduces sodium and water excretion, the effectiveness of drugs used in the treatment of hypertension may be reduced. Radix Glycyrrhizae should not be administered in conjunction with spironolactone or amiloride (*52*).

Carcinogenesis, mutagenesis, impairment of fertility

Radix Glycyrrhizae is not mutagenic *in vitro* (*53–55*).

Pregnancy: teratogenic effects

The drug is not teratogenic in animal models (*56*).

Pregnancy: non-teratogenic effects

The safety of Radix Glycyrrhizae preparations during pregnancy has not been established. As a precautionary measure the drug should not be used during pregnancy.

Nursing mothers

The safety of Radix Glycyrrhizae preparations during lactation has not been established. As a precautionary measure the drug should not be used during lactation except on medical advice.

Paediatric use

The safety and effectiveness of the drug in children have not been established.

Other precautions

No information available about drug and laboratory test interactions.

Adverse reactions

No adverse reactions have been associated with the drug when used within the recommended dosage and treatment period.

Prolonged use (>6 weeks) of excessive doses (>50 g/day) can lead to pseudoaldosteronism, which includes potassium depletion, sodium retention, oedema, hypertension, and weight gain (*9, 57, 58*). In rare cases, myoglobinuria and myopathy can occur (*59*).

Posology

Unless otherwise prescribed, average daily dose of crude plant material, 5–15 g, corresponding to 200–800 mg of glycyrrhizin. Doses of other preparations should be calculated accordingly (*29*). Radix Glycyrrhizae should not be used for longer than 4–6 weeks without medical advice.

References

1. *African pharmacopoeia, Vol. 1*, 1st. ed. Lagos, Organization of African Unity, Scientific Technical & Research Commission, 1985:131–134.
2. *European pharmacopoeia*, 2nd ed. Strasbourg, Council of Europe, 1995.
3. *British pharmacopoeia*. London, Her Majesty's Stationery Office, 1988.
4. *Deutsches Arzneibuch 1996*. Stuttgart, Deutscher Apotheker Verlag, 1996.
5. *Pharmacopoeia helvetica VII*. Berne, Département fédéral de l'intérieur, 1994.
6. *Pharmacopoeia of the People's Republic of China* (English ed.). Guangzhou, Guangdong Science and Technology Press, 1992.
7. *The pharmacopoeia of Japan XII*. Tokyo, The Society of Japanese Pharmacopoeia, 1991.
8. *Farmakope Indonesia*, 4th ed. Jakarta, Departemen Kesehatan, Republik Indonesia, 1995.
9. Bradley PR, ed. *British herbal compendium, Vol. 1*. Bournemouth, British Herbal Medicine Association, 1992:145–148.
10. Kapoor LD. *Handbook of Ayurvedic medicinal plants*. Boca Raton, FL, CRC Press, 1990:194–195.
11. *The Indian pharmaceutical codex. Vol. I. Indigenous drugs*. New Delhi, Council of Scientific & Industrial Research, 1953:112–113.

12. Ghazanfar SA. *Handbook of Arabian medicinal plants.* Boca Raton, FL, CRC Press, 1994:110–111.
13. Chin WY, Keng H. *An illustrated dictionary of Chinese medicinal herbs.* Singapore, CRCS Publications, 1992.
14. Hsu HY. *Oriental materia medica, a concise guide.* Long Beach, CA, Oriental Healing Arts Institute, 1986:532–535.
15. Farnsworth NR, ed. *NAPRALERT database.* University of Illinois at Chicago, IL, August 21, 1995 production (an on-line database available directly through the University of Illinois at Chicago or through the Scientific and Technical Network (STN) of Chemical Abstracts Services).
16. *Medicinal plants in China.* Manila, World Health Organization, 1989 (WHO Regional Publications, Western Pacific Series, No. 2).
17. Keys JD. *Chinese herbs, their botany, chemistry and pharmacodynamics.* Rutland, VT, CE Tuttle, 1976:120–121.
18. *Quality control methods for medicinal plant materials.* Geneva, World Health Organization, 1998.
19. *Deutsches Arzneibuch 1996. Vol. 2. Methoden der Biologie.* Stuttgart, Deutscher Apotheker Verlag, 1996.
20. *European pharmacopoeia*, 3rd ed. Strasbourg, Council of Europe, 1997.
21. *Guidelines for predicting dietary intake of pesticide residues*, 2nd rev. ed. Geneva, World Health Organization, 1997 (unpublished document WHO/FSF/FOS/97.7; available from Food Safety, WHO, 1211 Geneva 27, Switzerland).
22. Takino Y et al. Quantitative determination of glycyrrhizic acid in liquorice roots by TLC-densitometry studies on the evaluation of crude drugs. VI. *Planta medica*, 1979, 36:74–78.
23. Vanhaelen M, Vanhaelen-Fastré R. Quantitative determination of biologically active constituents in medicinal plant crude extracts by thin-layer chromatography densitometry. *Journal of chromatography*, 1983, 281:263–271.
24. Sticher O, Soldati F. Glycyrrhizinsäure-Bestimmung in Radix Liquiritiae mit Hochleistungs-flüssigkeitschromatographie (HPLC). *Pharmaceutica acta Helvetica*, 1978, 53:46–52.
25. Sagara K. Determination of glycyrrhizin in pharmaceutical preparations by ion-pair high-performance liquid chromatography. *Shoyakugaku zasshi*, 1986, 40:77–83.
26. Okada K et al. High-speed liquid chromatographic analysis of constituents in licorice root. I. Determination of glycyrrhizin. *Yakugaku zasshi*, 1981, 101:822–828.
27. Hikino H. Recent research on Oriental medicinal plants. In: Wagner H, Hikino H, Farnsworth NR, eds. *Economic and medicinal plant research.* Vol. 1. London, Academic Press, 1985:53–85.
28. Bruneton J. *Pharmacognosy, phytochemistry, medicinal plants.* Paris, Lavoisier, 1995:549–554.
29. German Commission E Monograph, Liquiritiae radix. *Bundesanzeiger*, 1985, 90:15 May
30. Schambelan M. Licorice ingestion and blood pressure regulating hormones. *Steroids*, 1994, 59:127–130.
31. Dehpour AR et al. The protective effect of liquorice components and their derivatives against gastric ulcer induced by aspirin in rats. *Journal of pharmacy and pharmacology*, 1994, 46:148–149.
32. Dehpour AR et al. Antiulcer activities of liquorice and its derivatives in experimental gastric lesion induced by ibuprofen in rats. *International journal of pharmaceutics*, 1995, 119:133–138.
33. Morgan RJ et al. The protective effect of deglycyrrhinized liquorice against aspirin and aspirin plus bile acid-induced gastric mucosal damage, and its influence

on aspirin absorption in rats. *Journal of pharmacy and pharmacology*, 1983, 35:605–607.

34. Russell RI, Morgan RJ, Nelson LM. Studies on the protective effect of deglycyrrhinized liquorice against aspirin (ASA) and ASA plus bile acid-induced gastric mucosal damage, and ASA absorption in rats. *Scandinavian journal of gastroenterology*, 1984, 19(Suppl.):97–100.
35. Takagi K, Harada M. Pharmacological studies on herb Peony root. III. Effects of peoniflorin on circulatory and respiration system and isolated organs. *Yakugaku zasshi*, 1969, 89:893–896.
36. Wrocinski T. Determination of the activity of spasmolytic drugs with reference to the papaverine standard. *Biuletyn Instytutu Roslin Leczniczych*, 1960, 6:236.
37. Shihata M, Elghamry MI. Experimental studies in the effect of *Glycyrrhiza glabra*. *Planta medica*, 1963, 11:37.
38. Chandler RF. Licorice, more than just a flavour. *Canadian pharmaceutical journal*, 1985, 118:420–424.
39. Wang GS, Han ZW. The protective action of *Glycyrrhiza* flavonoids against tetrachloride hepatotoxicity in mice. *Yao hsueh hsueh pao*, 1993, 28:572–576.
40. Sabahi T et al. Screening of plants from the southeast of Iran for antimicrobial activity. *International journal of crude drug research*, 1987, 25:72–76.
41. Grange JM, Davey RW. Detection of antituberculous activity in plant extracts. *Journal of applied bacteriology*, 1990, 68:587–591.
42. Toanun C, Sommart T, Rakvidhyasastra V. Effect of some medicinal plants and spices on growth of *Aspergillus. Proceedings of the 11th Conference of Science and Technology*. Bangkok, Kasetsart University, 1985:364–365.
43. Mitscher LA et al. Antimicrobial agents from higher plants. Antimicrobial isoflavonoids and related substances from *Glycyrrhiza glabra* L. var. *typica. Journal of natural products*, 1980, 43:259–269.
44. Chaturvedi GN. Some clinical and experimental studies on whole root of *Glycyrrhiza glabra* L. (Yashtimadhu) in peptic ulcer. *Indian medical gazette*, 1979, 113:200–205.
45. Baker ME, Fanestil DD. Liquorice as a regulator of steroid and prostaglandin metabolism. *Lancet*, 1991, 337:428–429.
46. Rask-Madsen J et al. Effect of carbenoxolone on gastric prostaglandin E_2 levels in patients with peptic ulcer disease following vagal and pentagastrin stimulation. *European journal of clinical investigation*, 1983, 13:875–884.
47. Kassir ZA. Endoscopic controlled trial of four drug regimens in the treatment of chronic duodenal ulceration. *Irish medical journal*, 1985, 78:153–156.
48. Molhuysen JA et al. A liquorice extract with deoxycortone-like action. *Lancet*, 1950, ii:381–386.
49. Groen J et al. Extract of licorice for the treatment of Addison's disease. *New England journal of medicine*, 1951, 244:471–475.
50. Card WI et al. Effects of liquorice and its derivatives on salt and water metabolism. *Lancet*, 1953, i:663–667.
51. Groen J et al. Effect of glycyrrhizinic acid on the electrolyte metabolism in Addison's disease. *Journal of clinical investigation*, 1952, 31:87–91.
52. Doll R. Treatment of gastric ulcer with carbenoxolone: antagonistic effect of spironolactone. *Gut*, 1968, 9:42–45.
53. Sakai Y et al. Effects of medicinal plant extracts from Chinese herbal medicines on the mutagenic activity of benzo[a]pyrene. *Mutation research*, 1988, 206:327–334.
54. Lee HK et al. Effect of bacterial growth-inhibiting ingredients on the Ames mutagenicity of medicinal herbs. *Mutation research*, 1987, 192:99–104.
55. Yamamoto H, Mizutani T, Nomura H. Studies on the mutagenicity of crude drug extracts. I. *Yakugaku zasshi*, 1982, 102:596–601.

56. Leslie GB, Salmon G. Repeated dose toxicity studies and reproductive studies on nine Bio-Strath herbal remedies. *Swiss medicine*, 1979, 1:1–3.
57. Epistein MT et al. Effects of eating liquorice on the renin-angiotensin aldosterone axis in normal subjects. *British medical journal*, 1977, 1:488–490.
58. Stewart PM et al. Mineralocorticoid activity of liquorice: 11-β hydroxysteroid dehydrogenase deficiency comes of age. *Lancet*, 1987, ii:821–824.
59. Caradonna P et al. Acute myopathy associated with chronic licorice ingestion: Reversible loss of myoadenylate deaminase activity. *Ultrastructural pathology*, 1992, 16:529–535.

Radix Paeoniae

Definition

Radix Paeoniae is the dried root of *Paeonia lactiflora* Pallas (Paeonaceae) (*1*, *2*).[1]

Synonyms

Paeonia albiflora Pallas., *P. edulis* Salisb., *P. officinalis* Thunb. (*5*, *6*).

Selected vernacular names

Báisháo, bo-báisháo, chuan-báisháo, hang-báisháo, mu-shaoyao, mudan, paeoniae alba, paeony, pai shao yao, pe-shou, peony, peony root, Pfingstrose, shakuyaku, shaoyao, syakuyaku, white peony, white-flowered peony (*2*, *4*, *6–8*).

Description

Paeonia lactiflora Pallas is a perennial herb, 50–80 cm high, with a stout branched root. Leaves alternate and biternately compound, the ultimate segments red-veined, oblong-elliptical. The leaflets are narrow-ovate or elliptical, 8–12 cm long and 2–4 cm wide. The petioles are 6–10 cm long. Flowers large (5–10 cm in diameter), solitary, and red, white, or purple. Sepals 4, herbaceous, persistent. Petals 5–10, larger than sepals. Stamens numerous and anthers yellow; carpels 3–5, many-seeded. Fruit, 3–5 coriaceous few-seeded follicles. Seeds large, subglobose; testa thick (*4*, *6*).

Plant material of interest: dried root

General appearance

Radix Paeoniae is cylindrical, straight or slightly curved, two ends truncate, 5–20 cm long and 1–2.5 cm in diameter; externally light greyish brown to reddish brown, glossy or with longitudinal wrinkles, rootlet scars and occasional remains of brown cork, and with laterally elongated lenticels; texture compact, easily broken, fracture relatively even, internally whitish or pale brownish red. Cambium ring distinct and rays radial (*1*, *2*).

---

[1] *Paeoniae veitchii* is described in the monograph "Radix Paeoniae Rubra" in the Chinese pharmacopoeia (*2*). Moutan Cortex, the root bark of *Paeonia moutan* Sims. (= *P. suffruticosa* Andr.) is also used in traditional medicine (*3–5*), and is listed as "Moutan Bark" in the Japanese pharmacopoeia (*1*).

Organoleptic properties

Odour, slight; taste, slightly sweet at first, followed by a sour or astringent taste and a slight bitterness (*1, 2*).

Microscopic characteristics

Literature description not available; to be established in accordance with national requirements.

Powdered plant material

Light greyish brown powder; masses of gelatinized starch granules fairly abundant, 5–25 μm in diameter; clusters of calcium oxalate 11–35 μm in diameter, packed in parenchyma cells in rows or singly; bordered, pitted, or reticulate vessels 20–65 μm in diameter, walls thickened and slightly lignified (*1, 2*).

Geographical distribution

China, India, and Japan (*6*).

General identity tests

Macroscopic, microscopic, and microchemical examinations; thin-layer chromatographic analysis for the presence of the monoterpene glycoside paeoniflorin (*1, 2*).

Purity tests

Microbiology

The test for *Salmonella* spp. in Radix Paeoniae products should be negative. The maximum acceptable limits of other microorganisms are as follows (*9–11*). For preparation of decoction: aerobic bacteria—not more than 10^7/g; fungi—not more than 10^5/g; *Escherichia coli*—not more than 10^2/g. Preparations for internal use: aerobic bacteria—not more than 10^5/g or ml; fungi—not more than 10^4/g or ml; enterobacteria and certain Gram-negative bacteria—not more than 10^3/g or ml; *Escherichia coli*—0/g or ml.

Total ash

Not more than 6.5% (*1, 2*).

Acid-insoluble ash

Not more than 0.5% (*1*).

Pesticide residues

To be established in accordance with national requirements. Normally, the maximum residue limit of aldrin and dieldrin for Radix Paeoniae is not more than 0.05 mg/kg (*11*). For other pesticides, see WHO guidelines on quality control methods for medicinal plants (*9*) and guidelines for predicting dietary intake of pesticide residues (*12*).

Heavy metals

Recommended lead and cadmium levels are not more than 10 and 0.3 mg/kg, respectively, in the final dosage form of the plant material (*9*).

Radioactive residues

For analysis of strontium-90, iodine-131, caesium-134, caesium-137, and plutonium-239, see WHO guidelines on quality control methods for medicinal plants (*9*).

Other purity tests

Alcohol-soluble extractive, chemical, foreign organic matter, moisture and water-soluble extractive tests to be established in accordance with national requirements.

Chemical assays

Contains not less than 2.0% of paeoniflorin (*1*, *2*), assayed by a combination of thin-layer chromatographic–spectrophotometric methods (*2*) or by high-performance liquid chromatography (*1*).

Major chemical constituents

Paeoniflorin, a monoterpene glycoside that is the major active constituent (*5*, *13*), is present in the range of 0.05–6.01% (*14*, *15*).

paeoniflorin

Dosage forms

Crude plant material, powder, and decoction. Store in a ventilated dry environment protected from light (*2*).

197

Medicinal uses

Uses supported by clinical data

None.

Uses described in pharmacopoeias and in traditional systems of medicine

As an analgesic, anti-inflammatory and antispasmodic drug in the treatment of amenorrhoea, dysmenorrhoea, and pain in the chest and abdomen (2). Radix Paeoniae is also used to treat dementia, headache, vertigo, spasm of the calf muscles (2, 4, 5), liver disease, and allergies, and as an anticoagulant (8, 13).

Uses described in folk medicine, not supported by experimental or clinical data

The treatment of atopic eczema, boils, and sores (5); to reduce fevers, induce sterility, and treat burns (8).

Pharmacology

Experimental pharmacology

The primary pharmacological effects of Radix Paeoniae are antispasmodic, anti-inflammatory, and analgesic. A decoction of the drug had antispasmodic effects on the ileum and uterus when administered orally to mice, rabbits, and guinea-pigs (13). Similar effects were observed with a methanol extract in rat uterus (16), but an ethanol extract had uterine stimulant activity in rabbits (17). Radix Paeoniae extracts tested *in vitro* relaxed smooth muscles in both rat stomach and uterine assays (13).

Intragastric administration of a hot-water extract of Radix Paeoniae to rats inhibited inflammation in adjuvant-induced arthritis (18) and carrageenin-induced paw oedema (19). The major active constituent of the drug, paeoniflorin, a monoterpenoid glycoside, has sedative, analgesic, antipyretic, anti-inflammatory and vasodilatory effects *in vivo*. Hexobarbital-induced hypnosis was potentiated and acetic acid-induced writhing was inhibited in mice after intragastric administration of paeoniflorin (20, 21).

Intragastric administration of hot-water or ethanol extracts of Radix Paeoniae to rats inhibited ADP-, arachidonic acid- and collagen-induced platelet aggregation, as well as endotoxin-induced disseminated intravascular coagulation (22–24). Similar effects were observed in rabbits and mice after intraperitoneal administration of the drug (25). When tested by the standard fibrin plate method, ethanol and hot-water extracts of the drug had antifibrinolytic activity *in vitro* (26). Paeoniflorin had anticoagulant activity both *in vitro* (24), and *in vivo* (in mice) (27).

Intragastric administration of extracts of Radix Paeoniae protected the liver against carbon tetrachloride-induced hepatotoxicity in mice and rats (28).

Oral administration of water extracts of Radix Paeoniae or its major constituent, paeoniflorin, attenuated the scopolamine-induced impairment of radial maze performance in rats (*29, 30*). Paeoniflorin prevented the scopolamine-induced decrease in acetylcholine content in the striatum, but not in the hippocampus or cortex (*30*). Oral administration of paeoniflorin further attenuated learning impairment of aged rats in operant brightness discrimination tasks (*31*). The results of this study suggest that further research to explore the therapeutic potential of paeoniflorin in cognitive disorders such as senile dementia may be promising (*31*).

Contraindications

Reports of traditional use indicate that Radix Paeoniae may have abortifacient activity; therefore, the use of Radix Paeoniae in pregnancy is contraindicated (*32*).

Warnings

No information available.

Precautions

Drug interactions

Radix Paeoniae should not be combined with *Fritillaria verticillata*, *Cuscuta japonica*, and *Rheum officinale* (*7*).

Carcinogenesis, mutagenesis, impairment of fertility

Hot-water or methanol extracts of Radix Paeoniae are not mutagenic *in vitro* (*33, 34*).

Pregnancy: non-teratogenic effects

See Contraindications.

Nursing mothers

Excretion of the drug into breast milk and its effects on the newborn have not been established; therefore, use of the drug during lactation is not recommended.

Paediatric use

No information available; therefore, use of Radix Paeoniae in children is not recommended.

Other precautions

No information available about general precautions, drug and laboratory test interactions, or teratogenic effects on pregnancy.

Adverse reactions

No information available.

Posology

Maximum daily oral dose of crude plant material, 6–15 g (2), standardized for paeoniflorin.

References

1. *The pharmacopoeia of Japan XII*. Tokyo, The Society of Japanese Pharmacopoeia, 1996.
2. *Pharmacopoeia of the People's Republic of China* (English ed.). Guangzhou, Guangdong Science and Technology Press, 1992.
3. Hsu HY. *Oriental materia medica, a concise guide*. Long Beach, CA, Oriental Healing Arts Institute, 1986:144–145.
4. National Institute for the Control of Pharmaceutical and Biological Products, ed. *Color atlas of Chinese traditional drugs, Vol. 1*. Beijing, Science Press, 1987:88–91; 131–133.
5. Bruneton J. *Pharmacognosy, phytochemistry, medicinal plants*. Paris, Lavoisier, 1995:400–404.
6. *Medicinal plants in China*. Manila, World Health Organization, 1989 (WHO Regional Publications, Western Pacific Series, No. 2).
7. Keys JD. *Chinese herbs, their botany, chemistry and pharmacodynamics*. Rutland, VT, CE Tuttle, 1976.
8. Farnsworth NR, ed. *NAPRALERT database*. Chicago, University of Illinois at Chicago, IL, March 15, 1995 production (an on-line database available directly through the University of Illinois at Chicago or through the Scientific and Technical Network (STN) of Chemical Abstracts Services).
9. *Quality control methods for medicinal plant materials*. Geneva, World Health Organization, 1998.
10. *Deutsches Arzneibuch 1996. Vol. 2. Methoden der Biologie*. Stuttgart, Deutscher Apotheker Verlag, 1996.
11. *European pharmacopoeia*, 3rd ed. Strasbourg, Council of Europe, 1997.
12. *Guidelines for predicting dietary intake of pesticide residues*, 2nd rev. ed. Geneva, World Health Organization, 1997 (unpublished document WHO/FSF/FOS/97.7; available from Food Safety, WHO, 1211 Geneva 27, Switzerland).
13. Hikino H. Oriental medicinal plants. In: Wagner H, Hikino H, Farnsworth NR, eds. *Economic and medicinal plant research Vol. 1*. London, Academic Press, 1985.
14. He LY. Assay of paeoniflorin. *Yao hsueh t'ung pao*, 1983, 18:230–231.
15. Yamashita Y et al. Studies on the good varieties of Paeoniae Radix. I. Yield of root, paeoniflorin and tannin contents in Paeoniae Radix. *Shoyakugaku zasshi*, 1993, 47:434–439.
16. Lee EB. The screening of biologically active plants in Korea using isolated organ preparation. IV. Anticholinergic and oxytocic actions in rat's ileum and uterus. *Korean journal of pharmacognosy*, 1982, 13:99–101.
17. Harada M, Suzuki M, Ozaki Y. Effect of Japanese *Angelicia* root and *Paeonia* root on uterine contraction in rabbit *in situ*. *Journal of pharmacobiological dynamics*, 1984, 7:304–311.
18. Cho S, Takahashi M, Toita S, Cyong JC. Suppression of adjuvant arthritis on rat by Oriental herbs. *Shoyakugaku zasshi*, 1982, 36:78–81.

19. Arichi S et al. Studies on Moutan Cortex. III. On anti-inflammatory activities. Part I. *Shoyakugaku zasshi*, 1979, 33:178–184.
20. Takagi K, Harada M. Pharmacological studies on herb Peony root. I. Central effects of paeoniflorin and combined effects with licorice component FM 100. *Yakugaku zasshi*, 1969, 89:879.
21. Sugishita E, Amagaya S, Ogihara Y. Studies on the combination of Glycyrrhizae Radix in Shakuyakukanzo-to. *Journal of pharmacobiological dynamics*, 1984, 7:427–435.
22. Kim JH et al. Effects of some combined crude drug preparations against platelet aggregations. *Korean journal of pharmacognosy*, 1990, 21:126–129.
23. Kubo M, Matsuda H, Matsuda R. Studies on Moutan Cortex VIII. Inhibitory effects on the intravascular coagulation (Part II). *Shoyakugaku zasshi*, 1984, 38:307–312.
24. Kubo M et al. Studies on Moutan Cortex VI. Inhibitory effects on the intravascular coagulation (Part I). *Shoyakugaku zasshi*, 1982, 36:70–77.
25. Wang HF et al. Radiation-protective and platelet aggregation inhibitory effects of five traditional Chinese drugs and acetylsalicylic acid following high-dose gamma-irradiation. *Journal of ethnopharmacology*, 1991, 34:215–219.
26. Kawashiri N et al. Effects of traditional crude drugs on fibrinolysis by plasmin: antiplasmin principles in eupolyphaga. *Chemical and pharmaceutical bulletin*, 1986, 34:2512–2517.
27. Ishida H et al. Studies on active substances in herbs used for Oketsu (Stagnant Blood) in Chinese medicine. VI. On the anticoagulative principle in Paeoniae Radix. *Chemical and pharmaceutical bulletin*, 1987, 35:849–852.
28. Yun HS, Chang IM. Liver protective activities of Korean medicinal plants. *Korean journal of pharmacognosy*, 1980, 11:149–152.
29. Ohta H et al. Peony and its major constituent, paeoniflorin, improve radial maze performance impaired by scopolamine in rats. *Pharmacology, biochemistry and behavior*, 1993, 45:719–723.
30. Ohta H et al. Involvement of $\alpha 1$- but not $\alpha 2$-adrenergic systems in the antagonizing effect of paeoniflorin on scopolamine-induced deficit in radial maze performance in rats. *Japan journal of pharmacology*, 1993, 62:199–202.
31. Ohta H et al. Paeoniflorin attenuates learning impairment of aged rats in operant brightness discrimination task. *Pharmacology, biochemistry and behavior*, 1994, 49:213–217.
32. Woo WS et al. A review of research on plants for fertility regulation in Korea. *Korean journal of pharmacognosy*, 1981, 12:153–170.
33. Chang IM et al. Assay of potential mutagenicity and antimutagenicity of Chinese herbal drugs by using SOS Chromotest (*E. coli* PQ37) and SOS UMU test (*S. typhimurium* TA 1535/ PSK 1002). *Proceedings of the first Korea–Japan Toxicology Symposium, Safety Assessment of Chemicals in Vitro*, 1989:133–145.
34. Morimoto I et al. Mutagenicity screening of crude drugs with *Bacillus subtilis* rec-assay and *Salmonella*/microsome reversion assay. *Mutation research*, 1982, 97:81–102.

Semen Plantaginis

Definition

Semen Plantaginis is the dried, ripe seed of *Plantago afra* L., *P. indica* L., *P. ovata* Forsk., or *P. asiatica* L. (Plantaginaceae) (*1–4*).

Synonyms

Plantago afra L.
P. psyllium L. (*2*).

Plantago asiatica
None.

Plantago indica L.
P. arenaria Waldstein et Kitaibel, *P. ramosa* Asch. (*1, 2, 5*).

Plantago ovata Forsk.
P. ispaghula Roxb. (*4*).

Selected vernacular names

Psyllium seed, plantain seed, flea seed, Flohsamen, semences de psyllium (*6*).

P. afra L.
Flohsamen, Spanish psyllium (*6*).

P. asiatica
Shazen-shi, Che-qian-zi.

P. indica L.
Flashsamen, fleavort plantago, French psyllium, Spanish psyllium seed, whorled plantago (*6*).

P. ovata Forsk.
Ashwagolam, aspaghol, aspagol, bazarqutuna, blond psyllium, ch'-ch'ientzu, ghoda, grappicol, Indian plantago, Indische Psylli-samen, isabgol, isabgul,

202

isabgul gola, ispaghula, isphagol, vithai, issufgul, jiru, obeko, psyllium, plantain, spogel seeds (*1, 6–9*).

Description
Plantago afra L.

An annual, erect, glandular-hairy caulescent herb, with an erect branching stem (0.2–0.4 m in height); it possesses whorls of flattened linear to linear-lanceolate leaves from the upper axils of which flowering stalks as long as the leaves arise. The stalks terminate in ovate-elliptical spikes up to 12 mm long. The upper bracts ovate-lanceolate up to 4 mm in length and somewhat similar in character to the lower bracts, but with chloroplastids fewer in the midrib of the proximal portion. The flowers are tetramerous with a calyx of 4 similar persistent, lanceolate sepals, each with green midrib and hyaline lamina, a hypo-crateriform corolla of 4 gamopetalous hyaline petals inserted below the ovary, the tube surrounding the ovary and a portion of the filiform, hairy style, the limb with 4-lanceolate, acuminate lobes. The fruit is membranous, 2-celled and 2-seeded (*6*).

Plantago asiatica L.

Usually wrinkled and contracted leaf and spike, greyish green to dark yellow-green in colour; when soaked in water and smoothed out, the lamina is ovate or orbicular-ovate, 4–15 cm in length, 3–8 cm in width; apex acute, and base sharply narrowed; margin slightly wavy, with distinct parallel veins; glabrous or nearly glabrous; petiole is rather longer than the lamina, and its base is slightly expanded with thin-walled leaf-sheath; scape is 10–50 cm in length, one-third to one-half of the upper part forming the spike, with dense florets; the lower part of inflorescence often shows pyxidia; roots usually removed, but, if any, fine roots are closely packed (*6*).

Plantago indica L.

An annual caulescent herb attaining a height of 0.3–0.5 m with an erect or diffuse, hairy, frequently branched stem with whorls of linear to filiform leaves, from the axils of the upper ones of which spring peduncles, which are longer than the leaves and more or less umbellate. The lower bracts are trans-versely obovate below, lanceolate above, with a herbaceous midrib and hyaline margin, glandular hairy; the upper bracts broadly ovate with obtuse summits and also have herbaceous midribs and hyaline margins. The calyx is persistent, hairy, of 2 large spatulate anterior segments and 2 smaller, lateroposterior, lanceolate segments. The corolla is hypocrateriform of 4 petals, the limbs oblong with acute to mucronate summits; the tube of the corolla covering the pyxis and portions of the style. The pyxis is membranous, 2-celled, 2-seeded, and dehisces about or slightly below the middle (*6*).

Plantago ovata Forsk.

An annual, acaulescent herb, the stem of which is very ramified and bears linear leaves that are lanceolate, dentate, and pubescent. The flowers are white and grouped into cylindrical spikes. The sepals are characterized by a distinct midrib extending from the base to the summit; the petal lobes are oval with a mucronate summit. The seeds are oval and clearly carinate, measure 2–3 mm, and are a light grey-pink with a brown line running along their convex side (*6, 7*).

Plant material of interest: seeds

General appearance

Plantago afra L.

Hemianatropous, silky to the touch; ovate to ovate-elongate, larger at one end than the other; concavo-convex; light to moderate brown, dark brown along the margin, very glossy. Length 1.3–2.7 mm, rarely up to 3 mm, and width 0.6–1.1 mm; the convex dorsal surface somewhat transparent, exhibiting a longitudinal brown area extending nearly the length of the seed and representing the embryo lying beneath the seed coat, and a transverse groove nearer the broader than the narrower end and over the point of union of the hypocotyl and cotyledons; the concave ventral surface with a deep excavation, in the centre of the base of which is an oval yellowish white hilum (*1, 6*).

Plantago asiatica L.

Flattened ellipsoidal seed, 2–2.25 mm in length, 0.7–1 mm in width, 0.3–0.5 mm in thickness; externally brown to yellow-brown and lustrous. Under a magnifying glass, the surface of the seed is practically smooth; the dorsal side protrudes like a bow and the ventral side is somewhat dented; micropyle and raphe not observable. A hundred seeds weigh about 0.05 g (*3*).

Plantago indica L.

Ovate-oblong to elliptical; dark brown to maroon, often dull, rough and reticulate, 1.6–3.0 mm in length and 1.0–1.5 mm in width; concavo-convex, the dorsal surface has a longitudinal light brown area extending lengthwise along the centre and beneath the seed coat and has a median transverse groove, dent, or fissure; the ventral surface with a deep concavity, the edge of which is somewhat flattened and frequently forms a sharp indented angle with the base of the cavity, the latter showing a pale brown to occasionally whitish oval hilum (*1, 6*).

Plantago ovata Forsk.

Boat-shaped with ovate outline, pinkish grey to brown in colour along the margin with opaque reticulate surface, 2–2.3 mm long, 1–1.5 mm wide and

1 mm thick, usually with central reddish brown oval patch extending about a third of the length of the seed. The convex dorsal surface has a longitudinal brown area extending nearly along the length of the seed that represents the position of the embryo lying beneath the seed-coat, and a transverse groove nearer to the broader than to the narrower extremity and over the points of union of the hypocotyl and cotyledons. The ventral surface shows a deep brown furrow that does not reach to either end of the seeds, in the centre of which is an oval yellowish white hilum, from which extends to the chalazal end a slightly elevated dark brown raphe. The seed is albuminous with oily endosperm; the embryo is straight, formed of two large plano-convex cotyledons and a small radicle in the narrow end and directed towards the micropyle. The seed is mucilaginous and upon soaking in water, the seed-coat swells and the seed becomes enveloped with a colourless mucilage. The weight of 100 seeds is about 0.1 g. A longitudinal cut, perpendicular to the ventral surface and passing through the hilum, shows a thin dark brown testa within which is a narrow endosperm surrounding a large oval lanceolate cotyledon and large pyramidal radicle directed towards the micropyle (*1, 4, 6*).

Organoleptic properties
Odourless with mucilage-like taste.

Microscopic characteristics
Plantago afra L.
The transverse sections of the seed cut through the central region possess a reniform outline and present for examination a spermoderm, endosperm, and embryo. The spermoderm shows an outer epidermis of mucilaginous epidermal cells with more or less obliterated walls in glycerine mounts; the radial and inner walls swell and disintegrate to form a clear mucilage upon irrigation of the mount with water; and a pigment layer with brown amorphous content. The endosperm composed of irregular-shaped, thick-walled cells with walls of reserve cellulose. The outer layer of this region consists of palisade cells 15–40 µm in height. Aleurone grains and fixed oils are found in the endosperm cells (*5*).

Plantago asiatica L.
Transverse section reveals a seed-coat consisting of three layers of epidermis composed of cells containing mucilage, a vegetative layer, and a pigment layer of approximately equidiameter cells; in the interior, endosperm thicker than seed-coat, enclosing 2 cotyledons (*6*).

Plantago indica L.
The transverse section of the seed shows a similar structure to that described above for *P. afra*, but the palisade cells of the endosperm are up to 52 µm in height (*6*).

P. ovata Forsk.

The transverse cut through the central region possesses a reniform or a concave-convex outline and shows a testa, an endosperm, and 2 plano-convex cotyledons. Each cotyledon shows aleurone strands. On the convex surface a small raphe. The testa formed of one integument showing outer epidermis consisting of polygonal tabular cells with straight thin anticlinal walls covered with smooth cuticle. They are 52–68 µm long, 30–52 µm wide and 27–32 µm thick. The middle (nutrient) layer is formed of collapsed thin cellulosic parenchyma, usually more than one layer, about 5 or 6 rows. The inner epidermis consists of polygonal cells with straight thin anticlinal walls, containing reddish brown contents; they are 16–38 µm long, and 11–20 µm wide and 2–3 µm thick. The endosperm is formed of irregularly shaped thick cellulosic parenchyma showing an epidermis which is palisade-like, cells containing aleurone grains without inclusion, and fixed oil. The embryo formed of thin-walled cellulosic parenchyma containing fixed oil and aleurone grains. Each cotyledon shows 3 pleurone strands (4).

Powdered plant material

The most commonly used *P. ovata* powder is greyish brown showing glossy particles, colourless and with mucilage-like taste, characterized by fragments of epidermis formed of thin-walled polygonal cells with smooth cuticle and containing mucilage in the outer tangential and anticlinal walls, staining red with ruthenium red and blue with methylene blue; fragments of the pigment layer which is formed of polygonal cells with thin straight anticlinal walls with brown content traversed by collapsed colourless parenchyma; abundant fragments of endosperm with aleurone grains which are free of content and fixed oil; fragments of embryo tissues showing thin-walled parenchyma containing fixed oil and aleurone grains; few fragments showing spiral vessels attaining 11–15 µm width and few fibres which are elongated with thin pitted walls and pointed ends attaining 80–180 µm in length and 8–12 µm in width (4).

Geographical distribution

P. afra and *P. indica*, west Mediterranean countries (6); *P. asiatica,* Japan (3). *P. ovata*, Asia and the Mediterranean countries; the plant is cultivated extensively in India and Pakistan and adapts to western Europe and subtropical regions (4, 6, 8–10).

General identity tests

Macroscopic and microscopic examination (1–4); determining the swelling index (1–4); and test for reducing sugars (3, 4).

Purity tests

Microbiology

The test for *Salmonella* spp. in Semen Plantaginis products should be negative. The maximum acceptable limits of other microorganisms are as follows (*11–13*). Preparations for internal use: aerobic bacteria—not more than 10^5/g; fungi—not more than 10^4/g; enterobacteria and certain Gram-negative bacteria—not more than 10^3/g; *Escherichia coli*—0/g.

Chemical

Swelling index of *P. afra* and *P. ovata*, not less than 10 (*2*); of *P. indica*, not less than 8 (*1*); of *P. asiatica*, to be established in accordance with national requirements.

Foreign organic matter

Not more than 0.5% (*1*).

Total ash

Not more than 4.0% (*1*).

Acid-insoluble ash

Not more than 1.0% (*1*).

Moisture

Not more than 14% (*2*).

Pesticide residues

To be established in accordance with national requirements. Normally, the maximum residue limit of aldrin and dieldrin in Semen Plantaginis is not more than 0.05 mg/kg (*2*). For other pesticides, see WHO guidelines on quality control methods for medicinal plants (*11*) and guidelines for predicting dietary intake of pesticide residues (*13*).

Heavy metals

Recommended lead and cadmium levels are not more than 10 and 0.3 mg/kg, respectively, in the final dosage form of the plant material (*11*).

Radioactive residues

For analysis of strontium-90, iodine-131, caesium-134, caesium-137, and plutonium-239, see WHO guidelines on quality control methods for medicinal plants (*11*).

Other purity tests

Tests for water-soluble extractive to be established in accordance with national requirements.

Chemical assays

Mucilage (10–30%) (*14*). *Plantago* products can be assayed for their fibre content by the method described by the Association of Official Analytical Chemists (*14*).

Major chemical constituents

Plantago seeds contain 10–30% mucilaginous hydrocolloid, which is localized in the outer seed-coat (husk) and is the major, active principle. The mucilage is composed of a soluble polysaccharide fraction containing mainly arabinoxylans (85%). The polymer backbone is a xylan with 1 → 3 and 1 → 4 linkages, with no apparent regularity in their distribution. The monosaccharides in this main chain are substituted on C-2 or C-3 by L-arabinose, D-xylose, and α-D-galacturonyl-(1 → 2)-L-rhamnose. In addition, secondary metabolites in the seed include sterols, triterpenes, and aucubin glycosides (*4–7, 15*).

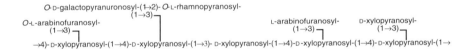

Dosage forms

Seeds, powder, and granules. Store in well-closed containers, in a cool dry place, protected from light (*1–4*).

Medicinal uses

Uses supported by clinical data

As a bulk-forming laxative used to restore and maintain regularity (*2, 4, 16–20*). Semen Plantaginis is indicated in the treatment of chronic constipation, temporary constipation due to illness or pregnancy, irritable bowel syndrome, constipation related to duodenal ulcer or diverticulitis (*17–22*). It is also used to soften the stools of those with haemorrhoids, or after anorectal surgery (*16, 17*).

Uses described in pharmacopoeias and in traditional systems of medicine

While Semen Plantaginis is primarily used in the treatment of constipation, it has also been used effectively in the short-term symptomatic treatment of diarrhoea of various etiologies (*23, 24*).

Uses described in folk medicine, not supported by experimental or clinical data

Other medical uses claimed for Semen Plantaginis include use as an expectorant and antitussive, an antibacterial agent, and a diuretic and in the treatment of rheumatic and gouty afflictions, glandular swelling, and bronchitis (*8*).

Pharmacology
Clinical pharmacology
Constipation

Semen Plantaginis increases the volume of the faeces by absorbing water in the gastrointestinal tract, which stimulates peristalsis (*25*, *26*). The intraluminal pressure is decreased, colon transit is increased, and the frequency of defecation is increased (*15*, *16*, *25*).

When mixed with water, the therapeutic efficacy of the drug is due to the swelling of the mucilaginous seed coat which gives bulk and lubrication (*7*). Semen Plantaginis increases stool weight and water content owing to the water-bound fibre residue and an increased faecal bacterial mass. Clinical studies have demonstrated that ingestion of 18 g of Semen Plantaginis significantly increases faecal fresh and dry weights as compared with weights obtained with placebo (*15*).

Antidiarrhoeal activity

The antidiarrhoeal effects of Semen Plantaginis have been extensively investigated in patients with acute and chronic diarrhoea (*23*, *24*). An increase in the viscosity of the intestinal contents due to the binding of fluid and an increased colonic transit time (decreased frequency of defecation) were observed in patients treated with the drug (*23*, *24*).

Contraindications

Known hypersensitivity or allergy to the plant; faecal impaction or intestinal obstruction; diabetes mellitus where insulin adjustment is difficult (*27*).

Warnings

Semen Plantaginis products should always be taken with sufficient amounts of liquid, and at least half an hour after other medications to prevent delayed absorption of the latter. If bleeding or no response occurs after ingesting the drug, or if abdominal pain occurs 48 hours after treatment, treatment should be stopped and medical advice sought. If diarrhoea persists longer than 3 or 4 days, medical attention should be sought (*28*).

To prevent the generation of airborne dust, users should spoon the product from the container directly into a drinking glass and then add liquid (*28*). To minimize the potential for allergic reaction, health professionals who frequently dispense powdered Semen Plantaginis should avoid inhaling airborne dust while handling these products.

Precautions
General
Semen Plantaginis should be taken with adequate volumes of fluid. It should never be taken orally as the dried powder, because of the possibility of bowel obstruction. In patients who are confined to bed or do little physical exercise, a medical examination may be necessary prior to treatment with the drug.

Drug interactions
Bulking agents have been reported to diminish the absorption of some minerals (calcium, magnesium, copper, and zinc), vitamin B_{12}, cardiac glycosides, and coumarin derivatives (*29–31*). The co-administration of Semen Plantaginis with lithium salts has been reported to reduce the plasma concentrations of the lithium salts and may inhibit their absorption from the gastrointestinal tract (*32*). Semen Plantaginis has also been reported to decrease both the rate and extent of carbamazepine absorption, inducing subclinical levels of the drug (*33*). Therefore, ingestion of lithium salts or carbamazepine and Semen Plantaginis should be separated in time as far as possible (*33*). Individual monitoring of the plasma levels of the drug in patients taking Semen Plantaginis products is also recommended. Insulin-dependent diabetic people may require less insulin (*27*).

Other precautions
No information available concerning carcinogenesis, mutagenesis, impairment of fertility; drug and laboratory test interactions; nursing mothers, paediatric use, or teratogenic or non-teratogenic effects on pregnancy.

Adverse reactions
Sudden increases in dietary fibre may cause temporary gas and bloating. These side-effects may be reduced by gradually increasing fibre intake, starting at one dose per day and gradually increasing to three doses per day (*28*). Occasional flatulence and bloating may be reduced by decreasing the amount of Semen Plantaginis taken for a few days (*28*).

Allergic reactions to *Plantago* products in response to ingestion or inhalation have been reported, especially after previous occupational exposure to these products (*34–36*). These reactions range from urticarial rashes to anaphylactic reactions (rare). One case of fatal bronchospasm has been reported in a *Plantago*-sensitive patient with asthma (*34*).

Posology

The suggested average dose is 7.5 g dissolved in 240 ml water or juice taken orally 1–3 times daily depending on the individual response. The recommended dose for children aged 6–12 years is one-half the adult dose. For children under 6 years, a physician should be consulted. An additional glass of liquid is recommended after ingestion of the drug and generally provides an optimal response. Continued use for 2 or 3 days is needed for maximum laxative benefit.

References

1. *The United States pharmacopeia XXIII*. Rockville, MD, US Pharmacopeial Convention, 1995.
2. *European pharmacopoeia*, 3rd ed. Strasbourg, Council of Europe, 1997.
3. *The pharmacopoeia of Japan XIII*. Tokyo, The Society of Japanese Pharmacopoeia, 1996.
4. *African pharmacopoeia*, 1st ed. Lagos, Organization of African Unity, Scientific, Technical & Research Commission, 1985.
5. Bruneton J. *Pharmacognosy, phytochemistry, medicinal plants*. Paris, Lavoisier, 1995.
6. Youngken HW. *Textbook of pharmacognosy*, 6th ed. Philadelphia, Blakiston, 1950.
7. Tyler VE, Brady LR, Robbers JE, eds. *Pharmacognosy*, 9th ed. Philadelphia, Lea & Febiger, 1988:52–53.
8. Kapoor LD. *Handbook of Ayurvedic medicinal plants*. Boca Raton, FL, CRC Press, 1990:267.
9. Farnsworth NR, ed. *NAPRALERT database*. Chicago, University of Illinois at Chicago, IL, August 8, 1995 production (an on-line database available directly through the University of Illinois at Chicago or through the Scientific and Technical Network (STN) of Chemical Abstracts Services).
10. Mossa JS, Al-Yahya MA, Al-Meshal IA. *Medicinal plants of Saudi Arabia*, Vol. 1. Riyadh, Saudi Arabia, King Saud University Libraries, 1987:262–265.
11. *Quality control methods for medicinal plant materials*. Geneva, World Health Organization, 1998.
12. *Deutsches Arzneibuch 1996. Vol. 2. Methoden der Biologie*. Stuttgart, Deutscher Apotheker Verlag, 1996.
13. *Guidelines for predicting dietary intake of pesticide residues*, 2nd rev. ed. Geneva, World Health Organization, 1997 (unpublished document WHO/FSF/FOS/97.7; available from Food Safety, WHO, 1211 Geneva 27, Switzerland).
14. Prosky L et al. Determination of total dietary fiber in food and food products: collaborative study. *Journal of the Association of Official Analytical Chemists*, 1985, 68:677–679.
15. Marteau P et al. Digestibility and bulking effect of ispaghula husks in healthy humans. *Gut*, 1994, 35:1747–1752.
16. Sölter H, Lorenz D. Summary of clinical results with Prodiem Plain, a bowel regulating agent. *Today's therapeutic trends*, 1983, 1:45–59.
17. Marlett JA et al. Comparative laxation of psyllium with and without senna in an ambulatory constipated population. *American journal of gastroenterology*, 1987, 82:333–337.
18. Lennard-Jones JE. Clinical management of constipation. *Pharmacology*, 1993, 47:216–223.
19. Reynolds JEF, ed. *Martindale, the extra pharmacopoeia*, 30th ed. London, Pharmaceutical Press, 1993.

20. *Goodman and Gilman's the pharmacological basis of therapeutics*, 8th ed. New York, Pergamon Press, 1996.
21. Edwards C. Diverticular disease of the colon. *European journal of gastroenterology and hepatology*, 1993, 5:583–586.
22. Ligny G. Therapie des Colon irritabile; Kontrollierte Doppelblindstudie zur Prüfung der Wirksamkeit einer hemizellulosehaltigen Arzneizubereitung. *Therapeutikon*, 1988, 7:449–453.
23. Qvitzau S, Matzen P, Madsen P. Treatment of chronic diarrhea: loperamide versus ispaghula husk and calcium. *Scandinavian journal of gastroenterology*, 1988, 23:1237–1240.
24. Harmouz W. Therapy of acute and chronic diarrhea with Agiocur ®. *Medizinische Klinik*, 1984, 79:32–33.
25. Read NW. Dietary fiber and bowel transit. In: Vahouny GV, Kritchevsky D, eds. *Dietary fiber. Basic and clinical aspects*. New York, Plenum Press, 1986.
26. Stevens J et al. Comparison of the effects of psyllium and wheat bran on gastrointestinal transit time and stool characteristics. *Journal of the American Dietetic Association*, 1988, 88:323–326.
27. Bradley PR, ed. *British herbal compendium, Vol. 1*. Bournemouth, British Herbal Medicine Association, 1983:199–203.
28. *Physicians' desk reference*, 45th ed. Montvale, NJ, Medical Economics Company, 1991:1740–1741.
29. Gattuso JM, Kamm MA. Adverse effects of drugs used in the management of constipation and diarrhea. *Drug safety*, 1994, 10:47–65.
30. Hänsel R et al., eds. *Hagers Handbuch der Pharmazeutischen Praxis, Vol. 6*, 5th ed. Berlin, Springer-Verlag, 1994.
31. Drews L, Kies C, Fox HM. Effect of dietary fiber on copper, zinc, and magnesium utilization by adolescent boys. *American journal of clinical nutrition*, 1981, 32:1893–1897.
32. Pearlman BB. Interaction between lithium salts and ispaghula husks. *Lancet*, 1990, 335:416.
33. Etman MA. Effect of a bulk forming laxative on the bioavailability of carbamazepine in man. *Drug development and industrial pharmacy*, 1995, 21:1901–1906.
34. Hubert DC et al. Fatal bronchospasm after oral ingestion of ispaghula. *Postgraduate medical journal*, 1995, 71:305–306.
35. Freeman GL. Psyllium hypersensitivity. *Annals of allergy*, 1994, 73:490–492.
36. Knutson TW et al. Intestinal reactivity in allergic and nonallergic patients; an approach to determine the complexity of the mucosal reaction. *Journal of allergy and clinical immunology*, 1993, 91:553–559.

Radix Platycodi

Definition

Radix Platycodi is the root of *Platycodon grandiflorum* (Jacq.) A. DC. (Campanulaceae) (*1, 2*).

Synonyms

Platycodon chinensis Lindl, *P. autumnalis* Decne., *P. sinensis* Lem., *P. stellatum*, *Campanula grandiflora* Jacq., *Campanula glauca* Thunb., *Campanula gentianoides* Lam. (*3, 4*).

Selected vernacular names

Balloon-flower, chieh keng, Chinese bell flower, gil gyeong, Japanese bell-flower, jiegeng, jieseng, kikiyou, kikyo, kikyokon, kikyou, platycodon radix (*3–8*).

Description

Perennial herb wholly glabrous, slightly glaucescent; root white, fleshy, radish-shaped, finger-thick, with abundant milky juice; stems ascending from base or straight, simple, 40–50 cm, herbaceous, glabrous or smooth, longitudinally striate in lower part; radical leaves alternate or sometimes nearly opposite, arranged along the lower half of stem or even higher, ovate-lanceolate, sessile, tapering at base, 2.5–3.4 cm long, 2–3 cm wide, rather large-toothed, pale beneath, glaucescent, upper leaves reduced. Flowers usually 1, sometimes 2, large, lengthily pedunculate, broadly campanulate or deeply saucer-shaped; calyx in 5 segments; corolla 5-lobed, violet-blue, 4 cm long; stamens 5; ovary many-celled. Fruit an ovoid capsule dehiscent at the top; seeds ovoid, compressed, obtuse, first violet then brown; albumen fleshy (*3, 9*).

Plant material of interest: dried root

General appearance

The root is irregular, somewhat thin and long fusiform, tapering, conical, often branched; externally greyish brown, light brown, or white; main root 10–15 cm in length, 1–3 cm in diameter at the upper end, with dented scars of removed stems, fine lateral wrinkles and longitudinal furrows, and slightly constricted;

the remaining part of the root, except the crown, covered with coarse longitudinal wrinkles, lateral furrows and lenticel-like lateral lines; hard in texture, but brittle; fractured surface not fibrous, often with cracks. Under a magnifying glass, a transverse section reveals cambium and its neighbourhood often brown in colour; cortex slightly thinner than xylem, almost white and with scattered cracks; xylem white to light brown and the tissue slightly denser than cortex (*2*).

Organoleptic properties
Odour, odourless; taste, tasteless at first, later bittersweet and pungent; colour, greyish brown (*1, 2*).

Microscopic characteristics
In transverse section of whole peeled root, cork cells occasionally remain; unpeeled roots show cork layers. Cork cells contain calcium oxalate prisms. Cortex narrow, often with clefts. Phloem scattered with laticiferous tube groups, walls somewhat thickened; contains yellowish brown granules. Cambium in a ring. Xylem vessels singly scattered or aggregated in groups arranged radially. Parenchymatous cells contain inulin (*1*).

Powdered plant material
Light greyish yellow to light greyish brown powder containing numerous fragments of colourless parenchyma cells; fragments of reticulate vessels and scalariform vessels; fragments of sieve tubes and lactiferous tubes; fragments of cork layer are sometimes observed. Starch grains are not usually observed, but very rarely simple grains are present, ellipsoid to irregular spheroid, 12–25 μm in diameter (*2*).

Geographical distribution
Northern Asia, China, the Democratic People's Republic of Korea, Japan, the Republic of Korea, the Russian Federation (east Siberia) (*3, 7, 9*).

General identity tests
Macroscopic and microscopic examinations; microchemical tests for saponins (*1, 2*), thin-layer chromatographic analysis for characteristic saponin profile (*10*).

Purity tests
Microbiology
The test for *Salmonella* spp. in Radix Platycodi should be negative. The maximum acceptable limits of other microorganisms are as follows (*11–13*). For preparation of decoction: aerobic bacteria—not more than 10^7/g; fungi—not

more than 10^5/g; *Escherichia coli*—not more than 10^2/g. Preparations for internal use: aerobic bacteria—not more than 10^5/g or ml; fungi—not more than 10^4/g or ml; enterobacteria and certain Gram-negative bacteria—not more than 10^3/g or ml; *Escherichia coli*—0/g or ml.

Total ash

Not more than 4.0% (*2*).

Acid-insoluble ash

Not more than 1.0% (*2*).

Alcohol-soluble extractive

Not less than 25% (*2*).

Pesticide residues

To be established in accordance with national requirements. Normally, the maximum residue limit of aldrin and dieldrin in Radix Platycodi is not more than 0.05 mg/kg (*13*). For other pesticides, see WHO guidelines on quality control methods for medicinal plants (*11*) and guidelines for predicting dietary intake of pesticide residues (*14*).

Heavy metals

Recommended lead and cadmium levels are not more than 10 and 0.3 mg/kg, respectively, in the final dosage form of the plant material (*11*).

Radioactive residues

For analysis of strontium-90, iodine-131, caesium-134, caesium-137, and plutonium-239, see WHO guidelines on quality control methods for medicinal plants (*11*).

Other purity tests

Chemical, foreign organic matter, moisture, and water-soluble extractive tests to be established in accordance with national requirements.

Chemical assays

Triterpene saponins, not less than 2% (*6*). Saponin content of the root can be evaluated by thin-layer chromatography–densitometry (*10*).

Major chemical constituents

The major chemical constituents of Radix Platycodi root are triterpene saponins based on the sapogenins platycodigenin and polygalacic acid; examples are platycodins A–I and polygalacins D and D_2 (*6, 15*).

	R1	R2	R3	R4
platycodin A	H	CH₂OH	H	CO-CH₃
platycodin C	H	CH₂OH	CO-CH₃	H
platycodin D	H	CH₂OH	H	H
platycodin D₂	glc *	CH₂OH	H	H
polygalacin D	H	CH₃	H	H
polygalacin D₂	glc *	CH₃	H	H

* glc = β-D-glucopyranosyl

Dosage forms

Dried roots, extracts, and other preparations.

Medicinal uses

Uses supported by clinical data

None.

Uses described in pharmacopoeias and in traditional systems of medicine

As an expectorant and antitussive (*1, 3–5*) used to treat coughs, colds, upper respiratory infections, sore throats, tonsillitis, and chest congestion (*1, 7*). In Chinese traditional medicine, Radix Platycodi has been used to treat cough with sputum, tonsillitis, pertussis, and asthma (*16*). Also used to treat stomatitis, peptic ulcers, and chronic inflammatory diseases (*17, 18*).

Uses described in folk medicine, not supported by experimental or clinical data

Other medical uses for Radix Platycodi include the treatment of viral infections and high blood pressure (*6*).

Pharmacology

Experimental pharmacology

Anti-inflammatory activity

The anti-inflammatory activity of Radix Platycodi has been attributed to the platycodins (*17, 19, 20*). *In vivo* studies have shown that intragastric administration of the drug antagonized carrageenin- and acetic acid-induced swelling of rat paws, and oral administration markedly inhibited cotton pledget-induced granulation in rats (*21*). Platycodins also effectively inhibited adjuvant-induced arthritis in rats (*22*). Researchers investigating some Japanese Kampo medicines concluded that Radix Platycodi was at least partly responsible for the anti-inflammatory activity of these preparations (*17*).

Expectorant and antitussive activity

Radix Platycodi has both antitussive and expectorant activities (*18, 20*). The expectorant effects include the promotion of salivary and bronchial secretions (*6*). Oral administration of a decoction of the drug (1 g/kg) to anaesthetized dogs increased mucus secretions in the respiratory tract with a potency similar to that of ammonium chloride (*23*). A similar response was observed in cats (*24*). The platycodins are believed to be the active components. Oral doses of platycodins irritated the pharyngeal and gastric mucosa, increasing mucosal secretions in the respiratory tract and diluting sputum for easy expectoration (*25*).

In vivo studies have demonstrated the effectiveness of platycodins as an antitussive drug. When administered to guinea-pigs, platycodins reduced the frequency of coughing; the median effective dose was 6.4 mg/kg given intra-peritoneally (*5, 26*). A 20% decoction of Radix Platycodi was also effective in treating coughing induced by ammonia in mice (*6*).

Antipeptic ulcer activity

Platycodins have been reported to inhibit gastric secretion and prevent peptic ulcer in rats (*5*). A dose of 100 mg/kg inhibited gastric secretion in rats induced by ligation of the pylorus and stress ulceration (*18*).

Antihypercholesterolaemic and antihyperlipidaemic activity

An effect of Radix Platycodi on serum and liver lipid concentrations has been demonstrated. Rats with diet-induced hyperlipidaemia were fed diets containing 5% and 10% Radix Platycodi. The rats fed with the 5% diet had significantly lower concentrations of total cholesterol and triglycerides in serum and of liver lipids than did controls (*27*).

Toxicity

The median lethal dose of a decoction of Radix Platycodi given orally was 24 g/kg in mice (*5*). The median lethal doses of platycodins in mice and rats were 420 and 800 mg/kg (oral), or 22.3 and 14.1 mg/kg (intraperitoneal), respectively (*5*). Crude platycodins have been reported to have sedative side-effects in mice, such as inhibition of movement and a decrease in respiration after both intraperitoneal and oral administration (*18*). These side-effects were less pronounced after oral administration, suggesting that platycodins are poorly absorbed through the gastrointestinal tract (*18*).

Crude platycodins have a highly haemolytic effect in mice, of which the haemolytic index is 1.2 times that of a commercial reagent-grade saponin used as a reference (*5, 18*). Radix Platycodi preparations should therefore be given only orally, after which the drug loses its haemolytic effect owing to decomposition in the alimentary tract (*18*).

Clinical pharmacology

Crude powdered drug or decoctions of Radix Platycodi have been used to treat the symptoms of lung abscesses, lobar pneumonia, and pharyngitis with reported success (*5*). However, the details of these clinical studies were not available.

Contraindications

No information available.

Warnings

Playtcodon extracts have a very pronounced haemolytic effect, and therefore the drug should not be administered by injection (*5*).

Precautions

General

Radix Platycodi reportedly depresses central nervous system (CNS) activity (*5*). Patients should avoid using alcohol or other CNS depressants in conjunction with this drug. Patients should be cautioned that the combination of the drug and alcohol may impair their ability to drive a motor vehicle or operate hazardous machinery.

Drug interactions

Because of the CNS depressant activity (*5*), Radix Platycodi may act synergistically with other CNS depressants such as alcohol, tranquillizers, and sleeping medications. Radix Platycodon is also reported to be incompatible with *Gentiana scabra* and *Bletilla hyacinthina* (*5*).

Carcinogenesis, mutagenesis, impairment of fertility

To date, no genotoxic effects have been reported. *Platycodon* root extracts were not mutagenic in the *Bacillus subtilis* rec-assay or the *Salmonella*/microsome reversion assay (*28*). Nor were they mutagenic in the SOS chromotest (*E. coli* PQ37) and in the SOS *umu* test (*S. typhimurium* TA 1535/pSK 1002) (*29*).

Pregnancy: teratogenic effects

Platycodon extracts are not teratogenic *in vivo* (*30*).

Pregnancy: non-teratogenic effects

No data available; therefore Radix Platycodi should not be administered during pregnancy.

Nursing mothers

Excretion of the drug into breast milk and its effects on the newborn infant have not been established; therefore the use of the drug during lactation is not recommended.

Other precautions

No information available on drug and laboratory test interactions or on paediatric use.

Adverse reactions

No information available.

Posology

The usual dose range is 2–9 g daily (*1, 3, 6*).

References

1. *Pharmacopoeia of the People's Republic of China* (English ed.). Guangzhou, Guangdong Science and Technology Press, 1992.
2. *The pharmacopoeia of Japan XII*. Tokyo, The Society of Japanese Pharmacopoeia, 1991.
3. Keys JD. *Chinese herbs, their botany, chemistry and pharmacodynamics*. Rutland, VT, CE Tuttle, 1976.
4. Bailey LH, Lawrence GHM. *The garden of bellflowers in North America*. New York, MacMillan, 1953.
5. Chang HM, But PPH, eds. *Pharmacology and applications of Chinese materia medica, Vol. 2*. World Scientific Publishing, Singapore, 1987.
6. Hsu H-Y. *Oriental materia medica, a concise guide*. Long Beach, CA, Oriental Healing Arts Institute, 1986.
7. *Medicinal plants in China*. Manila, World Health Organization, 1989 (WHO Regional Publications, Western Pacific Series, No. 2).
8. Farnsworth NR, ed. *NAPRALERT database*. Chicago, University of Illinois at Chicago, IL, March 15, 1995 production (an on-line database available directly through the University of Illinois at Chicago or through the Scientific and Technical Network (STN) of Chemical Abstracts Services).
9. Shishkin BK, ed. *Flora of the USSR, Vol. XXIV. Dipsacaceae, Cucurbitaceae, Campanulaceae*. Jerusalem, Israel Program for Scientific Translation, 1972 (published for the Smithsonian Institution and the National Science Foundation, Washington, DC).
10. Hosoda K et al. Studies on the cultivation and preparation of *Platycodon* root. III. Effect of picking flower and fruit on the quality of skin peeled root. *Chemical and pharmaceutical bulletin*, 1992, 40:1946–1947.
11. *Quality control methods for medicinal plant materials*. Geneva, World Health Organization, 1998.
12. *Deutsches Arzneibuch 1996. Vol. 2. Methoden der Biologie*. Stuttgart, Deutscher Apotheker Verlag, 1996.
13. *European pharmacopoeia*, 3rd ed. Strasbourg, Council of Europe, 1997.
14. *Guidelines for predicting dietary intake of pesticide residues*, 2nd rev. ed. Geneva, World

Health Organization, 1997 (unpublished document WHO/FSF/FOS/97.7; available from Food Safety, WHO, 1211 Geneva 27, Switzerland).

15. Tada A et al. Studies on the saponins of the root of *Platycodon grandiflorum* A. De Candolle. I. Isolation and the structure of platycodin-D. *Chemical and pharmaceutical bulletin*, 1975, 23:2965–2972.

16. Lee EB. Pharmacological studies on *Platycodi radix. Korean journal of pharmacognosy*, 1974, 5:49–60.

17. Ozaki Y. Studies of antiinflammatory effect of Japanese oriental medicines (Kampo medicines) used to treat inflammatory diseases. *Biological and pharmaceutical bulletin*, 1995, 18:559–562.

18. Lee EB. Pharmacological activities of crude platycodin. In: Woo ES, ed. *Terpenoids Symposium proceedings*. Seoul, Natural Products Research Institute, Seoul National University, 1975:52–64.

19. Kakimoto M et al. Anti-inflammatory and anti-allergic effects of a preparation of crude drugs, a remedy for nasal disease (fujibitol). *Pharmacometrics*, 1984, 28:555–565.

20. Shibata S. Medicinal chemistry of triterpenoid saponins and sapogenins. In: *Proceedings of the 4th Asian Symposium on Medicinal Plants and Spices*. Bangkok, 1981.

21. Takagi T. Metabolism and disease. In: *Foreign references on Chinese Materia Medica.* Hunan, Hunan Institute of Medical and Pharmaceutical Industry, 1975, 10:474.

22. Takagi K, Lee EB. Pharmacological studies on *Platycodon grandiflorum* A.DC. II. Anti-inflammatory activity of crude platycodin, its activities on isolated organs and other pharmacological activities. *Journal of the Pharmaceutical Society of Japan (Tokyo)*, 1972, 92:961–968.

23. Tang RY et al. *Chinese medical journal*, 1952, 38:4–5.

24. Gao YD et al. *Chinese medical journal*, 1954, 46:331.

25. Zhu Y. *Pharmacology and applications of Chinese medicinal materials*. Beijing, China, People's Medical Publishing House, 1958.

26. Takagi KJ, Lee EB. Pharmacological studies on *Platycodon grandiflorum* A.DC. III. Activities of crude platycodin, on respiratory and circulatory systems and other pharmacological activities. *Pharmaceutical Society of Japan (Tokyo)*, 1972, 92:969–973.

27. Kim K et al. Effects of *Platycodon grandiflorum* feeding on serum and liver lipid concentrations in rats with diet-induced hyperlipidemia. *Journal of nutritional science and vitaminology*, 1995, 41:485–491.

28. Morimoto I et al. Mutagenicity screening of crude drugs with *Bacillus subtilis* rec-assay and *Salmonella*/microsome reversion assay. *Mutation research*, 1982, 97:81–102.

29. Chang IM et al. Assay of potential mutagenicity and antimutagenicity of Chinese herbal drugs by using SOS Chromotest (*E. coli* PQ37) and SOS UMU test (*S. typhimurium* TA 1535/pSK 1002). *Proceedings of the first Korea–Japan Toxicology Symposium, Safety and Assessment of Chemicals in Vitro*. The Korean Society of Toxicology, 1989.

30. Lee EB. Tetratogenicity of the extracts of crude drugs. *Korean journal of pharmacognosy*, 1982, 13:116–121.

Radix Rauwolfiae

Definition

Radix Rauwolfiae is the dried root of *Rauvolfia serpentina* (L.) Benth. ex Kurz (Apocynaceae) (*1–4*).

Synonyms

Ophioxylon obversum Miq., *O. sautiferum* Salisb., *O. serpentinum* L., *Rauvolfia obversa* (Miq.) Baill., *R. trifoliata* (Gaertn.) Baill. (*3–5*).

Selected vernacular names

Most commonly called "rauwolfia". Acawerya, aika-wairey, akar-tikos, arsol, bhudra, bongmaiza, chandmaruwa, chandra, chandrika, chotachand, chota-chard, chundrika, chundrooshoora, churmuhuntree, chuvannayilpuri, covanamilpori, covannamipori, dhanbarua, dhannerna, dogrikme, eiya-kunda, ekaweriya, garudpathal, hadki, harkai, harkaya, ichneumon plant, Indian snakeroot, indojaboku, karai, karavi, karuvee, makeshwar chadrika, makeshwar churna, matavi-aloos, nogliever, nundunee, pagla-ka-dawa, palalganni, patala-agandhi, poelé pandak, poeleh pandak, pushoomehnunkarika, ra-yom, radix mungo, radix mustelae, raiz de mongo alba, rametul, ratekaweriya, rayom noi, rauvolfia, rauwalfia, rauwolfia, Rauwolfiawurzel, sanochado, sapasan, sarpagandha, sarpgandha, serpentina, sjouanna-amelpodi, snakeroot, sung, suvapaval-amepodi, talona, vasoopooshpa, vasura (*5–8*).

Description

Small, erect, glabrous shrub, 30–60 cm high. Leaves whorled, 7.5–17.5 cm long, lanceolate or oblanceolate, acute or acuminate, tapering gradually into the petiole, thin. Flowers white or pinkish; peduncles 5.0–7.5 cm long; pedicels and calyx red. Calyx lobes 2.5 mm long, lanceolate. Corolla about 1–1.3 cm long; tube slender; inflated slightly above middle; lobes much shorter than tube, obtuse. Drupes about 6 mm (diameter), single or didymous and more or less connate, purplish black when ripe (*1*).

Plant material of interest: root
General appearance
The root occurs as segments 5–15 cm in length and 3–20 mm in diameter, subcylindrical to tapering, tortuous or curved, rarely branched, occasionally bearing twisted rootlets, which are larger, more abundant, and more rigid and woody on the thicker parts of the roots. Externally light brown to greyish yellow to greyish brown, dull, rough or slightly wrinkled longitudinally, yet smooth to the touch, occasionally showing rootlet scars on the larger pieces, with some exfoliation of the bark in small areas that reveals the paler wood beneath. Bark separates easily from the wood on scraping. Fracture short but irregular, the longer pieces readily breaking with a snap, slightly fibrous marginally. The freshly fractured surfaces show a rather thin layer of greyish yellow bark, and the pale yellowish white wood constitutes about 80% of the radius. The smooth transverse surface of larger pieces shows a finely radiate stele with three or more clearly marked growth rings; a small knob-like protuberance is frequently noticeable in the centre. The wood is hard and of relatively low density (*1*).

Organoleptic properties
Root odour is indistinct, earthy, reminiscent of stored white potatoes, and the taste is bitter (*1*).

Microscopic characteristics
A transverse section of the root shows externally 2–8 alternating strata of cork cells, the strata with larger cells alternating with strata made up of markedly smaller cells. Each stratum composed of smaller cells includes 3–5 tangentially arranged cell layers. In cross-sectional view, the largest cells of the larger cell group measure 40–90 μm radially and up to 75 μm tangentially, while the cells of the smaller group measure 5–20 μm radially and up to 75 μm tangentially. The walls are thin and suberized. The secondary cortex consists of several rows of tangentially elongated to isodiametric parenchyma cells, most densely filled with starch grains; others (short latex cells) occur singly or in short series and contain brown resin masses. The secondary phloem is relatively narrow and is made up of phloem parenchyma (bearing starch grains and less commonly tabular to angular calcium oxalate crystals up to 20 μm in length; also, occasionally, with some brown resin masses in outer cells and phloem rays) interlaid with scattered sieve tissue and traversed by phloem rays 2–4 cells in width. Sclerenchyma cells are absent in root (a distinction from other *Rauvolfia* species). Cambium is indistinct, narrow, dark, and wavering. The secondary xylem represents the large bulk of the root and shows one or more prominent annual rings with a dense core of wood about 500 μm across at the centre. The xylem is composed of many wood wedges separated by xylem rays, and on closer examination reveals vessels in interrupted radial rows, much xylem paren-

chyma, many large-celled xylem rays, few wood fibres, and tracheids, all with lignified walls. The xylem fibres occur in both tangential and radial rows. The xylem rays are 1–12, occasionally up to 16 cells in width (*1, 3*).

Powdered plant material

Powdered Radix Rauwolfiae is brownish to reddish grey. Numerous starch grains (simple, 2- to 3-compound, occasionally 4-compound) present; simple grains spheroid, ovate, plano- to angular-convex, or irregular; hilum simple, Y-shaped, stellate, or irregularly cleft; unaltered grains 6–34 µm in diameter; altered grains up to about 50 µm; large unaltered grains clearly show polarization cross; calcium oxalate prisms and cluster crystals scattered, about 10–15 µm in size; brown resin masses and yellowish granular secretion masses occur occasionally; isolated cork cells elongated, up to 90 µm in length; phelloderm and phloem parenchyma cells similar in appearance; vessels subcylindrical, up to 360 µm in length and about 20–57 µm in diameter, the vessel end walls oblique to transverse, generally with openings in the end walls, some vessels showing tyloses; tracheids pitted, with moderately thick, tapering, beaded walls, with relatively broad lumina, polygonal in cross-section; xylem parenchyma cells with moderately thick walls with simple circular pits, cells polygonal in cross-section, bearing much starch, sometimes with brown resin masses; xylem fibres with thick heavily lignified walls showing small transverse and oblique linear pits and pointed simple to bifurcate ends, measuring about 200–750 µm in length. No phloem fibres or sclereids are present in root (colourless non-lignified pericycle or primary phloem fibres, single or in small groups, may be present from rhizome or stem tissues) (*1*).

Geographical distribution

The plant is found growing wild in the sub-Himalayan tracts in India and is also found in Indonesia, Myanmar, and Thailand (*3*).

Overcollection of Radix Rauwolfiae in India has significantly diminished supply and since 1997 there has been an embargo on export of this drug from India. Reserpine is currently either extracted from the roots of *Rauvolfia vomitoria* of African origin or produced by total synthesis.

General identity tests

Macroscopic and microscopic examinations (*1–3*) and thin-layer chromatographic analysis for the presence of characteristic indole alkaloids (*2, 3*).

Purity tests
Microbiology

The test for *Salmonella* spp. in Radix Rauwolfiae products should be negative. The maximum acceptable limits of other microorganisms are as follows (*9–11*).

For preparation of decoction: aerobic bacteria—not more than 10^7/g; moulds and yeast—not more than 10^4/g; *Escherichia coli*—not more than 10^2/g; other enterobacteria—not more than 10^4/g. Preparations for internal use: aerobic bacteria—not more than 10^5/g; moulds and yeast—not more than 10^3/g; *Escherichia coli*—not more than 10^1/g; other enterobacteria—not more than 10^3/g.

Foreign organic matter

Not more than 2.0% of stems, and not more than 3.0% of other foreign organic matter (*1*).

Total ash

Not more than 10% (*2*).

Acid-insoluble ash

Not more than 2.0% (*1*, *2*).

Moisture

Not more than 12% (*2*).

Pesticide residues

To be established in accordance with national requirements. Normally, the maximum residue limit of aldrin and dieldrin in Radix Rauwolfiae is not more than 0.05 mg/kg (*11*). For other pesticides, see WHO guidelines on quality control methods for medicinal plants (*9*) and guidelines for predicting dietary intake of pesticide residues (*12*).

Heavy metals

Recommended lead and cadmium levels are no more than 10 and 0.3 mg/kg, respectively, in the final dosage form of the plant material (*9*).

Radioactive residues

For analysis of strontium-90, iodine-131, caesium-134, caesium-137, and plutonium-239, see WHO guidelines on quality control methods for medicinal plants (*9*).

Other purity tests

Chemical, alcohol-soluble extractive and water-soluble extractive tests to be established in accordance with national requirements.

Chemical assays

Contains not less than 1% total alkaloids (*2*, *3*); and a minimum of 0.1% alkaloids of the reserpine–rescinnamine group (*3*).

Thin-layer chromatography to detect the presence of the reserpine–rescinnamine group of alkaloids (2, 3, 13). Quantitative analysis of total and reserpine–rescinnamine group of alkaloids can be performed by spectrophotometric analysis (2, 3) or by high-performance liquid chromatography (14, 15).

Major chemical constituents

Radix Rauwolfiae contains more than 60 indole alkaloids; the principal hypotensive alkaloids are identified as reserpine and rescinnamine (1, 6).

Dosage forms

Crude drug and powder. Package in well-closed containers and store at 15–25 °C (9) in a dry place, secure against insect attack (1).

Medicinal uses

Uses supported by clinical data

The principal use today is in the treatment of mild essential hypertension (16–22). Treatment is usually administered in combination with a diuretic agent to support the drug's antihypertensive activity, and to prevent fluid retention which may develop if Radix Rauwolfiae is given alone (18).

Uses described in pharmacopoeias and in traditional systems of medicine

As a tranquillizer for nervous and mental disorders (4, 5).

Uses described in folk medicine, not supported by experimental or clinical data

As a tonic in states of asthenia, a cardiotonic and antipyretic; against snake and insect bites; and for constipation, liver diseases, flatulence, insomnia, and rheumatism (8).

Pharmacology

Experimental pharmacology

It is well accepted that the pharmacological effects of Radix Rauwolfiae are due to its alkaloids, especially the reserpine–rescinnamine group. The experimental pharmacology of reserpine and related compounds has been well documented (*5, 16–18, 23*). Powdered Radix Rauwolfiae, as well as various forms of extracts (ethanolic, dried), has been reported to lower the blood pressure of experimental animals (dogs or cats) by various routes of administration (*5*).

Clinical pharmacology

Radix Rauwolfiae and its major alkaloids probably lower high blood pressure by depleting tissue stores of catecholamines (epinephrine and norepinephrine) from peripheral sites. By contrast, their sedative and tranquillizing properties are thought to be related to depletion of catecholamines and serotonin (5-hydroxytryptamine) from the brain. Following absorption from the gastrointestinal tract the active alkaloids concentrate in tissues with high lipid content. They pass the blood–brain barrier and the placenta. Radix Rauwolfiae products are characterized by slow onset of action and sustained effect. Both the cardiovascular and central nervous system effects may persist following withdrawal of the drug. The active alkaloids are metabolized in the liver to inactive compounds that are excreted primarily in the urine. Unchanged alkaloids are excreted primarily in the faeces (*16*).

Contraindications

Radix Rauwolfiae products are contraindicated in patients who have previously demonstrated hypersensitivity to the plant or its alkaloids. They are also contraindicated in patients with a history of mental depression (especially those with suicidal tendencies) during or shortly after therapy with monoamine oxidase inhibitors; active peptic ulcer, sinus node disorders, ulcerative colitis; epilepsy; or decreased renal function; and in patients receiving electroconvulsive therapy (*16, 18*).

Warnings

Radix Rauwolfiae products may cause mental depression (*24*). Recognition of depression may be difficult because this condition may often be disguised by somatic complaints (masked depression). The products should be discontinued at first signs of depression such as despondency, early morning insomnia, loss of appetite, impotence, or self-deprecation. Drug-induced depression may persist for several months after drug withdrawal and may be severe enough to result in suicide. Sensitivity reactions may occur in patients with or without a history of allergy or bronchial asthma. The use of Radix Rauwolfiae products may impair alertness and make it inadvisable to drive or operate heavy machinery (*16, 18*).

Precautions

General

Because Radix Rauwolfiae preparations increase gastrointestinal motility and secretion, they should be used cautiously in persons with a history of peptic ulcer, ulcerative colitis, or gallstones where biliary colic may be precipitated. Persons on high doses should be observed carefully at regular intervals to detect possible reactivation of peptic ulcer (*16*).

Caution should be exercised when treating hypertensive patients with renal insufficiency since they adjust poorly to lowered blood-pressure levels (*16*).

Drug interactions

When administered concurrently, the following drugs may interact with or potentiate Radix Rauwolfiae and its alkaloids (*16, 18*): alcohol or other central nervous system depressants, other antihypertensives or diuretics, digitalis glycosides or quinidine, levodopa, levomepromazine, monoamine oxidase inhibitors, sympathomimetics (direct-acting) and tricyclic antidepressants.

Concomitant use of Radix Rauwolfiae products and anaesthetics may provoke a fall in blood pressure (*4, 17, 25*) and add to the β-adrenoceptor–blocking activity of propranolol (*25*).

Drug and laboratory test interactions

Chronic administration of Radix Rauwolfiae preparations may increase serum prolactin levels and decrease excretion of urinary catecholamines and vanilmandelic acid. Therefore, any diagnostic tests performed for these determinations should be interpreted with caution (*16*).

Radix Rauwolfiae preparations slightly decrease absorbance readings obtained on urinary steroid colorimetric determinations (e.g. modified Glenn–Nelson technique or Holtorff Koch modification of Zimmermann reaction), and thus false low results may be reported (*16*).

Preoperative withdrawal of Radix Rauwolfiae products does not necessarily ensure circulatory stability during the procedure, and the anaesthetist must be informed of the patient's drug history (*4, 17, 25*).

Caution is indicated in elderly patients and also in those suffering from coronary and cerebral arteriosclerosis. Administration of products including Radix Rauwolfiae preparations at doses that might precipitate a sharp decrease in blood pressure should be avoided (*17*).

Carcinogenesis, mutagenesis, impairment of fertility

Animal carcinogenicity studies using reserpine at doses 50 times as high as the average human dose have been conducted with rats and mice. Carcinogenic effects associated with the administration of reserpine include an increased incidence of adrenal medullary phaeochromocytomas in male rats, unidentified carcinomas of the seminal vesicles in male mice, and mammary cancer in female mice; carcinogenic effects were not seen in female rats (*14, 23, 26*).

Bacteriological studies to determine mutagenicity using reserpine showed negative results (*16*). The extent of risk to humans is uncertain (*16, 26–28*).

Pregnancy: teratogenic effects

Reserpine, the major active alkaloid in Radix Rauwolfiae, administered parenterally has been shown to be teratogenic in rats at doses up to 2 mg/kg and to have an embryocidal effect in guinea-pigs at 0.5 mg daily (*27*). There are no adequate and well-controlled studies in pregnant women.

Pregnancy: non-teratogenic effects

Increased respiratory secretions, nasal congestion, cyanosis, hypothermia, and anorexia have occurred in neonates of mothers treated with Radix Rauwolfiae (*16, 28, 29*). Therefore, the use of Radix Rauwolfiae is not recommended during pregnancy.

Nursing mothers

Rauwolfia alkaloids are excreted in human milk. Because of the potential for serious adverse reactions in nursing infants, use of Radix Rauwolfiae during lactation is not recommended.

Paediatric use

Safety and effectiveness in children have not been established (*16*).

Adverse reactions

The following adverse reactions have been observed, but there are insufficient data to support an estimate of their frequency. The reactions are usually reversible and disappear when the Radix Rauwolfiae preparations are discontinued (*16, 18*).

Cardiovascular system: bradycardia, arrhythmias, particularly when used concurrently with digitalis or quinidine, angina-like symptoms. Water retention with oedema in persons with hypertensive vascular disease may occur rarely, but the condition generally clears with cessation of therapy, or the administration of a diuretic agent. Vasodilation produced by rauwolfia alkaloids may result in nasal congestion, flushing, a feeling of warmth, and conjunctival congestion.

Central nervous system: sensitization of the central nervous system manifested by optic atrophy, glaucoma, uveitis, deafness, and dull sensorium. Other reactions include depression, paradoxical anxiety, nightmares, nervousness, headache, dizziness, drowsiness. Large doses have produced parkinsonian syndrome, other extrapyramidal reactions, and convulsions.

Gastrointestinal system: hypersecretion and increased intestinal motility, diarrhoea, vomiting, nausea, anorexia, and dryness of mouth. Gastrointestinal bleeding has occurred in isolated cases.

Respiratory system: dyspnoea, epistaxis, nasal congestion.

Hypersensitivity: purpura, pruritus, rash.

Other: dysuria, muscular aches, weight gain, breast engorgement, pseudolactation, impotence or decreased libido, gynaecomastia.

Posology

Powder, 200 mg daily in divided doses for 1–3 weeks; maintenance 50–300 mg daily (*1*). Doses of other preparations should be calculated accordingly. Doses of Radix Rauwolfiae should be based on the recommended dosage of rauwolfia alkaloids, which must be adjusted according to the patient's requirements and tolerance in small increments at intervals of at least 10 days. Debilitated and geriatric patients may require lower dosages of rauwolfia alkaloids than do other adults (*18*). Rauwolfia alkaloids may be administered orally in a single daily dose or divided into two daily doses (*18*).

References

1. *National formulary XIV*. Washington, DC, National Formulary Board, American Pharmaceutical Association, 1975.
2. *Deutsches Arzneibuch 1996*. Stuttgart, Deutscher Apotheker Verlag, 1996.
3. *Pharmacopée française*. Paris, Adrapharm, 1996.
4. Reynolds JEF, ed. *Martindale, the extra pharmacopoeia*, 30th ed. London, Pharmaceutical Press, 1993.
5. Hänsel R, Henkler G. *Rauwolfia*. In: Hänsel R et al., eds. *Hagers Handbuch der Pharmazeutischen Praxis, Vol. 6*, 5th ed. Berlin, Springer-Verlag, 1994:361–384.
6. Monachino J. *Rauwolfia serpentina*: Its history, botany and medical use. *Economic botany*, 1954, 8:349–365.
7. *The Indian pharmaceutical codex. Vol. I. Indigenous drugs*. New Delhi, Council of Scientific & Industrial Research, 1953.
8. Farnsworth NR, ed. *NAPRALERT database*. Chicago, University of Illinois at Chicago, IL, March 15, 1995 production (an on-line database available directly through the University of Illinois at Chicago or through the Scientific and Technical Network (STN) of Chemical Abstracts Services).
9. *Quality control methods for medicinal plant materials*. Geneva, World Health Organization, 1998.
10. *Deutsches Arzneibuch 1996. Vol. 2. Methoden der Biologie*. Stuttgart, Deutscher Apotheker Verlag, 1996.
11. *European pharmacopoeia*, 3rd ed. Strasbourg, Council of Europe, 1997.
12. *Guidelines for predicting dietary intake of pesticide residues*, 2nd rev. ed. Geneva, World Health Organization, 1997 (unpublished document WHO/FSF/FOS/97.7; available from Food Safety, WHO, 1211 Geneva 27, Switzerland).
13. *Clarke's isolation and identification of drugs in pharmaceuticals, body fluids, and post-mortem material*, 2nd ed. London, Pharmaceutical Press, 1986.
14. Cieri UR. Identification and estimation of the alkaloids of *Rauwolfia serpentina* by high performance liquid chromatography and thin layer chromatography. *Journal of the Association of Official Analytical Chemists*, 1983, 66:867–873.
15. Cieri UR. Determination of reserpine and rescinnamine in *Rauwolfia serpentina* preparations by liquid chromatography with fluorescence detection. *Journal of the Association of Official Analytical Chemists*, 1987, 70:540–546.

16. *Physicians' desk reference.* 45th ed. Montvale, NJ, Medical Economics Company, 1991.
17. *Goodman and Gilman's the pharmacological basis of therapeutics*, 8th ed. New York, Pergamon Press, 1990.
18. *American Hospital Formulary Service drug information 94.* Bethesda, MD, American Society of Health System Pharmacists, 1994.
19. Bein HJ. The pharmacology of Rauwolfia. *Pharmacology review*, 1956, 8:435–483.
20. Vakil RJ. A clinical trial of *Rauwolfia serpentina* in essential hypertension. *British heart journal*, 1949, 11:350–355.
21. Wilkins RW, Judson WE. The use of *Rauwolfia serpentina* in hypertensive patients. *New England journal of medicine*, 1953, 248:48–53.
22. Kline NS. Use of *Rauwolfia serpentina* Benth. in neuropsychiatric conditions. *Annals of the New York Academy of Science*, 1954, 59:107–132.
23. Rand MJ, Jurevics H. The pharmacology of Rauwolfia alkaloids. In: Gross F, ed. *Antihypertensive agents.* New York, Springer-Verlag, 1977:77–159.
24. Howes LG, Louis WJ. *Rauwolfia* alkaloide (reserpine). In: Ganten D, Mulrow PJ, eds. *Pharmacology of antihypertensive therapeutics.* Berlin, Springer-Verlag, 1990:263–276.
25. *Physicians' desk reference*, 49th ed. Montvale, NJ, Medical Economics Company, 1995.
26. Shapiro S et al. Risk of breast cancer in relation to the use of Rauwolfia alkaloids. *European journal of clinical pharmacology*, 1984, 26:143–146.
27. Weiss RF. *Herbal medicine.* Gothenburg, Sweden, AB Arcanum, 1988.
28. Budnick IS et al. Effect in the new-born infant of reserpine administrated ante partum. *American journal of diseases of children*, 1955, 90:286–289.
29. Rogers SF. Reserpine and the new-born infant. *Journal of the American Medical Association*, 1956, 160:1090.

Rhizoma Rhei

Definition

Rhizoma Rhei consists of the underground parts (rhizome and root) of *Rheum officinale* Baill., or *R. palmatum* L. (Polygonaceae) (*1–7*).[1]

Synonyms

None.

Selected vernacular names

Akar kalembak, Chinese rhubarb, chuòng diêp dai hoàng, dai hoàng, daioh, daiou, kot nam tao, rawind, Rhabarberwurzel, rhabarbarum, rhubarb, rhubard de Chine, rhubarb root, turkey rhubarb, ta-huang (*8–10*).

Description

Rheum species are perennial herbs resembling the common garden rhubarb except for their lower growth and shape of their leaf blades; the underground portion consists of a strong vertical rhizome with fleshy, spreading roots; the portion above ground consists of a number of long petioled leaves that arise from the rhizome in the spring, and flower shoots bearing elongated leafy panicles that are crowded with greenish white, white, to dark purple flowers; the lamina is cordate to somewhat orbicular, entire or coarsely dentate (*Rheum officinale*) or palmately lobed (*R. palmatum*). The fruit is an ovoid-oblong or orbicular achene bearing 3 broad membranous wings and the remains of the perianth at the base (*9, 11*).

Plant material of interest: rhizomes and roots
General appearance

The appearance of the rhizomes and roots varies according to the plant's geographical origin (*12*). They occur on the market in subcylindrical, barrel-shaped, plano-convex or irregularly formed pieces, frequently showing a perfo-

---

[1] *Rheum tangutium* Max., *R. coreanum* Nakai, *R. palmatum* L., and *R. officinale* Baillow, or their interspecific hybrids, are also listed in the Japanese pharmacopoeia (*1*). *R. emodi* ("Indian rhubarb") is listed in the Indian pharmacopoeia (*7*).

ration, or in cubes or rectangular pieces, the last commonly known as "rhubarb fingers". They are hard and moderately heavy. The outer surfaces are smooth, longitudinally wrinkled or sunken, yellowish brown and mottled with alternating striae of greyish white parenchyma and brownish or reddish medullary rays, while here and there may be seen brown cork patches and branched scars, "star spots", of leaf trace fibrovascular bundles. The fracture is uneven and granular, the fractured surface pinkish brown. The smooth transverse surface of the rhizome exhibits a cambium line near the periphery traversed by radial lines that represent medullary rays that project for a short distance within it. The large area within this circle of medullary rays contains stellate vascular bundles 2–4mm in diameter that are arranged in a more or less continuous circle in *R. palmatum* or scattered irregularly in *R. officinale* (*9*).

Organoleptic properties

Odour, characteristic aromatic; taste, slightly astringent and bitter; when chewed, gritty between the teeth; colour, yellow-brown to light brown (*1, 2*).

Microscopic characteristics

The transverse section of the rhizome shows wavy medullary rays, 2–4 cells in width; the xylem consists of a matrix of wood parenchyma and resembles the phloem and cortex regions in that the cells possess either starch, tannin, or large cluster crystals of calcium oxalate. Large, reticulately thickened vessels occur singly or in small groups. Embedded in the parenchyma near the cambium line and mostly in the pith are a number of compound ("stellate") fibrovascular bundles, each of which consists of a small circle of open collateral bundles separated from each other by yellowish brown medullary rays containing anthraquinone derivatives. The bundles differ from the ordinary open collateral bundle in showing phloem inside and xylem outside the cambium. In *R. officinale* the compound bundles ("stellate spots") are scattered through the pith, whereas in *R. palmatum* they are mostly arranged in a ring, the remainder being scattered on either side of the ring (*1, 2, 9, 13*).

Powdered plant material

Powdered Rhizoma Rhei is dusky yellowish orange to moderate yellowish brown, and coloured red in the presence of alkali. Under the microscope, it shows numerous starch grains, spherical, single or 2–4-compound, 2–25μm in diameter; fragments of non-lignified, reticulate and spiral tracheae, vessels, parenchyma cells containing starch grains or tannin masses; large rosette aggregates of calcium oxalate, 30–60μm, frequently over 100μm, and occasionally attaining a diameter of 190μm; and medullary-ray cells containing an amorphous yellow substance, insoluble in alcohol but soluble in ammonia test solution with a reddish or pink colour; cork, sclerenchymatous cells, and fibres absent (*1, 2, 9, 10*).

Geographical distribution

Rheum officinale and *R. palmatum* are cultivated in China (Gansu, Sichuan, and Qinghai provinces), the Democratic People's Republic of Korea and the Republic of Korea. There are several commercial grades (rhizome with or without rootlets, peeled or unpeeled, in transverse or longitudinal cuts) (*9, 12, 14*).

General identity tests

Macroscopic and microscopic examinations; microchemical colour tests and thin-layer chromatographic analysis for the presence of anthraquinones (*1–7*).

Purity tests
Microbiology

The test for *Salmonella* spp. in Rhizoma Rhei products should be negative. The maximum acceptable limits of other microorganisms are as follows (*15–17*). For preparation of decoction: aerobic bacteria—not more than 10^7/g; fungi—not more than 10^5/g; *Escherichia coli*—not more than 10^2/g. Preparations for internal use: aerobic bacteria—not more than 10^5/g or ml; fungi—not more than 10^4/g or ml; enterobacteria and certain Gram-negative bacteria—not more than 10^3/g or ml; *Escherichia coli*—0/g or ml.

Foreign organic matter

Not more than 1.0% (*2–7*).

Total ash

Not more than 12% (*2, 3*).

Acid-insoluble ash

Not more than 2.0% (*2, 3*).

Dilute ethanol-soluble extractive

Not less than 30% (*1*).

Moisture

Not more than 12% (*2, 3*).

Pesticide residues

To be established in accordance with national requirements. Normally, the maximum residue limit of aldrin and dieldrin in Rhizoma Rhei is not more than 0.05 mg/kg (*17*). For other pesticides, see WHO guidelines on quality control methods for medicinal plants (*15*) and guidelines for predicting dietary intake of pesticide residues (*18*).

Heavy metals

Recommended lead and cadmium levels are no more than 10 and 0.3 mg/kg, respectively, in the final dosage form of the plant material (*15*).

Radioactive residues

For analysis of strontium-90, iodine-131, caesium-134, caesium-137, and plutonium-239, see WHO guidelines on quality control methods for medicinal plants (*15*).

Other purity tests

Chemical and water-soluble extractive tests to be established in accordance with national requirements.

Chemical assays

Contains not less than 2.2% hydroxyanthracene derivatives calculated as rhein (*2, 3*). Quantitative analysis of total hydroxyanthracene glycosides, calculated as rhein, performed by spectrophotometric analysis (*2–7*). High-performance liquid chromatography is also available (*19*) for quantitative analysis.

Thin-layer chromatography is employed for the qualitative analysis for the presence of emodin, physcione (emodin 3-methyl ether), chrysophanol (chrysophanic acid), rhein, and aloe-emodin (*2, 3*).

Major chemical constituents

The major constituents are hydroxyanthracene derivatives (2–5%) including emodin, physcione, aloe-emodin, and chrysophanol glycosides, along with di-*O*, *C*-glucosides of the monomeric reduced forms (rheinosides A–D), and dimeric reduced forms (sennosides A–F). The level of the oxidized forms is maximal in the summer and almost nil in the winter (*12*). Until the 1950s, chrysophanol and other anthraquinones were considered to be the constituents producing the purgative action of rhubarb. Current evidence indicates that the major active principles are the dimeric sennosides A–F (*20*).

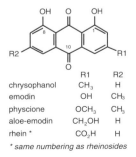

	R1	R2
chrysophanol	CH_3	H
emodin	OH	CH_3
physcione	OCH_3	CH_3
aloe-emodin	CH_2OH	H
rhein *	CO_2H	H

* same numbering as rheinosides

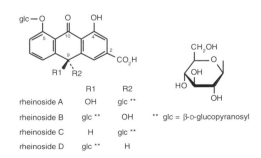

	R1	R2
rheinoside A	OH	glc **
rheinoside B	glc **	OH
rheinoside C	H	glc **
rheinoside D	glc **	H

** glc = β-D-glucopyranosyl

Dosage forms

Dried plant material and preparations standardized to contain 10–30 mg of hydroxyanthracene derivatives per dose (*21, 22*). Package in well-closed, light-resistant containers (*9, 11*).

Medicinal uses
Uses supported by clinical data

Short-term treatment of occasional constipation (*20, 23, 24*).

Uses described in pharmacopoeias and in traditional systems of medicine

None.

Uses described in folk medicine, not supported by experimental or clinical data

To treat hypotension, increase peripheral vasodilation, and inhibit blood coagulation (*8, 20*).

Pharmacology
Experimental pharmacology

As shown for senna, the mechanism of action is twofold: (1) stimulation of colonic motility, which augments propulsion and accelerates colonic transit (which in turn reduces fluid absorption from the faecal mass); and (2) an increase in the paracellular permeability across the colonic mucosa probably owing to an inhibition of Na^+/K^+-exchanging ATPase or to an inhibition of chloride channels (*25, 26*), which results in an increase in the water content in the large intestine (*27*). Purgation is followed by an astringent effect owing to the tannins present (*11, 12*).

Clinical pharmacology

The active constituents of Rhizoma Rhei are the anthraquinone glycosides, sennosides A–F and rheinosides A–D (*20*). The rheinosides are similar to aloin A and B, the main cathartic principles of *aloe*. The cathartic action of both the sennosides and rheinosides is limited to the large intestine, where they directly increase motor activity in the intestinal tract (*20, 23*). Consequently, they are seldom effective before 6 hours after oral administration, and they sometimes do not act before 24 hours.

The mechanism of action is similar to that of other anthraquinone stimulant laxatives. Both the sennosides and rheinosides are hydrolysed by intestinal bacteria and then reduced to the active anthrone metabolite, which acts as a stimulant and irritant to the gastrointestinal tract (*28*). Preparations of rhubarb are suitable as an occasional aperient, but should not be used in chronic constipation. A variable amount is absorbed and imparts a yellowish brown colour to the urine, which is changed to a purplish red on the addition of alkali (*11*). Rhizoma Rhei preparations have been employed occasionally for their astringent after effects, to check the diarrhoea produced by irritating substances in the intestines (*11*).

Toxicity

The major symptoms of overdose are griping and severe diarrhoea with consequent losses of fluid and electrolytes (*29*). Treatment should be supportive with generous amounts of fluid. Electrolytes, particularly potassium, should be monitored, especially in children and the elderly.

Contraindications

As with other stimulant laxatives, products containing Rhizoma Rhei should not be administered to patients with intestinal obstruction and stenosis, atony, severe dehydration states with water and electrolyte depletion, or chronic constipation. Rhizoma Rhei should not be used in patients with inflammatory intestinal diseases, such as appendicitis, Crohn disease, ulcerative colitis, or irritable bowel syndrome, or in children under 10 years of age. Rhizoma Rhei should not be used during pregnancy or lactation except under medical supervision after respective benefits and risks have been considered. As with other stimulant laxatives, Rhizoma Rhei is contraindicated in patients with cramps, colic, haemorrhoids, nephritis, or any undiagnosed abdominal symptoms such as pain, nausea, or vomiting (*23, 24*).

Warnings

Products containing Rhizoma Rhei should be used only if no effect can be obtained through a change of diet or use of bulk-forming laxatives. Stimulant laxatives should not be used when abdominal pain, nausea, or vomiting are present. Rectal bleeding or failure to have a bowel movement after the use of a laxative may indicate a serious condition (*29*). Use of stimulant laxatives for longer than the recommended short-term application may increase intestinal sluggishness (*28*).

The use of stimulant laxatives for more than 2 weeks requires medical supervision.

Chronic use may lead to pseudomelanosis coli (harmless) and to an aggravation of constipation with dependence and possible need for increased dosages.

Chronic abuse with diarrhoea and consequent fluid and electrolyte losses (mainly hypokalaemia) may cause albuminuria and haematuria, and it may result in cardiac and neuromuscular dysfunction, the latter particularly in case of concomitant use of cardiac glycosides (digoxin), diuretics, corticosteroids, or liquorice root (see below, Precautions).

Precautions
General
Laxatives containing anthraquinone glycosides should not be used for periods longer than 1–2 weeks continually, owing to the danger of electrolyte imbalance (29).

Drug interactions
Decreased intestinal transit time may reduce absorption of orally administered drugs (30).

Electrolyte imbalances such as increased loss of potassium may potentiate the effects of cardiotonic glycosides (digitalis, strophanthus). Existing hypokalaemia resulting from long-term laxative abuse can also potentiate the effects of antiarrhythmic drugs, such as quinidine, which affect potassium channels to change sinus rhythm. Simultaneous use with other drugs or herbs which induce hypokalaemia, such as thiazide diuretics, adrenocorticosteroids, or liquorice root, may exacerbate electrolyte imbalance (22).

Drug and laboratory test interactions
Anthranoid metabolites may not be detectable with standard methods. Thus results of measuring faecal excretion may not be reliable (31). Urinary excretion of certain anthranoid metabolites may discolour the urine, which is not clinically relevant but may cause false positive results for urinary urobilinogen and for estrogens when measured by the Kober procedure (30).

Carcinogenesis, mutagenesis, impairment of fertility
Data on the carcinogenicity of Rhizoma Rhei are not available. While chronic abuse of anthranoid-containing laxatives was hypothesized to play a role in colorectal cancer, no causal relationship between anthranoid laxative abuse and colorectal cancer has been demonstrated (32, 33).

Pregnancy: teratogenic effects
The teratogenic effects of Rhizoma Rhei have not been evaluated.

Pregnancy: non-teratogenic effects
Products containing Rhizoma Rhei should not be used by pregnant women because they have a pronounced action on the large intestine and have not undergone sufficient toxicological investigation (28).

Nursing mothers
Anthranoid metabolites appear in breast milk. Rhizoma Rhei should not be used during lactation as there are insufficient data available to assess the potential for pharmacological effects in the breast-fed infant (28).

Paediatric use

Use of Rhizoma Rhei for children under 10 years of age is contraindicated.

Adverse reactions

Single doses may cause cramp-like discomfort of the gastrointestinal tract, which may require a reduction of dosage. Overdoses can lead to colicky abdominal spasms and pain and the formation of thin, watery stools (*31*).

Chronic abuse of anthraquinone stimulant laxatives can lead to hepatitis (*34*). Long-term laxative abuse may lead to electrolyte disturbances (hypokalaemia, hypocalcaemia), metabolic acidosis, malabsorption, weight loss, albuminuria, and haematuria (*31, 35, 36*). Weakness and orthostatic hypotension may be exacerbated in elderly patients when stimulant laxatives are repeatedly used (*31*). Secondary aldosteronism may occur due to renal tubular damage after aggravated use. Steatorrhoea and protein-losing gastroenteropathy with hypoalbuminaemia have also been reported in laxative abuse (*37*). Melanotic pigmentation of the colonic mucosa (pseudomelanosis coli) has been observed in individuals taking anthraquinone laxatives for extended time periods (*29, 35*). The pigmentation is clinically harmless and usually reversible within 4–12 months after the drug has been discontinued (*30, 35*). Conflicting data exist on other toxic effects such as intestinal-neuronal damage after long-term use (*35*).

Posology

The individually correct dosage is the smallest dosage necessary to maintain a soft stool. The average dose is 0.5–1.5 g of dried plant material or in decoction; preparations standardized to contain 10–30 mg of hydroxyanthracene derivatives, usually taken at bedtime (*21, 22, 28*).

References

1. *The pharmacopoeia of Japan XII*. Tokyo, The Society of Japanese Pharmacopoeia, 1991.
2. *European pharmacopoeia*, 2nd ed. Strasbourg, Council of Europe, 1995.
3. *Pharmacopée française*. Paris, Adrapharm, 1996.
4. *British pharmacopoeia*. London, Her Majesty's Stationery Office, 1988.
5. *Deutsches Arzneibuch 1996*. Stuttgart, Deutscher Apotheker Verlag, 1996.
6. *Pharmacopoeia helvetica VII*. Berne, Département fédéral de l'intérieur, 1994.
7. *Pharmacopoeia of India*. New Delhi, The Controller of Publications, 1985.
8. Farnsworth NR, ed. *NAPRALERT database*. Chicago, University of Illinois at Chicago, IL, March 15, 1995 production (an on-line database available directly through the University of Illinois at Chicago or through the Scientific and Technical Network (STN) of Chemical Abstracts Services).
9. Youngken HW. *Textbook of pharmacognosy* 6th ed. Philadelphia, Blakiston, 1950.

10. *Vietnam materia medica*. Hanoi, Ministry of Health, 1972.
11. *The Indian pharmaceutical codex. Vol. I. Indigenous drugs*. New Delhi, Council of Scientific & Industrial Research, 1953.
12. Bruneton J. *Pharmacognosy, phytochemistry, medicinal plants*. Paris, Lavoisier, 1995.
13. Jackson BP, Snowden DW. *Atlas of microscopy of medicinal plants, culinary herbs and spices*. Boca Raton, FL, CRC Press, 1990.
14. Tyler VE, Brady LR, Robbers JE, eds. *Pharmacognosy*, 9th ed. Philadelphia, Lea & Febiger, 1988.
15. *Quality control methods for medicinal plant materials*. Geneva, World Health Organization, 1998.
16. *Deutsches Arzneibuch 1996. Vol. 2. Methoden der Biologie*. Stuttgart, Deutscher Apotheker Verlag, 1996.
17. *European pharmacopoeia*, 3rd ed. Strasbourg, Council of Europe, 1997.
18. *Guidelines for predicting dietary intake of pesticide residues*, 2nd rev. ed. Geneva, World Health Organization, 1997 (unpublished document WHO/FSF/FOS/97.7; available from Food Safety, WHO, 1211 Geneva 27, Switzerland).
19. Sagara K, Oshima T, Yoshida T. Rapid and simple determination of sennosides A and B in Rhei Rhizoma by ion-pair high-performance liquid chromatography. *Journal of chromatography*, 1987, 403:253–261.
20. Nishioka I. Biological activities and the active components of rhubarb. *International journal of Oriental medicine*, 1991, 16:193–212.
21. Bradley PR, ed. *British herbal compendium, Vol. 1*. Bournemouth, British Herbal Medicine Association, 1992.
22. German Commission E monograph, Rhei radix. *Bundesanzeiger*, 1993, 133:21 July.
23. Reynolds JEF, ed. *Martindale, the extra pharmacopoeia*, 30th ed. London, Pharmaceutical Press, 1993:903.
24. Bisset NG. *Max Wichtl's herbal drugs & phytopharmaceuticals*. Boca Raton, FL, CRC Press, 1994.
25. Leng-Peschlow E. Dual effect of orally administered sennosides on large intestine transit and fluid absorption in the rat. *Journal of pharmacy and pharmacology*, 1986, 36:230–236.
26. Yamauchi K et al. Suppression of the purgative action of rhein anthrone, the active metabolite of sennosides A and B, by calcium channel blockers, calmodulin antagonists and indomethacin. *Pharmacology*, 1993, 47(Suppl. 1):22–31.
27. de Witte P. Metabolism and pharmacokinetics of anthranoids. *Pharmacology*, 1993, 47(Suppl. 1):86–97.
28. *Physicians' desk reference*, 49th ed., Montvale, NJ, Medical Economics Company, 1995.
29. *Goodman and Gilman's the pharmacological basis of therapeutics*, 8th ed. New York, McGraw Hill, 1990.
30. *United States pharmacopeia, drug information*. Rockville, MD, US Pharmacopeial Convention, 1992.
31. *American hospital formulary service*. Bethesda, MD, American Society of Hospital Pharmacists, 1990.
32. Siegers CP. Anthranoid laxatives and colorectal cancer. *Trends in pharmacological sciences*, 1992, 13:229–231.
33. Patel PM et al. Anthraquinone laxatives and human cancer. *Postgraduate medical journal*, 1989, 65:216–217.
34. Beuers U, Spengler U, Pape GR. Hepatitis after chronic abuse of senna. *Lancet*, 1991, 337:472.
35. Muller-Lissner SA. Adverse effects of laxatives: facts and fiction. *Pharmacology*, 1993, 47(Suppl. 1):138–145.

36. Godding EW. Therapeutics of laxative agents with special reference to the anthraquinones. *Pharmacology*, 1976, 14(Suppl. 1):78–101.
37. Heizer WD et al. Protein-losing gastroenteropathy and malabsorption associated with factitious diarrhoea. *Annals of internal medicine*, 1968, 68:839–852.

Folium Sennae

Definition

Folium Sennae consists of the dried leaflets of *Cassia senna* L. (Fabaceae).[1]

Synonyms

Fabaceae are also referred to as Leguminosae.

Although recognized as two distinct species in many pharmacopoeias (*1–8*), *Cassia acutifolia* Delile and *C. angustifolia* Vahl. are considered botanically to be synonyms of the single species *Cassia senna* L. (*9*).

Selected vernacular names

Alexandria senna, Alexandrian senna, cassia, eshrid, falajin, fan xie ye, filaskon maka, hindisana, illesko, Indian senna, ma khaam khaek, makhaam khaek, mecca senna, msahala, nelaponna, nelatangedu, nilavaka, nilavirai, nubia senna, rinji, sanai, sand hijazi, sanjerehi, sen de alejandria, sen de la india, senna makki, senna, senamikki, sennae folium, sona-mukhi, Tinnevelly senna, true senna (*3, 10–14*).

Description

Low shrubs, up to 1.5 m high, with compound paripinnate leaves, having 3–7 pairs of leaflets, narrow or rounded, pale green to yellowish green. Flowers, tetracyclic, pentamerous, and zygomorphic, have quincuncial calyx, a corolla of yellow petals with brown veins, imbricate ascendent prefloration, and a partially staminodial androeceum. The fruit is a broadly elliptical, somewhat reniform, flattened, parchment-like, dehiscent pod, 4–7 cm long by 2 cm wide, with 6 to 10 seeds (*11, 14, 15*).

---

[1] *C. italica* Mill. is listed in the Malian pharmacopoeia.

Plant material of interest: leaflets
General appearance
Macroscopically, the leaflets are lanceolate or lanceolate-ovate, unequal at the base, with entire margin, acute-mucronate apex and short, stout petioles; sometimes broken; 1.5–5 cm in length and 0.5–1.5 cm in width, bearing a fine pubescence of appressed hairs, more numerous on the lower surface (1–7).

Organoleptic properties
The colour is weak yellow to pale olive (1, 2). The odour is characteristic, and the taste is mucilage-like and then slightly bitter (1, 3).

Microscopic characteristics
Epidermis with polygonal cells containing mucilage; unicellular thick-walled trichomes, length, up to 260 µm, slightly curved at the base, warty; paracytic stomata on both surfaces; under the epidermal cells a single row of palisade layer; cluster crystals of calcium oxalate distributed throughout the lacunose tissue; on the adaxial surface, sclerenchymatous fibres and a gutter-shaped group of similar fibres on the abaxial side containing prismatic crystals of calcium oxalate (1).

Powdered plant material
Light green to greenish yellow. Polygonal epidermal cells showing paracytic stomata. Unicellular trichomes, conical in shape, with warty walls, isolated or attached to fragments of epidermis. Fragments of fibrovascular bundles with a crystal sheath containing calcium oxalate prisms. Cluster crystals isolated or in fragments of parenchyma (2, 3).

Geographical distribution
The plant is indigenous to tropical Africa. It grows wild near the Nile river from Aswan to Kordofan, and in the Arabian peninsula, India and Somalia (15). It is cultivated in India, Pakistan, and the Sudan (11, 12, 14, 15).

General identity tests
Macroscopic, microscopic examinations, and microchemical analysis (1–6), and thin-layer chromatographic analysis for the presence of characteristic sennosides (sennosides A–D) (3–5).

Purity tests
Microbiology
The test for *Salmonella* spp. in Folium Sennae products should be negative. The maximum acceptable limits of other microorganisms are as follows (16–18). For

preparation of decoction: aerobic bacteria—10^7/g; moulds and yeast—10^5/g; *Escherichia coli*—10^2/g; other enterobacteria—10^4/g. Preparations for internal use: aerobic bacteria—10^5/g; moulds and yeast—10^4/g; *Escherichia coli*—0/g; other enterobacteria—10^3/g.

Foreign organic matter
Not more than 2.0% of stems (*1*) and not more than 1.0% of other foreign organic matter (*1, 4, 8*).

Total ash
Not more than 12% (*5*).

Acid-insoluble ash
Not more than 2.0% (*1, 8*).

Water-soluble extractive
Not less than 3% (*1*).

Moisture
Not more than 10% (*6*).

Pesticide residues
To be established in accordance with national requirements. Normally, the maximum residue limit of aldrin and dieldrin in Folium Sennae is not more than 0.05 mg/kg (*18*). For other pesticides, see WHO guidelines on quality control methods for medicinal plants (*16*) and guidelines for predicting dietary intake of pesticide residues (*19*).

Heavy metals
Recommended lead and cadmium levels are not more than 10 and 0.3 mg/kg, respectively, in the final dosage form of the plant material (*16*).

Radioactive residues
For analysis of strontium-90, iodine-131, caesium-134, caesium-137, and plutonium-239, see WHO guidelines on quality control methods for medicinal plants (*16*).

Other purity tests
Chemical tests and tests of alcohol-soluble extractive are to be established in accordance with national requirements.

Chemical assays

Contains not less than 2.5% of hydroxyanthracene glycosides, calculated as sennoside B (*1, 4, 5*). Quantitative analysis is performed by spectrophotometry (*1, 4–8*) and by high-performance liquid chromatography (*20*).

Thin-layer chromatography is employed for qualitative analysis for the presence of sennosides A and B (*3–5*).

Major chemical constituents

Folium Sennae contains a family of hydroxyanthracene glycosides, the most plentiful of which are sennosides A and B. There are also small amounts of aloe-emodin and rhein 8-glucosides, mucilage, flavonoids, and naphthalene precursors (*15*).

	R1	R2	9-9'
sennoside A	H	CO_2H	R^*, R^* (threo)
sennoside B	H	CO_2H	R^*, S^* (erythro)
sennoside C	H	CH_2OH	R^*, R^* (threo)
sennoside D	H	CH_2OH	R^*, S^* (erythro)
sennoside E	$CO\text{-}CO_2H$	CO_2H	R^*, R^* (threo)
sennoside F	$CO\text{-}CO_2H$	CO_2H	R^*, S^* (erythro)

Dosage forms

Crude plant material, powder, oral infusion, and extracts (liquid or solid) standardized for content of sennosides A and B (*15, 21, 22*). Package in well-closed containers protected from light and moisture (*1–8*).

Medicinal uses

Uses supported by clinical data

Short-term use in occasional constipation (*21–25*).

Uses described in pharmacopoeias and in traditional systems of medicine

None.

Uses described in folk medicine, not supported by experimental or clinical data

As an expectorant, a wound dressing, an antidysenteric, and a carminative agent; and for the treatment of gonorrhoea, skin diseases, dyspepsia, fever, and haemorrhoids (*11, 23, 25*).

Pharmacology

Experimental pharmacology

The effects of Folium Sennae are due primarily to the hydroxyanthracene glucosides, especially sennosides A and B. These β-linked glucosides are secretagogues that increase net secretion of fluids and specifically influence colonic motility and enhance colonic transit. They are not absorbed in the upper intestinal tract; they are converted by the bacteria of the large intestine into the active derivatives (rhein-anthrone). The mechanism of action is twofold: (1) effect on the motility of the large intestine (stimulation of peristaltic contractions and inhibition of local contractions), resulting in an accelerated colonic transit, thereby reducing fluid absorption, and (2) an influence on fluid and electrolyte absorption and secretion by the colon (stimulation of mucus and active chloride secretion), increasing fluid secretion (*24, 25*).

Clinical pharmacology

The time of action of senna is usually 8–10 hours, and thus the dose should be taken at night (*24*). The action of the sennosides augments, without disrupting, the response to the physiological stimuli of food and physical activity (*24*). The sennosides abolish the severe constipation of patients suffering from severe irritable bowel syndrome (*26*). In therapeutic doses, the sennosides do not disrupt the usual pattern of defecation times and markedly soften the stool (*24*). Sennosides significantly increase the rate of colonic transit (*27*) and increase colonic peristalsis, which in turn increase both faecal weight and dry bacterial mass (*24, 28*). Due to their colonic specificity, the sennosides are poorly absorbed in the upper gastrointestinal tract (*29*).

Toxicity

The major symptoms of overdose are griping and severe diarrhoea with consequent losses of fluid and electrolytes. Treatment should be supportive with generous amounts of fluid. Electrolytes, particularly potassium, should be monitored, especially in children and the elderly.

Contraindications

As with other stimulant laxatives, the drug is contraindicated in persons with ileus, intestinal obstruction, and stenosis, atony, undiagnosed abdominal symptoms, inflammatory colonopathies, appendicitis, abdominal pains of unknown cause, severe dehydration states with water and electrolyte depletion, or chronic constipation (*21, 30*). Folium Sennae should not be used in children under the age of 10 years.

Warnings

Stimulant laxative products should not be used when abdominal pain, nausea, or vomiting are present. Rectal bleeding or failure to have a bowel movement after use of a laxative may indicate a serious condition (*31*). Chronic abuse, with diarrhoea and consequent fluid electrolyte losses, may cause dependence and need for increased dosages, disturbance of the water and electrolyte balance (e.g. hypokalaemia), atonic colon with impaired function, albuminuria and haematuria (*29, 32*).

The use of stimulant laxatives for more than 2 weeks requires medical supervision.

Chronic use may lead to pseudomelanosis coli (harmless).

Hypokalaemia may result in cardiac and neuromuscular dysfunction, especially if cardiac glycosides (digoxin), diuretics, corticosteroids, or liquorice root are taken (*29*).

Precautions

General

Use for more than 2 weeks requires medical attention (*21, 31*).

Drug interactions

Decreased intestinal transit time may reduce absorption of orally administered drugs (*32, 33*).

The increased loss of potassium may potentiate the effects of cardiotonic glycosides (digitalis, strophanthus). Existing hypokalaemia resulting from long-term laxative abuse can also potentiate the effects of antiarrhythmic drugs, such as quinidine, which affect potassium channels to change sinus rhythm. Simultaneous use with other drugs or herbs which induce hypokalaemia, such as thiazide diuretics, adrenocorticosteroids, or liquorice root, may exacerbate electrolyte imbalance (*21, 22*).

Drug and laboratory test interactions

Urine discoloration by anthranoid metabolites may lead to false positive test results for urinary urobilinogen, and for estrogens measured by the Kober procedure (*32*).

Carcinogenesis, mutagenesis, impairment of fertility

No *in vivo* genotoxic effects have been reported to date (*34–37*). Although chronic abuse of anthranoid-containing laxatives was hypothesized to play a role in colorectal cancer, no causal relationship between anthranoid laxative abuse and colorectal cancer has been demonstrated (*38–40*).

Pregnancy: non-teratogenic effects

Use during pregnancy should be limited to conditions in which changes in diet or fibre laxatives are not effective (*41*).

Nursing mothers

Use during breast-feeding is not recommended owing to insufficient data on the excretion of metabolites in breast milk (*21*). Small amounts of active metabolites (rhein) are excreted into breast milk, but a laxative effect in breast-fed babies has not been reported (*21*).

Paediatric use

Contraindicated for children under 10 years of age (*21*).

Other precautions

No information available on teratogenic effects in pregnancy.

Adverse reactions

Senna may cause mild abdominal discomfort such as colic or cramps (*21, 22, 33*). A single case of hepatitis has been described after chronic abuse (*42*). Melanosis coli, a condition which is characterized by pigment-loaded macrophages within the submucosa, may occur after long-term use. This condition is clinically harmless and disappears with cessation of treatment (*33, 43, 44*).

Long-term laxative abuse may lead to electrolyte disturbances (hypokalaemia, hypocalcaemia), metabolic acidosis or alkalosis, malabsorption, weight loss, albuminuria, and haematuria (*21, 22, 33*). Weakness and orthostatic hypotension may be exacerbated in elderly patients when stimulant laxatives are repeatedly used (*21, 33*). Conflicting data exist on other toxic effects such as intestinal-neuronal damage due to long-term misuse (*45–54*).

Posology

The correct individual dose is the smallest required to produce a comfortable, soft-formed motion (*21*). Powder: 1–2 g of leaf daily at bedtime (*11*). Adults and children over 10 years: standardized daily dose equivalent to 10–30 mg sennosides (calculated as sennoside B) taken at night.

References

1. *The international pharmacopoeia*, 3rd ed. Vol. 3. *Quality specifications*. Geneva, World Health Organization, 1988.
2. *The United States Pharmacopeia XXIII*. Rockville, MD, US Pharmacopeial Convention, 1996.

3. *African pharmacopoeia*, 1st ed. Lagos, Organization of African Unity, Scientific, Technical & Research Commission, 1985.
4. *British pharmacopoeia*. London, Her Majesty's Stationery Office, 1988.
5. *European pharmacopoeia*, 2nd ed. Strasbourg, Council of Europe, 1995.
6. *Pharmacopoeia of the People's Republic of China* (English ed.). Guangzhou, Guangdong Science and Technology Press, 1992.
7. *Deutsches Arzneibuch 1996*. Stuttgart, Deutscher Apotheker Verlag, 1996.
8. *Pharmacopée française*. Paris, Adrapharm, 1996.
9. Brenan JPM. New and noteworthy Cassia from tropical Africa. *Kew bulletin*, 1958, 13:231–252.
10. Farnsworth NR, ed. *NAPRALERT database*. Chicago, University of Illinois at Chicago, IL, March 15, 1995 production (an on-line database available directly through the University of Illinois at Chicago or through the Scientific and Technical Network (STN) of Chemical Abstracts Services).
11. Youngken HW. *Textbook of pharmacognosy*, 6th ed. Philadelphia, Blakiston, 1950.
12. *Medicinal plants of India, Vol. 1*. New Delhi, Indian Council of Medical Research, 1976.
13. Huang KC. *The pharmacology of Chinese herbs*. Boca Raton, FL, CRC Press, 1994.
14. Farnsworth NR, Bunyapraphatsara N, eds. *Thai medicinal plants*. Bangkok, Prachachon, 1992.
15. Bruneton J. *Pharmacognosy, phytochemistry, medicinal plants*. Paris, Lavoisier, 1995.
16. *Quality control methods for medicinal plant materials*. Geneva, World Health Organization, 1998.
17. *Deutsches Arzneibuch 1996. Vol. 2. Methoden der Biologie*. Stuttgart, Deutscher Apotheker Verlag, 1996.
18. *European pharmacopoeia*, 3rd ed. Strasbourg, Council of Europe, 1997.
19. *Guidelines for predicting dietary intake of pesticide residues*, 2nd rev. ed. Geneva. World Health Organization, 1997 (unpublished document WHO/FSF/FOS/97.7; available from Food Safety, WHO, 1211 Geneva 27, Switzerland).
20. Duez P et al. Comparison between high-performance thin-layer chromatography-fluorometry and high-performance liquid chromatography for the determination of sennosides A and B in Senna (*Cassia* spp.) pods and leaves. *Journal of chromatography*, 1984, 303:391–395.
21. Core-SPC for Sennae Folium. *Coordinated review of monographs on herbal remedies*. Brussels, European Commission, 1994.
22. German Commission E Monograph, Senna folium. *Bundesanzeiger*, 1993, 133:21 July.
23. Leng-Peschlow E. Dual effect of orally administered sennosides on large intestine transit and fluid absorption in the rat. *Journal of pharmacy and pharmacology*, 1986, 38:606–610.
24. Godding EW. Laxatives and the special role of Senna. *Pharmacology*, 1988, 36(Suppl. 1):230–236.
25. Bradley PR, ed. *British herbal compendium, Vol. 1*. Bournemouth, British Herbal Medicine Association, 1992.
26. Waller SL, Misiewicz JJ. Prognosis in the irritable-bowel syndrome. *Lancet*, 1969, ii:753–756.
27. Ewe K, Ueberschaer B, Press AG. Influence of senna, fibre, and fibre + senna on colonic transit in loperamide-induced constipation. *Pharmacology*, 47(Suppl. 1):242–248.
28. Stephen AM, Wiggins HS, Cummings JH. Effect of changing transit time on colonic microbial metabolism in man. *Gut*, 1987, 28:610.
29. *Goodman and Gilman's the pharmacological basis of therapeutics*, 9th ed. New York, McGraw-Hill, 1996.

30. *Physicians' desk reference*, 49th ed. Montvale, NJ, Medical Economics Company, 1995.
31. *American hospital formulary service.* Bethesda, MD, American Society of Hospital Pharmacists, 1990.
32. *United States pharmacopeia, drug information.* Rockville, MD, US Pharmacopeial Convention, 1992.
33. *Martindale, the extra pharmacopoeia*, 30th ed. London, Pharmaceutical Press, 1993.
34. Heidemann A, Miltenburger HG, Mengs U. The genotoxicity of Senna. *Pharmacology*, 1993, 47(Suppl. 1):178–186.
35. Tikkanen L et al. Mutagenicity of anthraquinones in the *Salmonella* preincubation test. *Mutation research*, 1983, 116:297–304.
36. Westendorf et al. Mutagenicity of naturally occurring hydroxyanthraquinones. *Mutation research*, 1990, 240:1–12.
37. Sanders D et al. Mutagenicity of crude Senna and Senna glycosides in *Salmonella typhimurium*. *Pharmacology and toxicology*, 1992, 71:165–172.
38. Lyden-Sokolowsky A, Nilsson A, Sjoberg P. Two-year carcinogenicity study with sennosides in the rat: emphasis on gastrointestinal alterations. *Pharmacology*, 1993, 47(Suppl. 1):209–215.
39. Kune GA. Laxative use not a risk for colorectal cancer: data from the Melbourne colorectal cancer study. *Zeitschrift für Gasteroenterologie*, 1993, 31:140–143.
40. Siegers CP. Anthranoid laxatives and colorectal cancer. *Trends in pharmacological sciences*, 1992, 13:229–231.
41. Lewis JH et al. The use of gastrointestinal drugs during pregnancy and lactation. *American journal of gastroenterology*, 1985, 80:912–923.
42. Beuers U, Spengler U, Pape GR. Hepatitis after chronic abuse of Senna. *Lancet*, 1991, 337:472.
43. Loew D. Pseudomelanosis coli durch Anthranoide. *Zeitschrift für Phytotherapie*, 1994, 16:312–318.
44. Müller-Lissner SA. Adverse effects of laxatives: facts and fiction. *Pharmacology*, 1993, 47(Suppl. 1):138–145.
45. Godding EW. Therapeutics of laxative agents with special reference to the anthraquinones. *Pharmacology*, 1976, 14(Suppl. 1):78–101.
46. Dufour P, Gendre P. Ultrastructure of mouse intestinal mucosa and changes observed after long term anthraquinone administration. *Gut*, 1984, 25:1358–1363.
47. Dufour P et al. Tolérance de la muqueuse intestinale de la souris à l'ingestion prolongée d'une poudre de sené. *Annales pharmaceutiques françaises*, 1983, 41(6):571–578.
48. Kienan JA, Heinicke EA. Sennosides do not kill myenteric neurons in the colon of the rat or mouse. *Neurosciences*, 1989, 30(3):837–842.
49. Riemann JF et al. Ultrastructural changes of colonic mucosa in patients with chronic laxative misuse. *Acta hepato-gastroenterology*, 1978, 25:213–218.
50. Smith BA. Effect of irritant purgatives on the myenteric plexus in man and the mouse. *Gut*, 1968, 9:139–143.
51. Riemann JF et al. The fine structure of colonic submucosal nerves in patients with chronic laxative abuse. *Scandinavian journal of gastroenterology*, 1980, 15:761–768.
52. Rieken EO et al. The effect of an anthraquinone laxative on colonic nerve tissue: a controlled trial in constipated women. *Zeitschrift für Gasteroenterologie*, 1990, 28:660–664.
53. Riemann JF, Schmidt H. Ultrastructural changes in the gut autonomic nervous system following laxative abuse and in other conditions. *Scandinavian journal of gastroenterology*, 1982, 71(Suppl.):111–124.
54. Krishnamurti S et al. Severe idiopathic constipation is associated with a distinctive abnormality of the colonic myenteric plexus. *Gastroenterology*, 1985, 88:26–34.

Fructus Sennae

Definition

Fructus Sennae consists of the dried ripe fruit of *Cassia senna* L. (Fabaceae).[1]

Synonyms

Fabaceae are also referred to as Leguminosae.

Cassia acutifolia Delile and *Cassia angustifolia* Vahl. (*1*) are recognized as two distinct species in a number of pharmacopoeias as Alexandrian senna fruit and Tinnevelly senna fruit (*2–7*). Botanically, however, they are considered to be synonyms of the single species *Cassia senna* L. (*1*).

Selected vernacular names

Alexandria senna, Alexandrian senna, cassia, eshrid, falajin, fan xie ye, filaskon maka, hindisana, illesko, Indian senna, ma khaam khaek, makhaam khaek, Mecca senna, msahala, nelaponna, nelatangedu, nilavaka, nilavirai, nubia senna, rinji, sanai, sand hijazi, sanjerehi, sen de Alejandria, sen de la India, senna makki, senna, senna pod, senamikki, sona-mukhi, Tinnevelly senna, true senna (*8–11*).

Description

Low shrubs, up to 1.5 m high, with compound paripinnate leaves, having 3–7 pairs of leaflets, narrow or rounded, pale green to yellowish green. Flowers, tetracyclic, pentamerous and zygomorphic, have quincuncial calyx, a corolla of yellow petals with brown veins, imbricate ascendent prefloration, and a partially staminodial androeceum. The fresh fruit is a broadly elliptical, somewhat reniform, flattened, parchment-like, dehiscent pod, 4–7 cm long by 2 cm wide, with 6–10 seeds (*9, 12, 13*).

Plant material of interest: dried ripe fruit

General appearance

Fructus Sennae is leaf-like, has flat and thin pods, yellowish green to yellowish brown with a dark brown central area, oblong or reniform. Fruit is pale to greyish green, 3.5–6.0 cm in length, 1.4–1.8 cm in width; stylar point at one end,

---

[1] *Cassia italica* Mill. is listed in the Malian pharmacopoeia.

containing 6–10 obovate green to pale brown seeds with longitudinal prominent ridges on the testa (*2*).

Organoleptic properties

Colour is pale green to brown to greyish black (*2, 3*); odour, characteristic; taste,
mucilaginous and then slightly bitter (*2*).

Microscopic characteristics

Epicarp with very thick cuticularized isodiametrical cells, occasional
anomocytic or paracytic stomata, and very few unicellular and warty trichomes; hypodermis with collenchymatous cells; mesocarp with parenchymatous tissue containing a layer of calcium oxalate prisms; endocarp consisting of
thick-walled fibre, mostly perpendicular to the longitudinal axis of the fruit, but
the inner fibres running at an oblique angle or parallel to the longitudinal axis.
Seeds, subepidermal layer of palisade cells with thick outer walls; the endosperm has polyhedral cells with mucilaginous walls (*2*).

Powdered plant material

Brown; epicarp with polygonal cells and a small number of conical warty
trichomes and occasional anomocytic or paracytic stomata; fibres in two
crossed layers accompanied by a crystal sheath of calcium oxalate prisms;
characteristic palisade cells in the seeds and stratified cells in the endosperm;
clusters and prisms of calcium oxalate (*4*).

Geographical distribution

The plant is indigenous to tropical Africa. It grows wild near the Nile river from
Aswan to Kordofan, and in the Arabian peninsula, India, and Somalia (*12, 13*).
It is cultivated in India, Pakistan, and the Sudan (*8, 9, 11–14*).

General identity tests

Macroscopic, microscopic, and microchemical examinations (*2–7*), and thin-
layer chromatographic analysis for the presence of characteristic sennosides
(sennosides A–D).

Purity tests
Microbiology

The test for *Salmonella* spp. in Fructus Sennae products should be negative. The
maximum acceptable limits of other microorganisms are as follows (*15–17*). For
preparation of decoction: aerobic bacteria—10^7/g; moulds and yeast—10^5/g;
Escherichia coli—10^2/g; other enterobacteria—10^4/g. Preparations for internal use:
aerobic bacteria—10^5/g or ml; moulds and yeast—10^4/g or ml; *Escherichia coli*—
0/g or ml; other enterobacteria—10^3/g or ml.

251

Foreign organic matter
Not more than 1.0% (2).

Total ash
Not more than 6% (3).

Acid-insoluble ash
Not more than 2.0% (2, 4, 5).

Water-soluble extractive
Not less than 25% (2).

Moisture
Not more than 12% (5).

Pesticide residues
To be established in accordance with national requirements. Normally, the maximum residue limit of aldrin and dieldrin in Fructus Sennae is not more than 0.05 mg/kg (17). For other pesticides, see WHO guidelines on quality control methods for medicinal plants (15) and guidelines for predicting dietary intake of pesticide residues (18).

Heavy metals
Recommended lead and cadmium levels are not more than 10 and 0.3 mg/kg, respectively, in the final dosage form of the plant material (15).

Radioactive residues
For analysis of strontium-90, iodine-131, caesium-134, caesium-137, and plutonium-239, see WHO guidelines on quality control methods for medicinal plants (15).

Other purity tests
Chemical tests and tests of alcohol-soluble extractive to be established in accordance with national requirements.

Chemical assays
Contains not less than 2.2% of hydroxyanthracene glycosides, calculated as sennoside B (2–7). Quantitative analysis is performed by spectrophotometry (2, 5–7) or by high-performance liquid chromatography (19).

The presence of sennosides A and B (3–5) can be determined by thin-layer chromatography.

Major chemical constituents

Fructus Sennae contains a family of hydroxyanthracene glycosides, the most plentiful of which are sennosides A and B (for structures, see page 244). There are also small amounts of aloe-emodin and rhein 8-glucosides, mucilage, flavonoids, and naphthalene precursors (*12, 13, 20*).

Dosage forms

Crude plant material, powder, oral infusion, and extracts (liquid or solid, standardized for content of sennosides A and B) (*12, 20, 21*). Package in well-closed containers protected from light and moisture (*2–7*).

Medicinal uses

Uses supported by clinical data

Short-term use in occasional constipation (*21–25*).

Uses described in pharmacopoeias and in traditional systems of medicine

None.

Uses described in folk medicine, not supported by experimental or clinical data

As an expectorant, a wound dressing, an antidysenteric, and a carminative agent; and for the treatment of gonorrhoea, skin diseases, dyspepsia, fever, and haemorrhoids (*11, 23, 25*).

Pharmacology

Experimental pharmacology

The effects of Fructus Sennae are due primarily to the hydroxyanthracene glucosides, especially sennosides A and B. These β-linked glucosides are secretagogues that induce net secretion of fluids, and specifically influence colonic motility and enhance colonic transit. They are not absorbed in the upper intestinal tract; they are converted by the bacteria of the large intestine into the active derivatives (rhein-anthrone). The mechanism of action is twofold: an effect on the motility of the large intestine (stimulation of peristaltic contractions and inhibition of local contractions), which accelerates colonic transit, thereby reducing fluid absorption; and an influence on fluid and electrolyte absorption and secretion by the colon (stimulation of mucus and active chloride secretion), which increases fluid secretion (*24, 25*).

Clinical pharmacology

The time of action of Senna is usually 8–10 hours, and thus the dose should be taken at night (*24*). The action of the sennosides augments, without disrupting, the response to the physiological stimuli of food and physical activity (*24*). The sennosides abolish the severe constipation of patients suffering from severe irritable bowel syndrome (*26*). In therapeutic doses, the sennosides do not disrupt the usual pattern of defecation times and markedly soften stools (*24*). Sennosides significantly increase the rate of colonic transit (*27*) and increase colonic peristalsis, which in turn increases both faecal weight and dry bacterial mass (*24, 28*). Due to their colonic specificity, the sennosides are poorly absorbed in the upper gastrointestinal tract (*29*).

Toxicity

The major symptoms of overdose are griping and severe diarrhoea with consequent losses of fluid and electrolytes. Treatment should be supportive with generous amounts of fluid. Electrolytes, particularly potassium, should be monitored, especially in children and the elderly.

Contraindications

As with other stimulant laxatives, the drug is contraindicated in cases of ileus, intestinal obstruction, stenosis, atony, undiagnosed abdominal symptoms, inflammatory colonopathies, appendicitis, abdominal pains of unknown cause, severe dehydration states with water and electrolyte depletion, or chronic constipation (*20, 21, 30*). Fructus Sennae should not be used in children under the age of 10 years.

Warnings

Stimulant laxative products should not be used when abdominal pain, nausea, or vomiting are present. Rectal bleeding or failure to have a bowel movement after use of a laxative may indicate a serious condition (*31*). Chronic abuse with diarrhoea and consequent fluid and electrolyte losses may cause dependence and need for increased dosages, disturbance of the water and electrolyte balance (e.g. hypokalaemia), atonic colon with impaired function and albuminuria and haematuria (*21, 32*).

The use of stimulant laxatives for more than 2 weeks requires medical supervision.

Chronic use may lead to pseudomelanosis coli (harmless).

Hypokalaemia may result in cardiac and neuromuscular dysfunction, especially if cardiac glycosides (digoxin), diuretics, corticosteroids, or liquorice root are taken (*29*).

Precautions

General

Use for more than 2 weeks requires medical attention (*21, 31*).

Drug interactions

Decreased intestinal transit time may reduce absorption of orally administered drugs (*32, 33*).

The increased loss of potassium may potentiate the effects of cardiotonic glycosides (digitalis, strophanthus). Existing hypokalaemia resulting from long-term laxative abuse can also potentiate the effects of antiarrhythmic drugs, such as quinidine, which affect potassium channels to change sinus rhythm. Simultaneous use with other drugs or herbs which induce hypokalaemia, such as thiazide diuretics, adrenocorticosteroids, or liquorice root, may exacerbate electrolyte imbalance (*20*, *21*).

Drug and laboratory test interactions

Urine discoloration by anthranoid metabolites may lead to false positive test results for urinary urobilinogen and for estrogens measured by the Kober procedure (*32*).

Carcinogenesis, mutagenesis, impairment of fertility

No *in vivo* genotoxic effects have been reported to date (*34–37*). Although chronic abuse of anthranoid-containing laxatives was hypothesized to play a role in colorectal cancer, no causal relationship between anthranoid laxative abuse and colorectal cancer has been demonstrated (*38–40*).

Pregnancy: non-teratogenic effects

Use during pregnancy should be limited to conditions in which changes in diet or fibre laxatives are not effective (*41*).

Nursing mothers

Use during breast-feeding is not recommended owing to insufficient available data on the excretion of metabolites in breast milk (*21*). Small amounts of active metabolites (rhein) are excreted into breast milk, but a laxative effect in breast-fed babies has not been reported (*21*).

Paediatric use

Contraindicated for children under 10 years of age (*21*).

Other precautions

No information available concerning teratogenic effects on pregnancy.

Adverse reactions

Senna may cause mild abdominal discomfort such as colic or griping (*21*, *22*, *33*). A single case of hepatitis has been described after chronic abuse (*42*). Melanosis coli, a condition which is characterized by pigment-loaded macrophages within the submucosa, may occur after long-term use. This condition is clinically harmless and disappears with cessation of treatment (*33*, *43*, *44*).

Long-term laxative abuse may lead to electrolyte disturbances (hypokalaemia, hypocalcaemia), metabolic acidosis or alkalosis, malabsorption, weight loss, albuminuria, and haematuria (*21, 22, 33*). Weakness and orthostatic hypotension may be exacerbated in elderly patients who repeatedly use stimulant laxatives (*21, 33*). Conflicting data exist on other toxic effects such as intestinal-neuronal damage after long-term misuse (*45–54*).

Posology

The correct individual dose is the smallest required to produce a comfortable, soft-formed motion (*21*). Powder, 1–2 g of fruit daily at bedtime (*8, 19, 20*). Adults and children over 10 years: standardized daily dose equivalent to 10–30 mg sennosides (calculated as sennoside B) taken at night.

References

1. Brenan JPM. New and noteworthy *Cassia* from tropical Africa. *Kew bulletin*, 1958, 13:231–252.
2. *The international pharmacopoeia*, 3rd ed. *Vol. 3. Quality specifications.* Geneva, World Health Organization, 1988.
3. *African pharmacopoeia*, 1st ed. Lagos, Organization of African Unity, Scientific, Technical & Research Commission, 1985.
4. *British pharmacopoeia*. London, Her Majesty's Stationery Office, 1993.
5. *European pharmacopoeia*, 2nd ed. Strasbourg, Council of Europe, 1995.
6. *Deutsches Arzneibuch 1996.* Stuttgart, Deutscher Apotheker Verlag, 1991.
7. *Pharmacopée française*. Paris, Adrapharm, 1996.
8. Farnsworth NR, ed. *NAPRALERT database*. Chicago, University of Illinois at Chicago, IL, March 15, 1995 production (an on-line database available directly through the University of Illinois at Chicago or through the Scientific and Technical Network (STN) of Chemical Abstracts Services).
9. Youngken HW. *Textbook of pharmacognosy*, 6th ed. Philadelphia, Blakiston, 1950.
10. *Medicinal plants of India, Vol. 1.* New Delhi, Indian Council of Medical Research, 1976.
11. Huang KC. *The pharmacology of Chinese herbs*. Boca Raton, FL, CRC Press, 1994.
12. Farnsworth NR, Bunyapraphatsara N, eds. *Thai medicinal plants*. Bangkok, Prachachon, 1992.
13. Bruneton J. *Pharmacognosy, phytochemistry, medicinal plants.* Paris, Lavoisier, 1995.
14. Tyler VE, Brady LR, Robbers JE, eds. *Pharmacognosy*, 9th ed. Philadelphia, Lea & Febiger, 1988.
15. *Quality control methods for medicinal plant materials*. Geneva, World Health Organization, 1998.
16. *Deutsches Arzneibuch 1996. Vol. 2. Methoden der Biologie.* Stuttgart, Deutscher Apotheker Verlag, 1996.
17. *European pharmacopoeia*, 3rd ed. Strasbourg, Council of Europe, 1997.
18. *Guidelines for predicting dietary intake of pesticide residues*, 2nd rev. ed. Geneva, World Health Organization, 1997 (unpublished document WHO/FSF/FOS/97.7; available from Food Safety, WHO, 1211 Geneva 27, Switzerland).
19. Duez P et al. Comparison between high-performance thin-layer chromatography-fluorometry and high-performance liquid chromatography for the determination of sennosides A and B in Senna (*Cassia* spp.) pods and leaves. *Journal of chromatography*, 1984, 303:391–395.

20. Bisset NG. *Max Wichtl's herbal drugs and phytopharmaceuticals*. Boca Raton, FL, CRC Press, 1994.
21. Core-SPC for Sennae Fructus Acutifoliae/Fructus Angustifoliae. *Coordinated review of monographs on herbal remedies*. Brussels, European Commission, 1994.
22. German Commission E Monograph, Senna fructus. *Bundesanzeiger*, 1993, 133:21 July.
23. Leng-Peschlow E. Dual effect of orally administered sennosides on large intestine transit and fluid absorption in the rat. *Journal of pharmacy and pharmacology*, 1986, 38:606–610.
24. Godding EW. Laxatives and the special role of Senna. *Pharmacology*, 1988, 36(Suppl. 1):230–236.
25. Bradley PR, ed. *British herbal compendium, Vol. 1*. Bournemouth, British Herbal Medicine Association, 1992.
26. Waller SL, Misiewicz JJ. Prognosis in the irritable-bowel syndrome. *Lancet*, 1969, ii:753–756.
27. Ewe K, Ueberschaer B, Press AG. Influence of senna, fibre, and fibre + senna on colonic transit in loperamide-induced constipation. *Pharmacology*, 47(Suppl. 1):242–248.
28. Stephen AM, Wiggins HS, Cummings JH. Effect of changing transit time on colonic microbial metabolism in man. *Gut*, 1987, 28:610.
29. *Goodman and Gilman's the pharmacological basis of therapeutics*, 9th ed. New York, McGraw-Hill, 1996.
30. *Physicians' desk reference*, 49th ed. Montvale, NJ, Medical Economics Company, 1995.
31. *American hospital formulary service*. Bethesda, MD, American Society of Hospital Pharmacists, 1990.
32. *United States pharmacopeia, drug information*. Rockville, MD, US Pharmacopeial Convention, 1992.
33. Reynolds JEF, ed. *Martindale, the extra pharmacopoeia*, 30th ed. London, Pharmaceutical Press, 1993.
34. Heidemann A, Miltenburger HG, Mengs U. The genotoxicity of Senna. *Pharmacology*, 1993, 47(Suppl. 1):178–186.
35. Tikkanen L et al. Mutagenicity of anthraquinones in the *Salmonella* preincubation test. *Mutation research*, 1983, 116:297–304.
36. Westendorf et al. Mutagenicity of naturally occurring hydroxyanthraquinones. *Mutation research*, 1990, 240:1–12.
37. Sanders D et al. Mutagenicity of crude Senna and Senna glycosides in *Salmonella typhimurium*. *Pharmacology and toxicology*, 1992, 71:165–172.
38. Lyden-Sokolowsky A, Nilsson A, Sjoberg P. Two-year carcinogenicity study with sennosides in the rat: emphasis on gastrointestinal alterations. *Pharmacology*, 1993, 47(Suppl. 1):209–215.
39. Kune GA. Laxative use not a risk for colorectal cancer: data from the Melbourne colorectal cancer study. *Zeitschrift für Gasteroenterologie*, 1993, 31:140–143.
40. Siegers CP. Anthranoid laxatives and colorectal cancer. *Trends in pharmacological sciences (TIPS)*, 1992, 13:229–231.
41. Lewis JH et al. The use of gastrointestinal drugs during pregnancy and lactation. *American journal of gastroenterology*, 1985, 80:912–923.
42. Beuers U, Spengler U, Pape GR. Hepatitis after chronic abuse of Senna. *Lancet*, 1991, 337:472.
43. Loew D. Pseudomelanosis coli durch Anthranoide. *Zeitschrift für Phytotherapie*, 1994, 16:312–318.
44. Müller-Lissner SA. Adverse effects of laxatives: facts and fiction. *Pharmacology*, 1993, 47(Suppl. 1):138–145.
45. Godding EW. Therapeutics of laxative agents with special reference to the anthraquinones. *Pharmacology*, 1976, 14(Suppl. 1):78–101.

46. Dufour P, Gendre P. Ultrastructure of mouse intestinal mucosa and changes observed after long term anthraquinone administration. *Gut*, 1984, 25:1358–1363.
47. Dufour P et al. Tolérance de la muqueuse intestinale de la souris à l'ingestion prolongée d'une poudre de sené. *Annales pharmaceutiques françaises*, 1983, 41(6):571–578.
48. Kienan JA, Heinicke EA. Sennosides do not kill myenteric neurons in the colon of the rat or mouse. *Neurosciences*, 1989, 30(3):837–842.
49. Riemann JF et al. Ultrastructural changes of colonic mucosa in patients with chronic laxative misuse. *Acta hepato-gastroenterology*, 1978, 25:213–218.
50. Smith BA. Effect of irritant purgatives on the myenteric plexus in man and the mouse. *Gut*, 1968, 9:139–143.
51. Riemann JF et al. The fine structure of colonic submucosal nerves in patients with chronic laxative abuse. *Scandinavian journal of gastroenterology*, 1980, 15:761–768.
52. Rieken EO et al. The effect of an anthraquinone laxative on colonic nerve tissue: A controlled trial in constipated women. *Zeitschrift für Gasteroenterologie*, 1990, 28:660–664.
53. Riemann JF, Schmidt H. Ultrastructural changes in the gut autonomic nervous system following laxative abuse and in other conditions. *Scandinavian journal of gastroenterology*, 1982, 71(Suppl.):111–124.
54. Krishnamurti S et al. Severe idiopathic constipation is associated with a distinctive abnormality of the colonic myenteric plexus. *Gastroenterology*, 1985, 88:26–34.

Herba Thymi

Definition

Herba Thymi is the dried leaves and flowering tops of *Thymus vulgaris* L. or of *Thymus zygis* L. (Lamiaceae) (*1, 2*).

Synonyms

Lamiaceae are also known as Labiatae.

Selected vernacular names

Common thyme, farigola, garden thyme, herba timi, herba thymi, mother of thyme, red thyme, rubbed thyme, ten, thick leaf thyme, thym, Thymian, thyme, time, timi, tomillo, za'ater (*1, 3–7*).

Description

An aromatic perennial sub-shrub, 20–30 cm in height, with ascending, quadrangular, greyish brown to purplish brown lignified and twisted stems bearing oblong-lanceolate to ovate-lanceolate greyish green leaves that are pubescent on the lower surface. The flowers have a pubescent calyx and a bilobate, pinkish or whitish, corolla and are borne in verticillasters. The fruit consists of 4 brown ovoid nutlets (*5, 8, 9*).

Plant material of interest: dried leaves and flowering tops
General appearance
Thymus vulgaris

Leaf 4–12 mm long and up to 3 mm wide; it is sessile or has a very short petiole. The lamina is tough, entire, lanceolate to ovate, covered on both surfaces by a grey to greenish grey indumentum; the edges are markedly rolled up towards the abaxial surface. The midrib is depressed on the adaxial surface and is very prominent on the abaxial surface. The calyx is green, often with violet spots, and is tubular; at the end are 2 lips of which the upper is bent back and has 3 lobes on its end; the lower is longer and has 2 hairy teeth. After flowering, the calyx tube is closed by a crown of long, stiff hairs. The corolla, about twice as long as the calyx, is usually brownish in the dry state and is slightly bilabiate (*1*).

Thymus zygis

Leaf 1.7–6.5 mm long and 0.4–1.2 mm wide; it is acicular to linear-lanceolate and the edges are markedly rolled toward the abaxial surface. Both surfaces of the lamina are green to greenish grey and the midrib is sometimes violet; the edges, in particular at the base, have long, white hairs. The dried flowers are very similar to those of *Thymus vulgaris* (*1*).

Organoleptic properties

Odour and taste aromatic (*1–3, 5*).

Microscopic characteristics

In leaf upper epidermis, cells tangentially elongated in transverse section with a thick cuticle and few stomata, somewhat polygonal in surface section with beaded vertical walls and striated cuticle, the stoma being at a right angle to the 2 parallel neighbouring cells. Numerous unicellular, non-glandular hairs up to 30 μm in length with papillose wall and apical cell, straight, or pointed, curved, or hooked. Numerous glandular hairs of two kinds, one with a short stalk embedded in the epidermal layer and a unicellular head, the other with an 8- to 12-celled head and no stalk. Palisade parenchyma of 2 layers of columnar cells containing many chloroplastids; occasionally an interrupted third layer is present. Spongy parenchyma of about 6 layers of irregular-shaped chlorenchyma cells and intercellular air-spaces (*5*).

Powdered plant material

Grey-green to greenish brown powder; leaf fragments, epidermal cells prolonged into unicellular pointed, papillose trichomes, 60 μm long; trichomes of the lower surface uniseriate, 2–3 celled, sharp pointed, up to 300 μm in diameter, numerous labiate trichomes with 8–12 secretory cells up to 80 μm in diameter; broadly elliptical caryophyllaceous stomata. Six- to 8-celled uniseriate trichomes from the calyx up to 400 μm long; pollen grains spherical; pericyclic fibres of the stem (*1–3*).

Geographical distribution

Indigenous to southern Europe. It is a pan-European species that is cultivated in Europe, the United States of America and other parts of the world (*2, 3, 5, 10*).

General identity tests

Macroscopic and microscopic examinations (*1, 5*), and chemical and thin-layer chromatography tests for the characteristic volatile oil constituent, thymol [**1**].

Purity tests
Microbiology
The test for *Salmonella* spp. in Herba Thymi products should be negative. The maximum acceptable limits of other microorganisms are as follows (*11–13*). For preparation of infusion: aerobic bacteria—not more than 10^7/g; fungi—not more than 10^5/g; *Escherichia coli*—not more than 10^2/g. Preparations for oral use: aerobic bacteria—not more than 10^5/ml; fungi—not more than 10^4/ml; enterobacteria and certain Gram-negative bacteria—not more than 10^3/ml; *Escherichia coli*—0/ml.

Foreign organic matter
Not more than 10% of stem having a diameter up to 1 mm. Leaves with long trichomes at their base and with weakly pubescent other parts not allowed (*1*). The leaves and flowering tops of *Origanum creticum* or *O. dictamnus* are considered adulterants (*3, 5*). Other foreign organic matter, not more than 2% (*2*).

Total ash
Not more than 15% (*1*).

Acid-insoluble ash
Not more than 2.0% (*1*).

Moisture
Not more than 10% (*1*).

Pesticide residues
To be established in accordance with national requirements. Normally, the maximum residue limit of aldrin and dieldrin in Herba Thymi is not more than 0.05 mg/kg (*13*). For other pesticides, see WHO guidelines on quality control methods for medicinal plants (*11*) and guidelines for predicting dietary intake of pesticide residues (*14*).

Heavy metals
Recommended lead and cadmium levels are not more than 10 and 0.3 mg/kg, respectively, in the final dosage form of the plant material (*11*).

Radioactive residues
For analysis of strontium-90, iodine-131, caesium-134, caesium-137, and plutonium-239, see WHO guidelines on quality control methods for medicinal plants (*11*).

Other purity tests
Chemical, alcohol-soluble extractive, and water-soluble extractive tests to be established in accordance with national requirements.

Chemical assays

Herba Thymi contains not less than 1.0% volatile oil (*2, 3*), and not less than 0.5% phenols. Volatile oil is quantitatively determined by water/steam distillation (*1*), and the percentage content of phenols expressed as thymol is determined by spectrophotometric analysis (*1*). Thin-layer chromatographic analysis is used for thymol, carvacrol, and linalool (*1, 15*).

Major chemical constituents

Herba Thymi contains about 2.5% but not less than 1.0% of volatile oil. The composition of the volatile oil fluctuates depending on the chemotype under consideration. The principal components of Herba Thymi are thymol [1] and carvacrol [2] (up to 64% of oil), along with linalool, *p*-cymol, cymene, thymene, α-pinene, apigenin, luteolin, and 6-hydroxyluteolin glycosides, as well as di-, tri- and tetramethoxylated flavones, all substituted in the 6-position (for example 5,4′-dihydroxy-6,7-dimethoxyflavone, 5,4′-dihydroxy-6,7,3′-trimethoxyflavone and its 8-methoxylated derivative 5,6,4′-trihydroxy-7,8,3′-trimethoxyflavone) (*1, 3–6, 9*).

Dosage forms

Dried herb for infusion, extract, and tincture (*1*).

Medicinal uses

Uses supported by clinical data

None.

Uses described in pharmacopoeias and in traditional systems of medicine

Thyme extract has been used orally to treat dyspepsia and other gastrointestinal disturbances; coughs due to colds, bronchitis and pertussis; and laryngitis and tonsillitis (as a gargle). Topical applications of thyme extract have been used in the treatment of minor wounds, the common cold, disorders of the oral cavity, and as an antibacterial agent in oral hygiene (*3, 5, 8, 15, 16*). Both the essential oil and thymol are ingredients of a number of proprietary drugs including antiseptic and healing ointments, syrups for the treatment of respiratory disorders, and preparations for inhalation. Another species in the genus, *T. serpyllum* L., is used for the same indications (*8*).

Uses described in folk medicine, not supported by experimental or clinical data

As an emmenagogue, sedative, antiseptic, antipyretic, to control menstruation and cramps, and in the treatment of dermatitis (7).

Pharmacology

Experimental pharmacology

Spasmolytic and antitussive activities

The spasmolytic and antitussive activity of thyme has been most often attributed to the phenolic constituents thymol and carvacrol, which make up a large percentage of the volatile oil (17). Although these compounds have been shown to prevent contractions induced in the ileum and the trachea of the guinea-pig, by histamine, acetylcholine and other reagents, the concentration of phenolics in aqueous preparations of the drug is insufficient to account for this activity (18, 19). Experimental evidence suggests that the *in vitro* spasmolytic activity of thyme preparations is due to the presence of polymethoxyflavones (10). *In vitro* studies have shown that flavones and thyme extracts inhibit responses to agonists of specific receptors such as acetylcholine, histamine and L-norepinephrine, as well as agents whose actions do not require specific receptors, such as barium chloride (10). The flavones of thyme were found to act as non-competitive and non-specific antagonists (10); they were also shown to be Ca^{2+} antagonists and musculotropic agents that act directly on smooth muscle (10).

Expectorant and secretomotor activities

Experimental evidence suggests that thyme oil has secretomotoric activity (20). This activity has been associated with a saponin extract from *T. vulgaris* (21). Stimulation of ciliary movements in the pharynx mucosa of frogs treated with diluted solutions of thyme oil, thymol or carvacrol has also been reported (22). Furthermore, an increase in mucus secretion of the bronchi after treatment with thyme extracts has been observed (23).

Antifungal and antibacterial activities

In vitro studies have shown that both thyme essential oil and thymol have antifungal activity against a number of fungi, including *Cryptococcus neoformans*, *Aspergillus*, *Saprolegnia*, and *Zygorhynchus* species (24–27). Both the essential oil and thymol had antibacterial activity against *Salmonella typhimurium*, *Staphylococcus aureus*, *Escherichia coli*, and a number of other bacterial species (28, 29). As an antibiotic, thymol is 25 times as effective as phenol, but less toxic (30).

Contraindications

Pregnancy and lactation (See Precautions, below).

Warnings

No information available.

Precautions

General

Patients with a known sensitivity to plants in the Lamiaceae (Labiatae) should contact their physician before using thyme preparations. Patients sensitive to birch pollen or celery may have a cross-sensitivity to thyme (*31*).

Carcinogenesis, mutagenesis, impairment of fertility

Thyme essential oil did not have any mutagenic activity in the *Bacillus subtilis* *rec*-assay or the *Salmonella*/microsome reversion assay (*32, 33*). Recent investigations suggest that thyme extracts are antimutagenic (*34*) and that luteolin, a constituent of thyme, is a strong antimutagen against the dietary carcinogen Trp-P-2 (*35*).

Pregnancy: non-teratogenic effects

The safety of Herba Thymi preparations during pregnancy or lactation has not been established. As a precautionary measure, the drug should not be used during pregnancy or lactation except on medical advice. However, widespread use of Herba Thymi has not resulted in any safety concerns.

Nursing mothers

See Pregnancy: non-teratogenic effects, above.

Other precautions

No information available concerning drug interactions, drug and laboratory test interactions, paediatric use, or teratogenic effects on pregnancy.

Adverse reactions

Contact dermatitis has been reported. Patients sensitive to birch pollen or celery may have a cross-sensitivity to thyme (*31*).

Posology

Adults and children from 1 year: 1–2 g of the dried herb or the equivalent amount of fresh herb as an oral infusion several times a day (*30, 36*); children up to 1 year: 0.5–1 g (*36*). Fluid extract: dosage calculated according to the dosage of the herb (*37*). Tincture (1 : 10, 70% ethanol): 40 drops up to 3 times daily (*38*). Topical use: a 5% infusion as a gargle or mouth-wash (*30, 38*).

References

1. *European pharmacopoeia*, 2nd ed. Strasbourg, Council of Europe, 1995.
2. *Materia medika Indonesia*, Jilid. Jakarta, IV Departemen Kesehatan, Republik Indonesia, 1980.
3. *British herbal phamacopoeia*, Part 2. London, British Herbal Medicine Association, 1979.
4. *Deutsches Arzneibuch 1996*. Stuttgart, Deutscher Apotheker Verlag, 1996.
5. Youngken HW. *Textbook of pharmacognosy*, 6th ed. Philadelphia, Blakiston, 1950.
6. Ghazanfar SA. *Handbook of Arabian medicinal plants*. Boca Raton, FL, CRC Press, 1994:128.
7. Farnsworth NR, ed. *NAPRALERT database*. Chicago, University of Illinois at Chicago, IL, March 15, 1995 production (an on-line database available directly through the University of Illinois at Chicago or through the Scientific and Technical Network (STN) of Chemical Abstracts Services).
8. Bruneton J. *Pharmacognosy, phytochemistry, medicinal plants*. Paris, Lavoisier, 1995.
9. Mossa JS, Al-Yahya MA, Al-Meshal IA. *Medicinal plants of Saudi Arabia, Vol. 1*. Riyadh, Saudi Arabia, King Saud University Libraries, 1987.
10. Van den Broucke CO, Lemli JA. Spasmolytic activity of the flavonoids from *Thymus vulgaris*. *Pharmaceutisch Weekblad, scientific edition*, 1983, 5:9–14.
11. *Quality control methods for medicinal plant materials*. Geneva, World Health Organization, 1998.
12. *Deutsches Arzneibuch 1996. Vol. 2. Methoden der Biologie*. Stuttgart, Deutscher Apotheker Verlag, 1996.
13. *European pharmacopoeia*, 3rd ed. Strasbourg, Council of Europe, 1997.
14. *Guidelines for predicting dietary intake of pesticide residues*, 2nd rev. ed. Geneva, World Health Organization, 1997 (unpublished document WHO/FSF/FOS/97.7; available from Food Safety, WHO, 1211 Geneva 27, Switzerland).
15. Twetman S, Hallgren A, Petersson LG. Effect of antibacterial varnish on mutans *Streptococci* in plaque from enamel adjacent to orthodontic appliances. *Caries research*, 1995, 29:188–191.
16. Petersson LG, Edwardsson S, Arends J. Antimicrobial effect of a dental varnish, *in vitro*. *Swedish dental journal*, 1992, 16:183–189.
17. Reiter M, Brandt W. Relaxant effects on tracheal and ileal smooth muscles of the guinea pig. *Arzneimittel-Forschung*, 1985, 35:408–414.
18. Van Den Broucke CO. Chemical and pharmacological investigation on Thymi herba and its liquid extracts. *Planta medica*, 1980, 39:253–254.
19. Van Den Broucke CO, Lemli JA. Pharmacological and chemical investigation of thyme liquid extracts. *Planta medica*, 1981, 41:129–135.
20. Gordonoff T, Merz H. Über den Nachweis der Wirkung der Expektorantien. *Klinische Wochenschrift*, 1931, 10:928–932.
21. Vollmer H. Untersuchungen über Expektorantien und den Mechanismus ihrer Wirkung. *Klinische Wochenschrift*, 1932, 11:590–595.
22. Freytag A. Über den Einfluß von Thymianöl, Thymol und Carvacrol auf die Flimmerbewegung. *Pflügers Archiv, European journal of physiology*, 1933, 232:346–350.
23. Schilf F. Einfluss von Azetylcholin, Adrenalin, Histamin und Thymianextrakt auf die Bronchialschleimhautsekretion; zugleich ein Beitrag zur Messung der Bronchialschleimhautsekretion. *Naunyn-Schmiedebergs Archiv für Pharmakologie,* 1932, 166:22–25.
24. Vollon C, Chaumont JP. Antifungal properties of essential oils and their main components upon *Cryptococcus neoformans*. *Mycopathology*, 1994, 128:151–153.

25. Perrucci S et al. *In vitro* antimycotic activity of some natural products against *Saprolegnia ferax*. *Phytotherapy research*, 1995, 9:147–149.
26. Pasteur N et al. Antifungal activity of oregano and thyme essential oils applied as fumigants against fungi attacking stored grain. *Journal of food protection*, 1995, 58:81–85.
27. Tantaouielaraki A, Errifi A. Antifungal activity of essential oils when associated with sodium chloride or fatty acids. *Grasas-y-aceites*, 1994, 45:363–369.
28. Janssen AM, Scheffer JJC, Baerheim-Svendsen A. Antimicrobial activity of essential oils: A 1976–1986 literature review. Aspects of the test methods. *Planta medica*, 1987, 53:395–398.
29. Juven BJ, Kanner J, Schved F, Weisslowicz H. Factors that interact with the antibacterial action of thyme essential oil and its active constituents. *Journal of applied bacteriology*, 1994, 76:626–631.
30. Czygan C-F. Thymian, Thymi Herba. In: Wichtl M. ed. *Teedrogen*, 2nd ed. Stuttgart, Wissenschaftliche Verlagsgesellschaft, 1989:498–500.
31. Wüthrich B, Stäger P, Johannson SGO. Rast-specific IGE against spices in patients sensitized against birch pollen, mugwort pollen and celery. *Allergologie*, 1992, 15:380–383.
32. Zani F et al. Studies on the genotoxic properties of essential oils with *Bacillus subtilis* rec-assay and *Salmonella*/microsome reversion assay. *Planta medica*, 1991, 57:237–241.
33. Azizan A, Blevins RD. Mutagenicity and antimutagenicity testing of six chemicals associated with the pungent properties of specific spices as revealed by the Ames *Salmonella* microsomal assay. *Archives of environmental contamination and toxicology*, 1995, 28:248–258.
34. Natake M et al. Herb water-extracts markedly suppress the mutagenicity of Trp-P-2. *Agricultural and biological chemistry*, 1989, 53:1423–1425.
35. Samejima K et al. Luteolin, a strong antimutagen against dietary carcinogen, Trp-P-2, in peppermint, sage, and thyme. *Journal of agricultural and food chemistry*, 1995, 43:410–414.
36. Dorsch W et al. In: *Empfehlungen zu Kinderdosierungen von monographierten Arzneidrogen und ihren Zubereitungen*. Bonn, Kooperation Phytopharmaka, 1993:100–101.
37. Hochsinger K. Die Therapie des Krampf- und Reizhustens. *Wiener Medizinische Wochenschrift*, 1931, 13:447–448.
38. Van Hellemont J. *Fytotherapeutisch compendium*, 2nd ed. Bonn, Scheltema & Holkema, 1988:599–605.

Radix Valerianae

Definition

Radix Valerianae consists of the subterranean parts of *Valeriana officinalis* L. *(sensu lato)* (Valerianaceae)[1] including the rhizomes, roots, and stolons, carefully dried at a temperature below 40 °C (*1–6*).

Synonyms

Valeriana alternifolia Ledeb., *Valeriana excelsa* Poir., *Valeriana sylvestris* Grosch. (*1*).

Selected vernacular names

All heal, akar pulepandak, amantilla, balderbrackenwurzel, baldrian, Baldrianwurzel, cat's love, cat's valerian, fragrant valerian, garden heliotrope, great wild valerian, ka-no-ko-so, Katzenwurzel, kesso root, kissokon, kuanyexiccao, luj, nard, ntiv, racine de valeriane, St. George's herb, setwall, txham laaj, valerian fragrant, valerian, valeriana, valeriana extranjera, valeriana rhizome, valeriane, vandal root, waliryana, wild valerian (*8–11*).

Descriptions

A tall perennial herb whose underground portion consists of a vertical rhizome bearing numerous rootlets and one or more stolons. The aerial portion consists of a cylindrical hollow, channelled stem attaining 2 m in height, branched in the terminal region, bearing opposite exstipulate, pinnatisect, cauline leaves with clasping petioles. The inflorescence consists of racemes of cymes whose flowers are small, white, or pink. The fruits are oblong-ovate, 4-ridged, single-seeded achenes (*1, 9*).

Valeriana officinalis (*sensu lato*) is an extremely polymorphous complex of subspecies. The basic type is diploid, $2n = 14$, (*V. officinalis*) and other subspecies have very similar characteristics: *V. officinalis* ssp. *collina* (Wallr.) Nyman

---

[1] Approximately 200 *Valeriana* species are available, but only a few are or were used medicinally, such as *V. fauriei* Briquet (Japanese Valerian) (*7*), *V. wallichii* DC (Indian Valerian) and *V. edulis* Nutt ex. Torr. & Gray (*8*). In commerce, *V. edulis* Nutt. ex Torr. & Gray is known as "Valeriana mexicana". Plants bearing this common name should not be confused with *V. mexicana* DC., which is in fact *V. sorbifolia* H.B.K. var. *mexicana* (DC) F.G. Mey.

(2*n* = 28) has leaves with 15–27 folioles, all of the same width, and *V. officinalis* ssp. *sambucifolia* (Mikan f.) Celak, *V. excelsa* Poiret (2*n* = 56) has leaves with 5–9 folioles, with the apical one clearly larger than the others. In contrast to the other subspecies, the rhizome of the latter is clearly stoloniferous (epigenous and hypnogenous stolons). *V. repens* Host. (equivalent to *V. procurrens* Wallr.) could be considered a fourth species, according to the Flora Europaea. Often appended to this species are taxonomic groups of uncertain status and limited distribution (e.g. *V. salina* Pleigel or *V. versifolia* Brügger) (*12*).

Plant material of interest: dried roots, rhizomes and stolons

General appearance

Rhizome, erect, entire or usually cut into 2–4 longitudinal pieces, 2–5 cm long, 1–3 cm thick; externally, dull yellowish brown or dark brown, sometimes crowned by the remains of stem bases and scale leaves, and bears occasional, short, horizontal branches (stolons), and numerous rootlets or their circular scars; fracture, short and horny. Internally, whitish, with an irregular outline, occasionally hollow and exhibiting a comparatively narrow ark traversed, here and there, by root-traces, and separated by a dark line, the cambium, from a ring, small xylem bundles surrounding a central pith. Roots, numerous, slender, cylindrical, usually plump; 2–12 cm but mostly 8–10 cm long, 0.5–2 mm in diameter; externally, greyish brown to brownish yellow, longitudinally striated, with fibrous lateral rootlets; brittle; internally, showing a wide bark and a narrow central stele (*1*, *9*).

Organoleptic properties

Odour, characteristic, penetrating valeric acid-like, becoming stronger on aging; taste, sweetish initially, becoming camphoraceous and somewhat bitter (*1–5*, *9*).

Microscopic characteristics

Rhizome, with epidermis of polygonal cells, having the outer walls slightly thickened; cork, immediately below the epidermis, of up to 7 layers of slightly suberized, brownish, large polygonal cells; cortex, parenchymatous with rather thick-walled parenchyma, containing numerous starch granules and traversed by numerous root-traces; endodermis of a single layer of tangentially elongated cells containing globules of volatile oil; pericycle, parenchymatous; vascular bundles, collateral, in a ring and surrounding a very large parenchymatous pith, containing starch granules and occasional scattered groups of sclereids with thick pitted walls and narrow lumen; xylem, with slender, annular, spiral, and pitted vessels, in small numbers. Branches similar to rhizome but with a prominent endodermis and a well-defined ring of vascular bundles, showing secondary thickening.

Root, with piliferous layer, of papillosed cells, some developed into root hairs; exodermis, or a single layer of quadrangular to polygonal cells, with suberized walls, and containing globules of volatile oil; cortex, parenchymatous, with numerous starch granules, the outermost cells containing globules of volatile oil; endodermis, of 1 layer of cells with thickened radial walls; primary xylem, of 3–11 arches surrounding a small central parenchymatous pith containing starch granules, 5–15 µm in diameter, sometimes showing a cleft or stellate hilum; the compound granules, with 2–6 components, up to 20 µm in diameter. Older roots show a pith of starch-bearing parenchyma, vascular bundles with secondary thickening and a periderm originating in the piliferous layer (*1, 4, 9, 13*).

Powdered plant material

Light brown and characterized by numerous fragments of parenchyma with round or elongated cells and containing starch granules, 5–15 µm in diameter, sometimes showing a cleft or stellate hilum, the compound granules, with 2–6 components, up to 20 µm in diameter; cells containing light brown resin; rectangular sclereids with pitted walls, 5–15 µm thick; xylem, isolated or in noncompact bundles, 10–50 µm in diameter; some absorbing root hairs and cork fragments are also present (*4*).

Geographical distribution

Valeriana officinalis (*sensu lato*) is an extremely polymorphous complex of subspecies with natural populations dispersed throughout temperate and sub-polar Eurasian zones. The species is common in damp woods, ditches, and along streams in Europe, and is cultivated as a medicinal plant, especially in Belgium, England, eastern Europe, France, Germany, the Netherlands, the Russian Federation, and the United States of America (*1, 9, 10, 12*).

General identity tests

Macroscopic, microscopic, organoleptic, and microchemical examination (*1–6, 9, 13*); and by thin-layer chromatography for the presence of valerenic acid, acetoxyvalerenic acid, valtrate, and isovaltrate (*1–5*).

Purity tests
Microbiology

The test for *Salmonella* spp. in Radix Valerianae products should be negative. The maximum acceptable limits of other microorganisms are as follows (*14–16*). For preparation of decoction: aerobic bacteria—not more than 10^7/g; fungi—not more than 10^5/g; *Escherichia coli*—not more than 10^2/g. Preparations for internal use: aerobic bacteria—not more than 10^5/g or ml; fungi—not more than 10^4/g or ml; enterobacteria and certain Gram-negative bacteria—not more than 10^3/g or ml; *Escherichia coli*—0/g or ml.

Foreign organic matter
Not more than 5% (*1*).

Acid-insoluble ash
Not more than 7% (*1–5*).

Dilute ethanol-soluble extractive
Not less than 15% (*2–5*).

Pesticide residues
To be established in accordance with national requirements. Normally, the maximum residue limit of aldrin and dieldrin for Radix Valerianae is not more than 0.05 mg/kg (*16*). For other pesticides, see WHO guidelines on quality control methods for medicinal plants (*14*) and guidelines for predicting dietary intake of pesticide residues (*17*).

Heavy metals
Recommended lead and cadmium levels are no more than 10 and 0.3 mg/kg, respectively, in the final dosage form of the plant material (*14*).

Radioactive residues
For analysis of strontium-90, iodine-131, caesium-134, caesium-137, and plutonium-239, see WHO guidelines on quality control methods for medicinal plants (*14*).

Other purity tests
Chemical, moisture, total ash and water-soluble extractive tests are to be established in accordance with national standards.

Chemical assays
Contains not less than 0.5% v/w of essential oil (*3–5*), quantitatively determined by distillation (*2–5*). Content of individual constituents including valepotriates, valerenic acids and valerenal, determined by high-performance liquid (*18, 19*) or gas–liquid (*20*) chromatographic methods.

Major chemical constituents
The chemical composition of Radix Valerianae varies greatly depending on the subspecies, variety, age of the plant, growing conditions, and type and age of the extract. The volatile oil (ranges 0.2–2.8%) contains bornyl acetate and

bornyl isovalerate as the principal components. Other significant constituents include β-caryophyllene, valeranone, valerenal, valerenic acid, and other sesquiterpenoids and monoterpenes (*12*, *21*). The co-occurrence of three cyclopentane-sesquiterpenoids (valerenic acid, acetoxyvalerenic acid, and valerenal) is confined to *V. officinalis* and permits its distinction from *V. edulis* and *V. wallichii* (*12*). The various subspecies of *V. officinalis* have different compositions of volatile oil and, for example, average bornyl acetate content varies from 35% in *V. officinalis* ssp. *pratensis* to 0.45% in *V. officinalis* ssp. *illyrica* (*12*).

A second important group of constituents (0.05–0.67% range) is a series of non-glycosidic bicyclic iridoid monoterpene epoxy-esters known as the valepotriates. The major valepotriates are valtrate and isovaltrate (which usually represent more than 90% of the valepotriate content). Smaller amounts of dihydrovaltrate, isovaleroxy-hydroxydihydrovaltrate, 1-acevaltrate or others are present (*8*, *12*). The valepotriates are rather unstable owing to their epoxide structure, and losses occur fairly rapidly on storage or processing, especially if the drug is not carefully dried. Principal degradation products are baldrinal, homobaldrinal, and valtroxal (*8*).

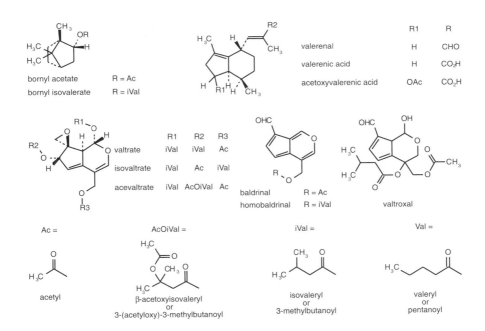

Dosage forms

Internal use as the expressed juice, tincture, extracts, and other galenical preparations (*8*, *22*). External use as a bath additive (*22*). Store in tightly closed containers, in a cool dry place, protected from light (*1–6*).

Medicinal uses

Uses supported by clinical data

As a mild sedative and sleep-promoting agent (*8, 12, 22–25*). The drug is often used as a milder alternative or a possible substitute for stronger synthetic sedatives, such as the benzodiazepines, in the treatment of states of nervous excitation and anxiety-induced sleep disturbances (*22–25*).

Uses described in pharmacopoeias and in traditional systems of medicine

As a digestive aid, and an adjuvant in spasmolytic states of smooth muscle and gastrointestinal pains of nervous origin (*8, 12*). When associated with papaverine, belladonna, and other spasmolytics, Radix Valerianae has been shown to be useful as an adjuvant in spastic states of smooth muscle such as spastic colitis (*8*).

Uses described in folk medicine, not supported by experimental or clinical data

To treat epilepsy, gum sores, headaches, nausea, sluggish liver, urinary tract disorders, vaginal yeast infections, and throat inflammations; and as an emmenagogue, antiperspirant, antidote to poisons, diuretic, anodyne, and a decoction for colds (*5, 8*).

Pharmacology

Experimental pharmacology

The sedative activity of *V. officinalis* has been demonstrated both *in vitro* and *in vivo*. *In vitro* studies have demonstrated the binding of valerian extracts to GABA (γ-aminobutyric acid) receptors, adenosine receptors and the barbiturate and benzodiazepine receptors (*8, 26*). Both hydroalcoholic and aqueous total extracts show affinity for the GABA-A receptors, but there is no clear correlation between any of the known chemical components isolated from Radix Valerianae and GABA-A binding activity (*8*). Aqueous extracts of the roots of *V. officinalis* inhibit re-uptake and stimulate the release of radiolabelled GABA in the synaptosomes isolated from rat brain cortex (*27, 28*). This activity may increase the extracellular concentration of GABA in the synaptic cleft, and thereby enhance the biochemical and behavioural effects of GABA (*8, 27*). Interestingly, GABA has been found in extracts of *V. officinalis* and appears to be responsible for this activity (*29*). The valtrates, and in particular dihydrovaltrate, also show some affinity for both the barbiturate receptors and the peripheral benzodiazepine receptors (*8*).

In vivo studies suggest that the sedative properties of the drug may be due to high concentrations of glutamine in the extracts (*29*). Glutamine is able to cross the blood–brain barrier, where it is taken up by nerve terminals and subsequently metabolized to GABA (29). The addition of exogenous glutamine stimulates GABA synthesis in synaptosomes and rat brain slices (29).

The spasmolytic activity of the valepotriates is principally due to valtrate or dihydrovaltrate (30). These agents act on centres of the central nervous system and through direct relaxation of smooth muscle (31), apparently by modulating Ca^{2+} entry into the cells or by binding to smooth muscle (8, 32).

Clinical pharmacology

A number of clinical investigations have demonstrated the effectiveness of Radix Valerianae as a sleep aid and minor sedative (8, 22–25). In a double-blind study, valerian (450 mg or 900 mg of an aqueous root extract) significantly decreased sleep latency as compared with a placebo (23). The higher dose of valerian did not further decrease sleep latency (23). Additional clinical studies have demonstrated that an aqueous extract of valerian root significantly increased sleep quality, in poor and irregular sleepers, but it had no effect on night awakenings or dream recall (24). The use of Radix Valerianae appears to increase slow-wave sleep in patients with low baseline values, without altering rapid eye movement (REM) sleep (24).

While extracts of the drug have been clearly shown to depress central nervous system activity, the identity of the active constituents still remains controversial. Neither the valepotriates, nor the sesquiterpenes valerenic acid and valeranone, nor the volatile oil alone can account for the overall sedative activity of the plant (8, 33). It has been suggested that the baldrinals, degradation products of the valepotriates, may be responsible (26). Currently, it is still not known whether the activity of Radix Valerianae extracts resides in one compound, a group of compounds, or some unknown compound, or is due to a synergistic effect.

Contraindications

Radix Valerianae should not be used during pregnancy or lactation (31, 34).

Warnings

No information available.

Precautions

General

May cause drowsiness. Those affected should not drive or operate machinery. Although no interaction between valerian and alcohol has been demonstrated clinically, as a precautionary measure patients should avoid consuming alcoholic beverages or other sedatives in conjunction with Radix Valerianae (31).

Carcinogenesis, mutagenesis, impairment of fertility

Some concern has been expressed over the cytotoxicity of the valepotriates. Cytotoxicity has been demonstrated *in vitro* but not *in vivo*, even in doses of 1350 mg/kg (*35*). Some of the valepotriates demonstrate alkylating activity *in vitro*. However, because the compounds decompose rapidly in the stored drug, there is no cause for concern (*35*). The valepotriates are also poorly absorbed and are rapidly metabolized to the baldrinals (*26*), which have better sedating effects. *In vitro*, the baldrinals are less toxic than the valepotriates, but *in vivo* they are more cytotoxic because they are more readily absorbed by the intestine. Baldrinals have been detected at levels up to 0.988 mg/dose in commercial preparations standardized with respect to the concentration of valepotriates and may be of cytotoxic concern (*36*).

Pregnancy: teratogenic effects

Prolonged oral administration of valepotriates did not produce any teratogenic effects (*8, 37*).

Pregnancy: non-teratogenic effects

The safety of Radix Valerianae during pregnancy has not been established; therefore it should not be administered during pregnancy.

Nursing mothers

Excretion of Radix Valerianae into breast milk and its effects on the newborn infant have not been established; therefore it should not be administered during lactation.

Paediatric use

Radix Valerianae preparations should not be used for children less than 12 years of age without medical supervision (*34*).

Other precautions

No information on general precautions or drug interactions or drug and laboratory test interactions was found.

Adverse reactions

Minor side-effects have been associated with chronic use of Radix Valerianae and include headaches, excitability, uneasiness, and insomnia. Very large doses may cause bradycardia and arrhythmias, and decrease intestinal motility (*38*). The recommended first aid is gastric lavage, charcoal powder, and sodium sulfate (*38*). Doses up to 20 times the recommended therapeutic dose have been reported to cause only mild symptoms which resolved within 24h (*38*). Four cases of liver damage have been associated with use of preparations containing

Radix Valerianae (*39*). However, in all cases the patients were taking a combination herbal product containing four different plant species and thus a causal relationship to the intake of valerian is extremely doubtful.

Posology

Dried root and rhizome, 2–3 g drug per cup by oral infusion, 1–5 times per day, up to a total of 10 g and preparations correspondingly (*6, 22*). Tincture (1:5, 70% ethanol), 0.5–1 teaspoon (1–3 ml), once to several times a day. External use, 100 g drug for a full bath (*22*).

References

1. *African pharmacopoeia*, 1st ed. Lagos, Organization of African Unity, Scientific, Technical & Research Commission, 1985.
2. *British pharmacopoeia*. London, Her Majesty's Stationery Office, 1988.
3. *Deutsches Arzneibuch 1996*. Stuttgart, Deutscher Apotheker Verlag, 1996.
4. *European pharmacopoeia*, 2nd ed. Strasbourg, Council of Europe, 1995.
5. *Pharmacopée française*. Paris, Adrapharm, 1996.
6. *Pharmacopoea hungarica VII*. Budapest, Medicina konyvkiado, 1986.
7. *The Japanese pharmacopoeia XIII*. Tokyo, Ministry of Health and Welfare, 1996.
8. Morazzoni P, Bombardelli E. *Valeriana officinalis*: traditional use and recent evaluation of activity. *Fitoterapia*, 1995, 66:99–112.
9. Youngken HW. *Textbook of pharmacognosy*, 6th ed. Philadelphia, Blakiston, 1950.
10. Bisset NG. *Max Wichtl's herbal drugs & phytopharmaceuticals*. Boca Raton, FL, CRC Press, 1994.
11. Farnsworth, NR. ed. *NAPRALERT database*. Chicago, University of Illinois at Chicago, IL, March 15, 1995 production (an on-line database available directly through the University of Illinois at Chicago or through the Scientific and Technical Network (STN) of Chemical Abstracts Services).
12. Bruneton J. *Pharmacology, phytochemistry, medicinal plants*. Paris, Lavoisier, 1995.
13. Jackson BP, Snowden DW. *Atlas of microscopy of medicinal plants, culinary herbs and spices*. Boca Raton, FL, CRC Press, 1990.
14. *Quality control methods for medicinal plant materials*. Geneva, World Health Organization, 1998.
15. *Deutsches Arzneibuch 1996. Vol. 2. Methoden der Biologie*. Stuttgart, Deutscher Apotheker Verlag, 1996.
16. *European pharmacopoeia*, 3rd ed. Strasbourg, Council of Europe, 1997.
17. *Guidelines for predicting dietary intake of pesticide residues*, 2nd rev. ed. Geneva, World Health Organization, 1997 (unpublished document WHO/FSF/FOS/97.7; available from Food Safety, WHO, 1211 Geneva 27, Switzerland).
18. Feytag WE. Bestimmung von Valerensäuren und Valerenal neben Valepotriaten in *Valeriana officinalis* durch HPLC. *Pharmazeutische Zeitung*, 1983, 128:2869–2871.
19. van Meer JH, Labadie RP. Straight-phase and reverse phase high-performance liquid chromatographic separations of valepotriate isomers and homologues. *Journal of chromatography*, 1981, 205:206–212.
20. Graf E, Bornkessel B. Analytische und pharmazeutisch-technologische Versuche mit Baldrian. *Deutsche Apotheker Zeitung*, 1978, 118:503–505.
21. Hänsel R, Schultz J. Valerensäuren und Valerenal als Leitstoffe des offizinellen Baldrians. Bestimmung mittels HPLC-Technik. *Deutsche Apotheker Zeitung*, 1982, 122:333–340.

22. Leathwood PD, Chauffard F. Quantifying the effects of mild sedatives. *Journal of psychological research*, 1982/1983, 17:115.
23. Leathwood PD, Chauffard F. Aqueous extract of valerian reduces latency to fall asleep in man. *Planta medica*, 1985, 2:144–148.
24. Schultz H, Stolz C, Muller J. The effect of valerian extract on sleep polygraphy in poor sleepers: a pilot study. *Pharmacopsychiatry*, 1994, 27:147–151.
25. Balderer G, Borbely A. Effect of valerian on human sleep. *Psychopharmacology*, 1985, 87:406–409.
26. Wagner H, Jurcic K, Schaette R. Comparative studies on the sedative action of *Valeriana* extracts, valepotriates and their degradation products. *Planta medica*, 1980, 37:358–362.
27. Santos MS et al. Synaptosomal GABA release as influenced by valerian root extract, involvement of the GABA carrier. *Archives of international pharmacodynamics*, 1994, 327:220–231.
28. Santos MS et al. An aqueous extract of valerian influences the transport of GABA in synaptosomes. *Planta medica*, 1994, 60:278–279.
29. Santos MS et al. The amount of GABA present in the aqueous extracts of valerian is sufficient to account for ^{3}H-GABA release in synaptosomes. *Planta medica*, 1994, 60:475–476.
30. Wagner H, Jurcic K. On the spasmolytic activity of *Valeriana* extracts. *Planta medica*, 1979, 37:84–89.
31. Houghton P. Herbal products: valerian. *Pharmacy journal*, 1994, 253:95–96.
32. Hazelhoff B, Malingre TM, Meijer DKF. Antispasmodic effects of *Valeriana* compounds: An *in vivo* and *in vitro* study on the guinea pig ileum. *Archives of international pharmacodynamics*, 1982, 257:274–278.
33. Krieglstein J, Grusla D. Zentraldämpfende Inhaltsstoffe im Baldrian. Valepotriate, Valerensäure, Valeranon und ätherisches Öl sind jedoch unwirksam. *Deutsche Apotheker Zeitung*, 1988, 128:2041–2046.
34. German Commission E Monograph, Valerianae radix. *Bundesanzeiger*, 1985, 90:15 May.
35. Tortarolo M et al. *In vitro* effects of epoxide-bearing valepotriates on mouse early hematopoietic progenitor cells and human T-lymphocytes. *Archives of toxicology*, 1982, 51:37–42.
36. Braun R. Valepotriates with an epoxide structure-oxygenating alkylating agents. *Planta medica*, 1982, 41:21–28.
37. Tufik S. Effects of a prolonged administration of valepotriates in rats on the mothers and their offspring. *Journal of ethnopharmacology*, 1985, 87:39–44.
38. Willey LB et al. Valerian overdose: a case report. *Veterinary and human toxicology*, 1995, 37:364–365.
39. MacGregor FB. Hepatotoxicity of herbal remedies. *British medical journal*, 1989, 299:1156–1157.

Rhizoma Zingiberis

Definition

Rhizoma Zingiberis is the dried rhizome of *Zingiber officinale* Roscoe (*Zingiberaceae*) (1–5).

Synonyms

Amomum zingiber L. (*1, 6*), *Zingiber blancoi* Massk. (*6*).

Selected vernacular names

Ada, adrak, adu, African ginger, ajenjibre, ale, alea, allam, allamu, ardak, ardraka, ardrakam, ardrakamu, asunglasemtong, ata-le jinja, baojiang, beuing, chiang, citaraho, cochin ginger, common ginger, djae, gember, gengibre, gingembre, ginger, ginger root, gnji, gung, halia bara, halia, halija, hli, inchi, Ingberwurgel, inguere, inguru, Ingwer, jahe, Jamaica ginger, janzabeil, kallamu, kan chiang, kanga, kerati, khenseing, khiang, khing, khing-daeng, khing klaeng, khing phueak, khuong, kintoki, jion, konga, lahja, lei, luya, mangawizi, ngesnges, niamaku, oshoga, palana, palu, rimpang jahe, sa-e, sakanjabir, sge u-gser, shengiang, shenjing, shoga, shonkyoh, shokyo, shouhkyoh, tangawizi, wai, zanjabeel, zangabil ee-e-tar, zingibil urratab, zingibil, zingiberis rhizoma, zinjabil, zingiber, zinam (*1, 4, 6–13*).

Description

A perennial herb with a subterranean, digitately branched rhizome producing stems up to 1.50 m in height with linear lanceolate sheathing leaves (5–30 cm long and 8–20 mm wide) that are alternate, smooth and pale green. Flower stems shorter than leaf stems and bearing a few flowers, each surrounded by a thin bract and situated in axils of large, greenish yellow obtuse bracts, which are closely arranged at end of flower stem forming collectively an ovate-oblong spike. Each flower shows a superior tubular calyx, split part way down one side; an orange yellow corolla composed of a tube divided above into 3 linear-oblong, blunt lobes; 6 staminodes in 2 rows, the outer row of 3 inserted at mouth of corolla; the posterior 2, small, horn-like; the anterior petaloid, purple and spotted and divided into 3 rounded lobes; an inferior, 3-celled ovary with tufted stigma. Fruit a capsule with small arillate seeds (*1, 7, 8*).

Plant material of interest: dried rhizome

General appearance

Ginger occurs in horizontal, laterally flattened, irregularly branching pieces; 3–16 cm long, 3–4 cm wide, up to 2 cm thick; sometimes split longitudinally; pale yellowish buff or light brown externally, longitudinally striated, somewhat fibrous; branches known as "fingers" arise obliquely from the rhizomes, are flattish, obovate, short, about 1–3 cm long; fracture, short and starchy with projecting fibres. Internally, yellowish brown, showing a yellow endodermis separating the narrow cortex from the wide stele, and numerous scattered fibrovascular bundles, abundant scattered oleoresin cells with yellow contents and numerous larger greyish points, vascular bundles, scattered on the whole surface (*1–5*).

Organoleptic properties

Odour, characteristic aromatic; taste, pungent and aromatic (*1–5*); colour, internally pale yellow to brown (*1, 4*).

Microscopic characteristics

Cortex of isodiametric, thin-walled parenchyma cells contains abundant starch granules, each with a pointed hilum up to 50 μm long and 25 μm wide and 7 μm thick, and showing scattered secretion cells with suberized walls and yellowish brown oleoresinous content, and scattered bundles of the leaf-traces accompanied by fibres; endodermis, of pale brown, thin-walled cells with suberized radial walls; stele, with parenchymatous ground tissue, numerous yellow oleoresin secretion cells and numerous scattered, closed collateral vascular bundles with nonlignified, reticulate, scalariform, and spiral vessels, often accompanied by narrow cells; containing a dark brown pigment, and supported by thin-walled fibres with wide lumen, small oblique slit-like pits, and lignified middle lamella; some of the fibres are septate (*1, 3, 4*).

Powdered plant material

Powdered ginger is yellowish white to yellowish brown; characterized by numerous fragments of thin-walled parenchyma cells containing starch granules; fragments of thin-walled septate fibres with oblique slit-like pits; fragments of nonlignified scalariform, reticulate, and spiral vessels, often accompanied by dark pigment cells; oleoresin in fragments or droplets with oil cells and resin cells scattered in parenchyma; numerous starch granules, simple, flat, oval, oblong with terminal protuberance, in which the hilum is pointed, 5–60 μm usually 15–30 μm long, 5–40 μm (usually 18–25 μm) wide, 6–12 μm (usually 8–10 μm) thick with somewhat marked fine transverse striations (*1–4*).

Geographical distribution

The plant is probably native to south-east Asia and is cultivated in the tropical regions in both the eastern and western hemispheres. It is commercially grown in Africa, China, India, and Jamaica; India is the world's largest producer (*1, 4, 6, 7, 10, 14*).

General identity tests

Rhizoma Zingiberis is identified by its macroscopic and organoleptic character-istics, including its characteristic form, colour, pungent taste, and volatile oil content; and by microchemical tests (*1–5*).

Purity tests
Microbiology

The test for *Salmonella* spp. in Rhizoma Zingiberis products should be negative. The maximum acceptable limits of other microorganisms are as follows (*15–17*). For preparation of decoction: aerobic bacteria—not more than 10^7/g; fungi—not more than 10^5/g; *Escherichia coli*—not more than 10^2/g. Preparations for internal use: aerobic bacteria—not more than 10^5/g or ml; fungi—not more than 10^4/g or ml; enterobacteria and certain Gram-negative bacteria—not more than 10^3/g or ml; *Escherichia coli*—0/g or ml.

Foreign organic matter

Not more than 2.0% (*1*). Powdered ginger is frequently adulterated with ex-hausted ginger (*8*).

Total ash

Not more than 6.0% (*2, 3*).

Acid-insoluble ash

Not more than 2.0% (*5*).

Water-soluble extractive

Not less than 10% (*3, 4*).

Alcohol-soluble extractive

Not less than 4.5% (*3*).

Pesticide residues

To be established in accordance with national requirements. Normally, the maximum residue limit of aldrin and dieldrin in Rhizoma Zingiberis is not more than 0.05 mg/kg (*17*). For other pesticides, see WHO guidelines on quality control methods for medicinal plants (*15*) and guidelines for predicting dietary intake of pesticide residue (*18*).

Heavy metals

Recommended lead and cadmium levels are not more than 10 and 0.3 mg/kg, respectively, in the final dosage form of the plant material (*15*).

Radioactive residues

For analysis of strontium-90, iodine-131, caesium-134, caesium-137, and plutonium-239, see WHO guidelines on quality control methods for medicinal plants (*15*).

Other purity tests

Chemical and moisture tests to be established in accordance with national requirements.

Chemical assays

Contains not less than 2% v/w of volatile oil (*1*), as determined by the method described in WHO guidelines (*15*). Qualitative analysis by thin-layer chromatography (*1*); qualitative and quantitative gas chromatography and high-performance liquid chromatography analyses of ginger oils for gingerols, shogaols, α-zingiberene, β-bisabolene, β-sesquiphellandrene, and *ar*-curcumene (*19*).

Major chemical constituents

The rhizome contains 1–4% essential oil and an oleoresin. The composition of the essential oil varies as a function of geographical origin, but the chief constituent sesquiterpene hydrocarbons (responsible for the aroma) seem to remain constant. These compounds include (−)-zingiberene, (+)-*ar*-curcumene, (−)-β-sesquiphellandrene, and β-bisabolene. Monoterpene aldehydes and alcohols are also present. The constituents responsible for the pungent taste of the drug and possibly part of its anti-emetic properties have been identified as 1-(3′-methoxy-4′-hydroxyphenyl)-5-hydroxyalkan-3-ones, known as [3–6]-, [8]-, [10]-, and [12]-gingerols (having a side-chain with 7–10, 12, 14, or 16 carbon atoms, respectively) and their corresponding dehydration products, which are known as shogaols (*1, 4, 6, 14, 19*). Representative structures of zingiberene, gingerols and shogaols are presented below.

gingerols

($n = 0, 2, 3, 4, 5, 7, 9$)

zingiberene

shogaols

($n = 4, 5, 7, 9, 10$)

Dosage forms

Dried root powder, extract, tablets and tincture (*2, 14*). Powdered ginger should be stored in well-closed containers (not plastic) which prevent access of moisture. Store protected from light in a cool, dry place (*4, 5*).

Medicinal uses

Uses supported by clinical data

The prophylaxis of nausea and vomiting associated with motion sickness (*20–23*), postoperative nausea (*24*), pernicious vomiting in pregnancy (*25*), and seasickness (*26, 27*).

Uses described in pharmacopoeias and in traditional systems of medicine

The treatment of dyspepsia, flatulence, colic, vomiting, diarrhoea, spasms, and other stomach complaints (*1, 2, 4, 9, 21*). Powdered ginger is further employed in the treatment of colds and flu, to stimulate the appetite, as a narcotic antagonist (*1, 2, 4, 6, 11, 12, 21*), and as an anti-inflammatory agent in the treatment of migraine headache and rheumatic and muscular disorders (*9, 11, 12, 28*).

Uses described in folk medicine, not supported by experimental or clinical data

To treat cataracts, toothache, insomnia, baldness, and haemorrhoids, and to increase longevity (*9, 10, 12*).

Pharmacology

Experimental pharmacology

Cholagogic activity

Intraduodenal administration of an acetone extract (mainly essential oils) of ginger root to rats increased bile secretion for 3 hours after dosing, while the aqueous extract was not active (*29*). The active constituents of the essential oil were identified as [6]- and [10]-gingerol (*29*).

Oral administration of an acetone extract of ginger (75 mg/kg), [6]-shogaol (2.5 mg/kg), or [6]-, [8]-, or [10]-gingerol enhanced gastrointestinal motility in mice (*30*), and the activity was comparable to or slightly weaker than that of metoclopramide (10 mg/kg) and domperidone (*30*). The [6]-, [8]-, or [10]-gingerols are reported to have antiserotoninergic activity, and it has been suggested that the effects of ginger on gastrointestinal motility may be due to this activity (*30, 31*). The mode of administration appears to play a critical role in studies on gastrointestinal motility. For example, both [6]-gingerol and [6]-shogaol inhibited intestinal motility when administered intravenously but accentuated gastrointestinal motility after oral administration (*6, 12, 32*).

Antiemetic activity

The emetic action of the peripherally acting agent copper sulfate was inhibited in dogs given an intragastric dose of ginger extract (33), but emesis in pigeons treated with centrally acting emetics such as apomorphine and digitalis could not be inhibited by a ginger extract (34). These results suggest that ginger's antiemetic activity is peripheral and does not involve the central nervous system (11). The antiemetic action of ginger has been attributed to the combined action of zingerones and shogaols (11).

Anti-inflammatory activity

One of the mechanisms of inflammation is increased oxygenation of arachidonic acid, which is metabolized by cyclooxygenase and 5-lipoxygenase, leading to prostaglandin E_2 and leukotriene B_4, two potent mediators of inflammation (28). *In vitro* studies have demonstrated that a hot-water extract of ginger inhibited the activities of cyclooxygenase and lipoxygenase in the arachidonic acid cascade; thus its anti-inflammatory effects may be due to a decrease in the formation of prostaglandins and leukotrienes (35). The drug was also a potent inhibitor of thromboxane synthase, and raised prostacyclin levels without a concomitant rise in prostaglandins E_2 or $F_{2\alpha}$ (36). *In vivo* studies have shown that oral administration of ginger extracts decreased rat paw oedema (37, 38). The potency of the extracts was comparable to that of acetylsalicylic acid. [6]-Shogaol inhibited carrageenin-induced paw oedema in rats by inhibiting cyclooxygenase activity (39). Recently, two labdane-type diterpene dialdehydes isolated from ginger extracts have been shown to be inhibitors of human 5-lipoxygenase *in vitro* (40).

Clinical pharmacology

Antinausea and antiemetic activities

Clinical studies have demonstrated that oral administration of powdered ginger root (940 mg) was more effective than dimenhydrinate (100 mg) in preventing the gastrointestinal symptoms of kinetosis (motion sickness) (22). The results of this study further suggested that ginger did not act centrally on the vomiting centre, but had a direct effect on the gastrointestinal tract through its aromatic, carminative, and absorbent properties, by increasing gastric motility and adsorption of toxins and acids (22).

In clinical double-blind randomized studies, the effect of powdered ginger root was tested as a prophylactic treatment for seasickness (26, 27). The results of one study demonstrated that orally administered ginger was statistically better than a placebo in decreasing the incidence of vomiting and cold sweating 4 hours after ingestion (27). The other investigation compared the effects of seven over-the-counter and prescription antiemetic drugs on prevention of seasickness in 1489 subjects. This study concluded that ginger was as effective as the other antiemetic drugs tested (26).

At least eight clinical studies have assessed the effects of ginger root on the symptoms of motion sickness. Four of these investigations showed that orally administered ginger root was effective for prophylactic therapy of nausea and vomiting. The other three studies showed that ginger was no more effective than a placebo in treating motion sickness (*23, 41, 42*). The conflicting results appear to be a function of the focus of these studies. Clinical studies that focused on the gastrointestinal reactions involved in motion sickness recorded better responses than those studies that concentrated primarily on responses involving the central nervous system.

The hypothesis that an increase in gastric emptying may be involved in the antiemetic effects of ginger has recently come under scrutiny. Two clinical studies demonstrated that oral doses of ginger did not affect the gastric emptying rate, as measured by sequential gastric scintigraphy (*43*) or the paracetamol absorption technique (*44*).

In a double-blind, randomized, cross-over trial, oral administration of powdered ginger (250 mg, 4 times daily) effectively treated pernicious vomiting in pregnancy (*25*). Both the degree of nausea and the number of vomiting attacks were significantly reduced (*25*). Furthermore, in a prospective, randomized, double-blind study, there were statistically significantly fewer cases of postoperative nausea and vomiting in 60 patients receiving ginger compared to a placebo (*24*). The effect of ginger on postoperative nausea and vomiting was reported to be as good as or better than that of metoclopramide (*24, 45*). In contrast, another double-blind randomized study concluded that orally administered ginger BP (prepared according to the British Pharmacopoeia) was ineffective in reducing the incidence of postoperative nausea and vomiting (*46*).

Anti-inflammatory activity

One study in China reported that 113 patients with rheumatic pain and chronic lower back pain, injected with a 5–10% ginger extract into the painful points or reaction nodules, experienced full or partial relief of pain, decrease in joint swelling, and improvement or recovery in joint function (*11*). Oral administration of powdered ginger to patients with rheumatism and musculoskeletal disorders has been reported to provide varying degrees of relief from pain and swelling (*28*).

Contraindications

No information available.

Warnings

No information available.

Precautions
General
Patients taking anticoagulant drugs or those with blood coagulation disorders should consult their physician prior to self-medication with ginger. Patients with gallstones should consult their physician before using ginger preparations (*21*).

Drug interactions
Ginger may affect bleeding times and immunological parameters owing to its ability to inhibit thromboxane synthase and to act as a prostacyclin agonist (*47, 48*). However, a randomized, double-blind study of the effects of dried ginger (2 g daily, orally for 14 days) on platelet function showed no differences in bleeding times in patients receiving ginger or a placebo (*49, 50*). Large doses (12–14 g) of ginger may enhance the hypothrombinaemic effects of anticoagulant therapy, but the clinical significance has yet to be evaluated.

Carcinogenesis, mutagenesis, impairment of fertility
The mutagenicity of ginger extracts is a controversial subject. A hot-water extract of ginger was reported to be mutagenic in B291I cells and *Salmonella typhimurium* strain TA 100, but not in strain TA 98 (*51*). A number of constituents of fresh ginger have been identified as mutagens. Both [6]-gingerol and shogaols have been determined to be mutagenic in a *Salmonella*/microsome assay (*52*), and increased mutagenesis was observed in an Hs30 strain of *Escherichia coli* treated with [6]-gingerol (*53*). However, the mutagenicity of [6]-gingerol and shogaols was suppressed in the presence of various concentrations of zingerone, an antimutagenic constituent of ginger (*52*). Furthermore, ginger juice was reported to be antimutagenic and suppressed the spontaneous mutations induced by [6]-gingerol, except in cases where the mutagenic chemicals 2-(2-furyl)-3-(5-nitro-2-furyl)acryl amide and *N*-methyl-*N*'-nitro-*N*-nitroso-guanidine were added to [6]-gingerol (*54*). Other investigators have also reported that ginger juice is antimutagenic (*54, 55*).

Pregnancy: teratogenic effects
In a double-blind randomized cross-over clinical trial, ginger (250 mg by mouth, 4 times daily) effectively treated pernicious vomiting in pregnancy (*25*). No teratogenic aberrations were observed in infants born during this study, and all newborn babies had Apgar scores of 9 or 10 after 5 minutes (*25*).

Paediatric use
Not recommended for children less than 6 years of age.

Other precautions
No information available concerning drug and laboratory test interactions, or non-teratogenic effects on pregnancy or nursing mothers.

Adverse reactions

Contact dermatitis of the finger tips has been reported in sensitive patients (*56*).

Posology

For motion sickness in adults and children more than 6 years: 0.5 g, 2–4 times daily. Dyspepsia, 2–4 g daily, as powdered plant material or extracts (*21*).

References

1. *Standard of ASEAN herbal medicine*, Vol. I. Jakarta, ASEAN Countries, 1993.
2. *Pharmacopoeia of the People's Republic of China* (English ed.). Guangzhou, Guangdong Science and Technology Press, 1992.
3. *British pharmacopoeia*. London, Her Majesty's Stationery Office, 1993.
4. *African pharmacopoeia*, Vol. *1*. 1st ed. Lagos, Organization of African Unity, Scientific, Technical & Research Commission, 1985.
5. *The Japanese pharmacopoeia XIII*. Tokyo, Ministry of Health and Welfare, 1996.
6. Bisset NG. *Max Wichtl's herbal drugs & phytopharmaceuticals*. Boca Raton, FL, CRC Press, 1994.
7. Keys JD. *Chinese herbs, their botany, chemistry and pharmacodynamics*. Rutland, VT, CE Tuttle, 1976.
8. Youngken HW. *Textbook of pharmacognosy*, 6th ed. Philadelphia, Blakiston, 1950.
9. Farnsworth NR, ed. *NAPRALERT database*. Chicago, University of Illinois at Chicago, IL, March 15, 1995 production (an on-line database available directly through the University of Illinois at Chicago or through the Scientific and Technical Network (STN) of Chemical Abstracts Services).
10. Kapoor LD. *Handbook of Ayurvedic medicinal plants*. Boca Raton, FL, CRC Press, 1990.
11. Ghazanfar SA. *Handbook of Arabian medicinal plants*. Boca Raton, FL, CRC Press, 1994.
12. Chang HM, But PPH, eds. *Pharmacology and applications of Chinese materia medica*, Vol. *1*. Singapore, World Scientific Publishing, 1986.
13. Farnsworth NR, Bunayapraphatsara N, eds. *Thai medicinal plants*. Bangkok, Prachachon, 1992.
14. Awang DVC. Ginger. *Canadian pharmaceutical journal*, 1982, 125:309–311.
15. *Quality control methods for medicinal plant materials*. Geneva, World Health Organization, 1998.
16. *Deutsches Arzneibuch 1996. Vol. 2. Methoden der Biologie*. Stuttgart, Deutscher Apotheker Verlag, 1996.
17. *European pharmacopoeia*, 3rd ed. Strasbourg, Council of Europe, 1997.
18. *Guidelines for predicting dietary intake of pesticide residues*, 2nd rev. ed. Geneva, World Health Organization, 1997 (unpublished document WHO/FSF/FOS/97.7; available from Food Safety, 1211 Geneva 27, Switzerland).
19. Yoshikawa M et al. Qualitative and quantitative analysis of bioactive principles in Zingiberis rhizoma by means of high performance liquid chromatography and gas liquid chromatography. *Yakugaku zasshi*, 1993, 113:307–315.
20. Reynolds JEF, ed. *Martindale, the extra pharmacopoeia*, 30th ed. London, Pharmaceutical Press, 1993:885.
21. German Commission E Monograph, Zingiberis rhizoma. *Bundesanzeiger*, 1988, 85:5 May.
22. Mowrey DB, Clayson DE. Motion sickness, ginger, and psychophysics. *Lancet*, 1982, i:655–657.
23. Holtmann S et al. The anti-motion sickness mechanism of ginger. A comparative study with placebo and dimenhydrinate. *Acta otolaryngology*, 1989, 108:168–174.

24. Bone ME et al. Ginger root, a new antiemetic. The effect of ginger root on postoperative nausea and vomiting after major gynaecological surgery. *Anaesthesia*, 1990, 45:669–671.
25. Fischer-Rasmussen W et al. Ginger treatment of hyperemesis gravidarum. *European journal of obstetrics, gynecology and reproductive biology*, 1991, 38:19–24.
26. Schmid R et al. Comparison of seven commonly used agents for prophylaxis of seasickness. *Journal of travel medicine*, 1994, 1:203–206.
27. Grontved A et al. Ginger root against seasickness. A controlled trial on the open sea. *Acta otolaryngology*, 1988, 105:45–49.
28. Srivastava KC, Mustafa T. Ginger (*Zingiber officinale*) in rheumatism and musculoskeletal disorders. *Medical hypotheses*, 1992, 39:342–348.
29. Yamahara J et al. Cholagogic effect of ginger and its active constituents. *Journal of ethnopharmacology*, 1985, 13:217–225.
30. Yamahara J et al. Gastrointestinal motility enhancing effect of ginger and its active constituents. *Chemical and pharmaceutical bulletin*, 1991, 38:430–431.
31. Yamahara J et al. Inhibition of cytotoxic drug-induced vomiting in suncus by a ginger constituent. *Journal of ethnopharmacology*, 1989, 27:353–355.
32. Suekawa M et al. Pharmacological studies on ginger. I. Pharmacological actions of pungent components, (6)-gingerol and (6)-shogaol. *Journal of pharmacobio-dynamics*, 1984, 7:836–848.
33. *Japan centra revuo medicina*, 1954, 112:669.
34. Zhou JG. *Tianjin medical journal*, 1960, 2:131.
35. Mustafa T, Srivastava KC, Jensen KB. Drug development report 9. Pharmacology of ginger, *Zingiber officinale*. *Journal of drug development*, 1993, 6:25–39.
36. Srivastava KC. Aqueous extracts of onion, garlic and ginger inhibit platelet aggregation and alter arachidonic acid metabolism. *Biomedica biochimica acta*, 1984, 43:335–346.
37. Mascolo N et al. Ethnopharmacologic investigation of ginger (*Zingiber officinale*). *Journal of ethnopharmacology*, 1989, 27:129–140.
38. Sharma JN, Srivastava KC, Gan EK. Suppressive effects of eugenol and ginger oil on arthritic rats. *Pharmacology*, 1994, 49:314–318.
39. Suekawa M, Yuasa K, Isono M. Pharmacological studies on ginger: IV. Effects of (6)-shogaol on the arachidonic cascade. *Folia pharmacologia Japan*, 1986, 88:236–270.
40. Kawakishi S, Morimitsu Y, Osawa T. Chemistry of ginger components and inhibitory factors of the arachidonic acid cascade. *American Chemical Society Symposium series*, 1994, 547:244–250.
41. Stott JR, Hubble MP, Spencer MB. A double-blind comparative trial of powdered ginger root, hyosine hydrobromide, and cinnarizine in the prophylaxis of motion sickness induced by cross coupled stimulation. *Advisory Group for Aerospace Research Development conference proceedings*, 1984, 39:1–6.
42. Wood CD et al. Comparison of the efficacy of ginger with various antimotion sickness drugs. *Clinical research practice and drug regulatory affairs*, 1988, 6:129–136.
43. Stewart JJ et al. Effects of ginger on motion sickness susceptibility and gastric function. *Pharmacology*, 1991, 42:111–120.
44. Phillips S, Hutchinson S, Ruggier R. *Zingiber officinale* does not affect gastric emptying rate. *Anaesthesia*, 1993, 48:393–395.
45. Phillips S, Ruggier R, Hutchinson SE. *Zingiber officinale* (Ginger), an antiemetic for day case surgery. *Anaesthesia*, 1993, 48:715–717.
46. Arfeen Z et al. A double-blind randomized controlled trial of ginger for the prevention of postoperative nausea and vomiting. *Anaesthesia and intensive care*, 1995, 23:449–452.
47. Backon J. Ginger: inhibition of thromboxane synthetase and stimulation of prostacyclin; relevance for medicine and psychiatry. *Medical hypotheses*, 1986, 20:271–278.

48. Backon J. Ginger as an antiemetic: possible side effects due to its thromboxane synthetase activity. *Anaesthesia*, 1991, 46:705–706.
49. Srivastava KC. Isolation and effects of some ginger components on platelet aggregation and eicosanoid biosynthesis. *Prostaglandins and leukotrienes in medicine*, 1986, 25:187–198.
50. Lumb AB. Effect of ginger on human platelet function. *Thrombosis and haemostasis*, 1994, 71:110–111.
51. Yamamoto H, Mizutani T, Nomura H. Studies on the mutagenicity of crude drug extracts. *Yakugaku zasshi*, 1982, 102:596–601.
52. Nagabhushan M, Amonkar AJ, Bhide SV. Mutagenicity of gingerol and shogoal and antimutagenicity of zingerone in *Salmonella*/microsome assay. *Cancer letters*, 1987, 36:221–233.
53. Nakamura H, Yamamoto T. Mutagen and anti-mutagen in ginger, *Zingiber officinale*. *Mutation research*, 1982, 103:119–126.
54. Kada T, Morita M, Inoue T. Antimutagenic action of vegetable factor(s) on the mutagenic principle of tryptophan pyrolysate. *Mutation research*, 1978, 53:351–353.
55. Morita K, Hara M, Kada T. Studies on natural desmutagens: screening for vegetable and fruit factors active in inactivation of mutagenic pyrolysis products from amino acids. *Agricultural and biological chemistry*, 1978, 42:1235–1238.
56. Seetharam KA, Pasricha JS. Condiments and contact dermatitis of the finger tips. *Indian journal of dermatology, venereology and leprology*, 1987, 53:325–328.

Annex
Participants in the WHO Consultation on Selected Medicinal Plants

Munich, Germany, 8–10 July 1996

Dr Keita Arouna, National Institute for Research in Public Health, Bamako, Mali

Professor Elaine Elisabetsky, Department of Pharmacology, Federal University of Rio Grande do Sul, Porto Alegre, Brazil

Professor Norman Farnsworth, University of Illinois at Chicago, College of Pharmacy, Chicago, IL, USA

Professor Harry Fong, University of Illinois at Chicago, College of Pharmacy, Chicago, IL, USA

Dr Abdel-Azim M. Habib, Professor of Pharmacognosy, Faculty of Pharmacy, University of Alexandria, Alexandria, Egypt

Dr Djoko Hargono, Former Head, Directorate General of Drugs and Food Control, Ministry of Health, Jakarta, Indonesia

Dr Konstantin Keller, Director, Federal Institute of Drug and Medicinal Products, Berlin, Germany

Professor Fritz H. Kemper, Umweltprobenbanken für Human-Organproben, University of Münster, Münster, Germany

Mr Eftychios Kkolos, Director, Pharmaceutical Services, Ministry of Health, Nicosia, Cyprus

Dr Mamadou Koumaré, School of Medicine and Pharmacy, Bamako, Mali

Dr Gail Mahady, University of Illinois at Chicago, College of Pharmacy, Chicago, IL, USA

Dr Satish Mallya, Representative, Bureau of Pharmaceutical Assessment, Health Protection Branch, Drugs Directorate, Ottawa, Ontario, Canada

Professor Tamas Paal, National Institute of Pharmacy, Budapest, Hungary

Dr Tharnkamol Reancharoen, Food and Drug Administration, Ministry of Public Health, Bangkok, Thailand

Dr Gillian Scott, National Botanical Institute, Conservation Biology Research Unit, Cape Town, South Africa

Dr Geoffrey N. Vaughan, National Manager, Therapeutic Goods Administration, Commonwealth Department of Health, Housing and Community Service, Woden, Australian Capital Territory, Australia

Mr Tuley De Silva, Special Technical Adviser, United Nations Industrial Development Organization, Vienna, Austria

WHO Secretariat

Dr Mary Couper, Medical Officer, Division of Drug Management and Policies, World Health Organization, Geneva, Switzerland

Dr Martijn ten Ham, Chief, Drug Safety, Division of Drug Management and Policies, World Health Organization, Geneva, Switzerland

288

Dr Jutta Schill, Technical Officer, Traditional Medicine Programme, Action Programme on Essential Drugs, World Health Organization, Geneva, Switzerland

Dr Xiaorui Zhang, Medical Officer, Traditional Medicine Programme, Action Programme on Essential Drugs, World Health Organization, Geneva, Switzerland